Manual of
histological techniques

Manual of
histological techniques

John D. Bancroft
Senior Chief Medical Laboratory Scientific Officer,
Histopathology Department, University Hospital, Queen's
Medical Centre, Nottingham, UK

Harry C. Cook
Senior Chief Medical Laboratory Scientific Officer,
Pathology Department, West Middlesex University Hospital,
Isleworth, Middlesex, UK

Foreword by
David R Turner
Professor of Pathology, University of
Nottingham Medical School, Nottingham, UK

CHURCHILL LIVINGSTONE
EDINBURGH LONDON MELBOURNE AND NEW YORK 1984

CHURCHILL LIVINGSTONE
Medical Division of Longman Group Limited

Distributed in the United States of America by Churchill
Livingstone Inc., 1560 Broadway, New York, N.Y. 10036, and
by associated companies, branches and representatives
throughout the world.

First published 1984

ISBN 0 443 02870 2

British Library Cataloguing in Publication Data
Bancroft, John D.
    Manual of histological techniques.
    1. Histology, Pathological — Technique
    I. Title   II. Cook, Harry C.
    616.07′583   RB43

Library of Congress Cataloging in Publication Data
Bancroft, John D.
    Manual of histological techniques,

    Includes indexes.
    1. Histology — Technique.   2. Histology — Laboratory
manuals.   I. Cook, Harry C.   II. Title. [DNLM: 1. Histology — Laboratory manuals. QS 525 B213m]
QM 556.B28   1984   616.07′583   83-26173

Printed in Great Britain by the Pitman Press, Bath

Foreword

Modern histopathology is making increasing demands on laboratory scientific staff both in the quality and quantity of specimens with which they have to deal. Histologists have always enjoyed the use of a wide range of dyes to produce both attractive and informative preparations. However, in more recent times, a more precise scientific logic has been applied particularly with the introduction of enzyme histochemical techniques and immunocytochemistry. The histopathologist now frequently sets out to identify more precisely a particular substance within a cell or tissue which has been suggested by an appearance within a haematoxylin and eosin preparation. Fortunately the trend has been for greater co-operation between the medical and technical staff in the investigation of such problems and indeed both can learn from each other. All the more reason, therefore, why workers in this field need to be able to use their knowledge of staining techniques to solve problems posed by the histopathologist. This book, which has been prepared by two experienced senior members of their profession, is arranged in such a way that each chapter attempts to provide the basic answers to a particular line of enquiry. It is intended to be, and certainly should be, used as a bench book. The fact that one of the authors is the Chief Examiner for the Institute of Medical Laboratory Sciences in Cellular Pathology, and that both are active teachers in their profession, should reassure those readers who are concerned with the acquisition of knowledge for examination purposes.

Nottingham, 1984

David R. Turner

Preface

In writing this book we have tried to meet three objectives. Firstly, to integrate two existing texts; Cook's *Manual of Histological Demonstration Techniques* and Bancroft's *Histochemical Techniques*. Within this integration one of our aims has been to produce a textbook suitable for courses in cellular pathology in the United Kingdom and similar histological courses elsewhere. The second objective was to produce a book that is an introduction to, and a practical companion of, Bancroft and Stevens: *Theory and Practice of Histological Techniques* (Churchill Livingstone 1982), which is designed as a comprehensive reference work. Our final and major aim has been to produce a laboratory manual containing standard and occasionally non-standard methods. In attempting to meet these objectives we have tried to appeal to qualified and non-qualified personnel alike and to anticipate the staining techniques required in a busy histological laboratory.

This manual is designed to cover demonstration techniques only; the other specialised techniques are to be found in *Theory and Practice*.

Whenever possible, the theoretical aspects of the topic have been discussed, and where relevant, the associated pathology has been included.

Nottingham and Isleworth, 1984   J.D.B.
     H.C.C.

Acknowledgements

The authors wish to acknowledge the assistance of the contributors to Bancroft and Stevens: *Theory and Practice of Histological Techniques* and other professional colleagues: in particular, Pat Chapman for helpful suggestions on clinical cytology, Dr Paul Forster and Dr James Lowe for comments on histology and pathology. Helpful advice resulted from discussions during the preparation of the text with Brian Chalk and Stanley Terras.

Secretarial assistance was provided by Audrey Cook, Flora Ottawa and Jane Burgass; we are grateful for their untiring efforts. Our thanks go to Dr Carol Tinkler for her patient proof reading and considerable help with the index.

We wish to thank colleagues in our departments for helpful advice and comment; additionally, thanks are due to Professor D. R. Turner and Dr A. Knudsen for their tolerance during the writing of the manuscript.

Contents

1

Fundamentals of normal histology and histopathology

A thorough preparation in normal histology is a prerequisite for the successful practice and study of histological technique. To achieve this it is necessary to have recourse to the appropriate text-books and more importantly, stained sections. The following pages are intended as a reminder of the basic elements that form the various organs and structures of the body and are intended to complement the demonstration techniques to be covered. Equally important, is an elementary knowledge of pathological terms and lesions so that the employment of the various demonstration techniques is firmly related to the diagnosis (see Table 1.2).

Because the techniques later described are those at light microscope level the ultrastructure of normal and pathological tissues will not be dealt with.

NORMAL HISTOLOGY

TYPES OF TISSUE

The following descriptions apply to formalin fixed paraffin sections stained by haematoxylin and eosin.

EPITHELIUM

This type of tissue forms glands, and lines surfaces (Table 1.1). There are three main subdivisions:

1. Simple (non-stratified)

Squamous (syn. pavement). There is an abundant flattened cytoplasm and in profile an elongated, central, darkly staining nucleus in an extended cytoplasm found, e.g. in loop of Henle in the kidney.

Two other cells have a similar histological appearance but are mesenchymal in origin (as opposed to endodermal or ectodermal as is usually the case); these are the endothelial and mesothelial cells found lining blood vessels and serous membranes respectively.

Cuboidal. These are small round cells with a central nucleus found, e.g. forming the walls of small, glandular intralobular ducts, also renal tubules.

Columnar. This can be found as either 'low' or 'high' columnar and is an elongated cell having a basal nucleus. It usually contains mucin and is found, e.g. as the lining epithelium for much of the alimentary tract (stomach onwards). In the

Table 1.1 Epithelium: summary of types and location

Type	Location
Simple	
Squamous	Lung, kidney
Cuboidal	Kidney, glandular ducts
Columnar	Stomach, large and small intestine
Ciliated	Fallopian tubes, endocervix
Pseudostratified columnar	Bronchus, trachea
Stratified	
Squamous keratinized	Epidermis of skin
Squamous nonkeratinized	Oesophagus, cervix
Transitional	Urinary bladder, ureters
Columnar	Large ducts, urethra
Mixed columnar-cuboidal	Epididymis
Glandular	
Tubular	Stomach, uterus
Acinar	Pancreas, salivary glands
Tubulo-acinar	Prostate

small intestine the free border of the columnar cells has a so-called 'brush border', which is a layer formed of microvilli, which appears as a darker staining line at the free surface.

Ciliated. Both cuboidal and columnar cells may carry on their free border fine hair-like processes termed *cilia*, and may be found lining organs such as the Fallopian tubes and uterus.

Pseudo-stratified ciliated columnar. This type of epithelium is synonymous with respiratory epithelium, and consists of somewhat misshapen ciliated columnar cells which, although they at first sight appear to be in layers, in reality extend from the basement membrane (basal lamina) to the free surface.

Goblet cells. A somewhat ubiquitous cell it is abundant wherever there is copious mucus production, e.g. mucous membranes of the respiratory tract and the small and large intestine. It is a large bulbous cell having a dilated cytoplasm filled with mucin and possesses a basal nucleus.

2. Stratified (multilayered)

Squamous keratinized. This forms the epidermis of skin and consists of a varying number of layers depending on the site, e.g. 'thin' skin as obtained from the inner aspect of the thigh, whilst 'thick' skin is exemplified by that from the solar aspect of the foot.

The deepest layer is columnar in type compared to the middle layers (the so-called 'prickle cell' layers) which are polyhedral in shape and bear desmosomal spines, a feature which is artefactually exaggerated in conditions of epidermal oedema. The superficial layers are more classically squamous in shape with an uppermost granular layer, the cells of which contain haematoxylophilic keratohyalin granules. Finally, there is a non-cellular keratinous layer, the stratum corneum. (There is also allegedly a 'stratum lucidum'; we have yet to see a convincing example in routinely prepared skin.) Also to be found in epidermis are melanoblasts, melanocytes and melanophores, together with Langerhans cells — a type of histiocyte.

Squamous non-keratinized. This is similar in structure to the foregoing but it lacks a keratinized layer and granular layer. It is found in a number of sites, e.g. ectocervix and oesophagus.

Transitional is composed of cuboidal-like cells. It resembles on casual inspection the stratified squamous epithelia, but more careful examination reveals more uniform cells, i.e. the basal cells are only slightly more columnar than the most superficial cells, in addition, 'prickle', granular and keratinized layers are lacking.

Columnar. True stratified columnar epithelium is only found in a few situations; these include the urethra and the major ducts of the salivary glands.

Mixed stratified. Occasionally a type of epithelium is seen which does not easily fit into one of the above categories. Such an epithelium occurs in the epididymis, where the tubules are lined by tall columnar cells, bearing stereocilia, with an underlying uniform layer of cuboidal-type cells.

3. Glandular

Tubular. These glands may be coiled or straight and have wide lumina lined by large columnar-type cells, with basal nuclei. This type of gland is found in the stomach and endometrium.

Acinar (syn. alveolar). The component cells have a broad base and narrow apex with the nucleus occupying a basal position. Each group of cells or acinus has an ill-defined central ductule which communicates with intra and extralobular ducts. The pancreas and the salivary glands are good examples.

Mixed tubulo-acinar. As the name indicates, these are formed of mixtures of both of the above gland elements. The prostate shows this type of feature well.

MUSCLE

Skeletal muscle (syn. striated, voluntary)

This is the main motor tissue of the body and is under the direct control of the central nervous system. Examination of H and E stained sections with the light microscope gives only limited information as to structure and composition, enzyme histochemistry and electron microscopy being necessary for systematic study. Skeletal muscle consists essentially of adjacent fibres varying in length from 1–40 mm, and in diameter from 10–100 μm. Each fibre is surrounded by a thin membrane, the sarcolemma, which encloses the cytoplasm or sarcoplasm. Nuclei are multiple and peripherally situated, a feature which is most easily seen when the fibres are in cross section.

Within the sarcoplasm are longitudinal myofibrils and transverse striations. The latter cross striations consist of alternating light I discs with a narrow central darker Z band, and darker A discs having a lighter central H band.

Skeletal muscle is rich in mitochondria and glycogen, and in H and E preparations usually stains a brighter red colour, compared to the other types of muscle.

Cardiac muscle

Under this heading may be considered two different muscle fibres, the contractile heart muscle per se and the specialized conductor muscle which initiates and propagates heart contraction. The former type of muscle is similar to skeletal in having longitudinal myofibrils and cross striations (although these are less evident in H and E type preparations), but differ in that they branch and anastomose and are somewhat shorter (100–150 μm). Present in the sarcoplasm in the Z band region are intercalated discs which mark the cell boundaries. The nuclei are single and centrally placed. Mitochondria and glycogen are again abundant, and granules of lipofuscin are usually present in older age groups. The conducting system of the heart comprises the SA node, AV node and bundles of His, also the interventricular Purkinje fibres. These are not easily seen in human heart and, indeed, careful dissection is needed in order to locate the various constituents (Hudson, 1963).

Broadly speaking the muscle cells of the nodes are somewhat smaller and more compact than the main cardiac muscle cells, whilst the Purkinje fibres are composed of larger somewhat ovoid muscle cells, which have a perinuclear centre rich in glycogen. But it must be stressed again, that experience (and patience) are needed to successfully visualize the conductor system of the heart.

Smooth muscle (syn. involuntary, nonstriated)

Muscle controlled by the autonomic nervous system has a wide distribution, being found in the walls of the alimentary, respiratory and genito-urinary tracts. As the name implies, there are no cross striations in the sarcoplasm of these cells, only longitudinal myofibrils. Typically smooth muscle cells are 'cigar' shaped in that the poles are somewhat tapered. The nuclei are single and centrally placed, and the sarcoplasm contains fewer mitochondria and glycogen granules compared to the other muscles. The overall size, too, is less being in the order of 20–100 μm in length.

NERVOUS TISSUE

The microscopic study of both the central (CNS) and peripheral (PNS) nervous systems is best carried out with the aid of special techniques — usually silver impregnation on frozen or celloidin embedded material. However, a certain amount of detail can be visualized in H and E stained paraffin sections and this will be described.

CNS

This comprises the brain and spinal cord.

Neurones. The larger neurones such as the Betz cells of the cerebrum, Purkinje cells of the cerebellum and the anterior horn cells of the spinal cord have well-marked characteristics. There is a large cell body with discrete granules of ribonucleic acid termed Nissl substance and, as with cardiac muscle fibres, granules of lipofuscin pigment may be present in tissue from the older age-groups. The nuclear membrane and chromatin are ill-defined but there is a prominent nucleolus. (Myelinated nerve fibres stain pink in the H and E unlike the non-myelinated which may hardly stain at all.)

Small or medium size neurones have comparatively indistinct cell bodies and are often shown solely by their nuclei which, compared to the large neurones, tend to have a more distinct chromatin pattern.

Neuroglia. There are several different types of glial cell having a variety of functions, varying from supportive (the astrocytes), ventricular lining cells (ependymal) to myelin formation (oligodendrocytes). Another cell, the microglial cell is, embryologically speaking, not a true neuroglial element being derived from mesenchyme and is usually included because of its possession of processes; it is a reticulo-endothelial (RE) cell and thus has a marked phagocytic function.

Astrocytes. The two members of this group — fibrous and protoplasmic — are indistinguishable in a routine H and E, and indeed, show virtually no cytoplasmic detail or evidence of processes. Their position is solely indicated by their round to ovoid moderately-sized nuclei, having a well marked chromatin structure. Special stains reveal abundant, substantial processes.

Ependyma. These cells are largely found lining the ventricles of the brain and appear as ciliated cuboidal-like cells. Unlike the other neuroglial cells, special methods do not materially assist in their identification.

Oligodendrocytes. These are the smallest cells of the neuroglial system and appear not unlike lymphocytes in an H and E stained section having a scanty cytoplasm and a small round pyknotic nucleus. Special methods reveal these cells to have scanty, relatively small processes.

Microglia. As is the case with the astrocytes, H and E staining shows only the nuclei to advantage which are intermediate in size between astrocytes and oligodendrocytes. Unlike those cells the microglial nucleus is more irregular in shape and usually more elongated. Special stains reveal a somewhat elongated cell body with short processes extending from each pole.

Axons. These are the nerve fibres which comprise the main substance of both grey and white matter. They vary considerably in both length and diameter; fine fibrils, the *neurofibrils* can often be demonstrated within the nerve fibre.

Axons of white matter are surrounded by a dense fatty sheath termed *myelin*. By contrast, the fibres in the grey matter are largely nonmyelinated.

PNS

The nerve fibre appearance is very much that found in the CNS excepting that they may be formed into discrete nerve bundles with accompanying specialized connective tissue. The nerve cell bodies or ganglion cells as they are termed in the PNS tend to be modelled on the larger type of CNS neurone, although the Nissl substance is less pronounced. Lipofuscin is often a prominent feature. Posterior root ganglia of the spinal cord

are formed of sensory neurones and their processes the nerve fibres, but unlike the CNS there is an abundant supporting framework of collagen fibres.

Nerve endings, either sensory or motor, are not usually distinguishable in H and E preparations. Exceptions to this rule are the Pacinian corpuscles, which are sensory end organs found prominently in the deeper layers of skin, and neuromuscular spindles, another form of sensory nerve ending found in the skeletal muscle.

The former nerve ending is often quite large (up to 3 mm in diameter) and fairly readily identified in that it is not unlike an onion in appearance, consisting as it does of concentric pale-staining layers of connective tissue surrounding a central nerve fibre. By contrast, neuromuscular spindles are much less easily found; they appear as a pale-staining area in muscle, which on closer inspection is made up of thin muscle cells and nerve cells, invested and surrounded by fine connective tissue.

CONNECTIVE TISSUE

The role of connective tissue is largely that of support, and because this supporting function is a variable one depending on the structure involved, so does the form vary in appearance, elasticity and strength. In addition to this supporting function there are certain types of connective tissue which have a distinct metabolic role, e.g. adipose tissue.

Associated with the tissue entities which comprise connective tissue, there are several different types of cell which are in environmental association. These cells are as follows:

Plasma cells are found in lymphoid tissue, spleen, bone marrow. The plasma cells have an ovoid cytoplasm and eccentric nucleus with prominent radial chromatin. They are derived from B lymphocytes and secrete immunoglobulins.

Mast cells. Occurring in loose connective tissue such as that of the wall of the large and small intestines, these cells are small with a large central nucleus and prominent cytoplasmic basophilic granules (note that human mast cell granules are not easily seen in H and E stained sections).

Fibroblasts. These cells occur wherever there are collagen fibres, e.g. dermis of skin and submucosa of the alimentary tract, and are relatively large elongated cells having an indistinct cytoplasm and a large elongated pale-staining nucleus. Fibroblasts produce the protein tropocollagen which is the precursor substance for collagen.

Histiocytes are found in similar situations to fibroblasts. These are round to oval cells intermediate in size between a fibroblast and a mast cell. The cytoplasm stains weakly as does the nucleus which in shape is typically oval or indented (kidney shaped). They have a phagocytic role.

Blood cells. In non-haemopoietic tissue these comprise neutrophils, lymphocytes and eosinophils and have the classical normal features of the circulating blood cells. They may be seen to greatest advantage in loose connective tissue such as the lamina propria of the alimentary tract.

TYPES OF CONNECTIVE TISSUE

Collagen and reticulin

Using special biochemical techniques it is current practice to classify collagen into subgroups I to V. So for example, conventional collagen found in dermis or colonic wall is type I, whilst reticulin is type III; this will be referred to again in subsequent chapters. However, purely from a standard morphological point of view, collagen presents as a non-branching coarse fibre (maximum diameter 100 μm) made up of fibrils which stain bright pink with eosin, whilst reticulin fibres are much finer (up to 1.5 μm) and branch freely, needing special silver staining to be clearly delineated.

The latter fibres whilst often present in association with collagen may be found as a separate entity lining the liver sinusoids or investing lymphoid tissue.

Elastic tissue

This connective tissue is formed of branching fibres of .varying diameter (1–10 μm). They possess the ability to expand or contract, and are thus to be found wherever this property is required, e.g. blood vessels, skin and lung. They stain intensely pink with eosin.

It is interesting that whilst the formative cells for most connective tissues are known, that for elastic fibres has yet to be firmly established, although the weight of opinion seems to favour a modified fibroblast.

Loose connective tissue (syn. areolar tissue)

Found as a 'filling' between muscles and fascia also as the lamina propria of alimentary tract, this is a composite tissue formed of fine collagen, elastic and reticulin fibres. Also present are the connective tissue cells described earlier and to a variable degree, a mucoprotein ground substance.

Cartilage

Essentially this is formed of polygonal chondrocytes which lie in varying sized groups in the lacunae (spaces) of a dense mucoprotein matrix. There is a varying fibre content. Three forms are recognised:

Hyaline. The matrix is low in fibre content which is principally collagenous. The articular cartilage of bone is comprised of this tissue.

Fibrous. The collagen fibre content of the matrix is high giving greater strength. Fibrocartilage forms the intervertebral discs.

Elastic. The main fibres present are elastic in this less common cartilage which forms the epiglottis and pinna of the ear.

Bone

Structurally, bone presents either as dense compact material such as is found forming the cortex of long bones, or as the cancellous (spongy) tissue of the medulla of the long bones. The latter encloses the cells of the bone marrow. In either case, bone is essentially collagen and ground substance termed osteoid impregnated by various calcium salts.

The mature bone cells are termed osteocytes, and have small dense round to elongated nuclei with an ill defined cytoplasm. These cells lie in bone spaces called lacunae, which interconnect by means of fine channels — the canaliculi.

Active or growing bone is evidenced by the presence of bone-forming cells — the osteoblasts — and multinucleated bone remodelling cells — the osteoclasts. Both cells are found principally at the interface of bone trabeculae with the bone marrow.

Adipose tissue

Depot fat of the body contains the major proportion of adipose tissue such as in the mesentery and omentum of the abdominal cavity, and the subcutaneous layer of the skin.

The individual fat cells have a large vacuolated (in paraffin sections) cytoplasm with a thin nucleus compressed to one side. Fine collagen or reticulin fibres surround the cells which are formed into lobules. Small blood vessels run in the somewhat denser collagen fibres of the interlobular tissue.

Lymphoid tissue

It is convenient to describe lymphoid tissue in this context, as while its function is far removed from that of being merely supportive many of the cellular elements of lymphoid tissue and the supportive connective tissue have a common origin. It is found to greatest extent in lymph nodes, spleen and large and small intestine.

The following necessarily oversimplified description of this complex and controversial tissue is merely an attempt to highlight the more important constituents. In addition it must be appreciated that many of these constituents are not readily identified if only conventional paraffin H and E preparations are available.

A typical lymph node exhibits the following structure:

Cortex. An inactive gland shows follicles containing small lymphocytes (B type) tingible body macrophages and dendritic reticulum cells; the former cells are round with pyknotic nuclei and the latter two cells are much greater in size with large irregular pale-staining nuclei.

An active gland will show in addition germinal centres. These are paler-staining zones compared to the primary follicles and contain histiocytic cells and different forms of B lymphocytes such as the cleaved (centrocyte) and noncleaved forms (centroblast) — the description referring to the nuclear presentation. Immunoblasts and plasma cells are also present, plus scanty T lymphocytes.

Paracortex. This occupies a position internal to the cortex, but external to the medullary cords, and is the domain of the T lymphocyte series.

Both cortex and paracortex are drained by a system of cortical sinuses having a reticulin fibre framework which lead into the medullary cords.

Medullary cords. The cortical sinuses drain into a system of medullary sinuses. These run between medullary cords which are formed of various lymphocytic cells, plasma cells and histiocytes.

Gross structure. The efferent lymph flow is from the medullary sinuses and the afferent lymphatics via channels in the fibroreticular membrane that covers the lymph node, and thence into subcapsular sinuses.

It should be noted that a dense reticulin pattern can be demonstrated throughout the lymph node, with the exception of the germinal centres where it is perifollicular in distribution.

GENERAL NOTES

Having set out the various tissue types and subtypes, it may be helpful to note the following points.

1. The structure of a tissue often mirrors its function or physiological role. For example epithelial cells lining an intralobular duct in an acinar gland are usually cuboidal in type, whereas those cells lining the extralobular, i.e. larger ducts will tend to be more columnar. The main duct for the gland may well be lined by stratified (layered) columnar cells. Similarly, stratified squamous epithelium forming external skin surfaces are keratinized to varying degrees, whereas the internal 'skin' surfaces such as the oesophagus lack a protective layer of keratin. Both of these examples exemplify the arrangement of cells according to their role; in the case of the ducts, the degree of secretion required and resistance to the flow-stress of the duct contents, and in the case of the skin layers the degree of surface protection required against trauma.

2. When comparing sections of tissues with descriptions or pictures in textbooks, remember that 'normal' is a relative word and that, of necessity, textbook illustrations show tissue under ideal conditions of fixation, preservation and demonstration. It is important to expect minor variations

in presentation due to these modifying factors.

3. In the authors' experience the important microscopy objectives for studying the normal histology of stained slides are a low-power scanning lens, e.g. × 2.5 and a higher power lens such as × 40.

The low-power lens should be initially employed so as to afford a general idea of the cellular arrangement followed by examination with the higher-power lens to confirm or resolve important fine structural details. A lens of intermediate magnification such as the × 10 is normally less useful than the objectives mentioned, whilst the × 100 oil-immersion objective is rarely called for.

BASIC HISTOPATHOLOGY

The type of pathological change to be discussed here is that which is most likely to be encountered in the routine diagnostic laboratory. It will be described in relation to the type of material most likely to be handled by such a laboratory.

NON-TUMOUR PATHOLOGY

Under this umbrella is to be found a wide spectrum of disorders involving tissue. Some degree of inflammation is usually involved either as the primary lesion, or as a secondary reaction to other disease processes.

The following explanation of some common terms may be found useful:

Aneurysm is a localized dilatation of an artery which may be a large vessel, e.g. aorta, or quite small, as found at the base of the brain. The media of the affected area is defective and there is associated degeneration of elastic fibres. There are various types, such as atheromatous, congenital, syphilitic and dissecting.

Embolism. There are various forms of embolus which usually consist of detached material which is transported from one part of the circulation to another. Examples of emboli are pieces of blood clot, fat or tumour.

Diverticulum. The large intestine is most commonly involved in diverticula formation which is the presence of a pouch-like dilatation of the bowel wall. The diverticular wall is usually thin with a scanty muscle coat. The condition is known as diverticulosis, and if inflammation is present, is termed diverticulitis.

Endometriosis. When normal tissue is found in an abnormal situation it is termed 'ectopic', and ectopic endometrium gives rise to the condition of endometriosis where nodular lesions occur in a number of sites including the ovary, umbilicus and gut. The wall of the uterus commonly shows this condition where it is known as 'adenomyosis'.

Granuloma. Inflammatory reactions may take many forms and a granulomatous reaction is one where there is a marked proliferation of abnormal histiocytes called 'epithelioid' cells plus their conglomerates the giant cells. Examples of this type of reaction are tuberculosis and sarcoidosis.

Infarct. Infarction is a localized area of tissue necrosis caused by an interruption to the blood supply (resulting in haemorrhage to the area). Whilst this can occur to almost any situation, it is seen to greatest advantage in placenta, heart (myocardial infarction), brain, lung, kidney and spleen.

Inflammation. In purely histological terms an acute inflammatory reaction involves to varying degrees, hyperaemia, oedema and neutrophil proliferation. This reaction gradually lessens until the chronic stage is reached when lymphocytes, and to a lesser degree, histiocytes and fibroblasts are predominant. The final stage is one of collagen overgrowth (fibrosis).

Ischaemia. Sometimes the blood supply to a given tissue is decreased because of partial obstruction or narrowing of the relevant blood vessel. This partial occlusion commonly occurs in the heart muscle due to coronary artery deficiency, and results over a period of time in fibrotic diseases in the myocardium. A similar diminution of blood supply can occur in the large intestine — a condition termed 'ischaemic colitis'.

Metaplasia denotes a change in differentiation of tissue from one mature type to another and is thought to be due to the proliferation and differentiation of totipotential cells. Metaplastic change can be nonspecific or as a result of inflammation. Examples are squamous metaplasia of bronchial mucosa in chronic bronchitis, the appearance of bony areas in scar tissue, and intestinal metaplasia of the stomach. In certain tumours squamous metaplasia is often present, particularly adenocarcinoma of the uterus and transitional cell carcinoma of the bladder.

Necrosis. Implied in this term is death of cells or tissues and, as would be expected, a loss of normal cellular detail and architecture. Nuclear changes are evident including pyknosis (condensation of chromatin), and karyorrhexis (nuclear breakdown). Calcification is often present so that this type of tissue change is less than popular with the microtomist!

There are different types of necrotic change; infarction (see above) is one such, as is the caseation necrosis associated with tuberculous lesions.

Disturbances of growth

Anaplasia. The term anaplastic implies immaturity or lack of differentiation and cells showing anaplasia often present as highly malignant tumours.

Atrophy. Atrophic change is applied to the macroscopic appearance of shrinkage of a structure and can be due to a decrease in number or size of the component cells. Examples are disuse atrophy of muscle, and renal atrophy due to ureteric blockage.

Dysplasia denotes an abnormal growth pattern.

Hyperplasia/hypoplasia. Denotes an increase or decrease, respectively in the number of component cells. Endocrine glands such as the thyroid or pituitary may exhibit these features; also haemopoietic bone marrow in a variety of diseases, and tumour cells generally.

Hypertrophy. This is the converse of atrophy and denotes an increase in cell volume. An example is ventricular hypertrophy of heart muscle in hypertension.

TUMOUR PATHOLOGY

A benign tumour differs in a number of significant respects when compared to a malignant tumour. This is true not only clinically but histologically too, and the following few guidelines may be found useful. It is important to bear in mind that there is not infrequently overlap as regards the histological parameters of benign and malignant tumours, and that type of situation calls for long experience and/or high interpretative skills.

Benign tumours. These may be small or large, but the component cells are distinguished by a relatively uniform appearance with very little variation in size and shape of both nucleus and cytoplasm. Important is the lack of invasion into deeper structure. Examples are squamous cell papillomas of the skin and uterine fibromyomata ('fibroids').

Malignant tumours. Most malignant tumours arise from epithelium and are termed 'carcinoma' and thus commonly arise in glands and lining surfaces.

Microscopically the cells exhibit some or all of the following features.

1. Pleomorphism (variation in size and shape of nuclei and cytoplasm)
2. Invasion of deeper structures
3. Nuclear immaturity (abnormal chromatin clumping, prominent nucleoli)
4. Mitotic activity.

The other, less common, type of malignant tumour is the sarcoma and consists of tissue elements of mesenchymal origin. This is a complex group and tends to present the pathologist with greater diagnostic problems. The names of the individual sarcomata reflect the type of tissue from which they spring, e.g. fibrosarcoma, myosarcoma, osteosarcoma, liposarcoma, etc. The sarcomas affect all age groups, unlike the carcinomas which have a predeliction for the older age groups.

The following explanations of some commonly employed terms may be found useful:

Adenoma is a benign tumour of glandular or secretory tissue. Common examples are to be found in rectum, skin appendages and thyroid. The malignant variant is known as an adenocarcinoma and is the commonest type of tumour in the gastro-intestinal tract.

Neoplasm refers to an abnormal growth or tumour which can be benign or malignant.

Papilloma. A papillomatous growth is one where there are finger-like projections of tissue. It is most commonly a benign tumour and examples are squamous papillomas of the skin and villous adenomas of the rectum. In each case there is an epithelial lining overlying a connective tissue core of the papillary projections.

Polyp. 'Polyps' (or more correctly 'polypi') are round, usually benign growths which often have a connecting stalk and are 'pedunculated'; a non-pedunculated polyp is termed 'sessile'. Occasionally malignant change takes place, more particularly in those arising in the gastro-intestinal tract. The cervix uteri and rectum are common site for polyps.

Tumour differentiation. When one refers to a given malignant tumour as being histologically *well* — or *poorly* — differentiated, it denotes the degree to which the malignant tissue resembles the normal parent tissue. Thus a 'well differentiated' adenocarcinoma of the colon will show a well marked glandular structure often with mucin secretion. A 'poorly differentiated' adenocarcinoma, on the other hand, will consist of cell masses with little or no glandular structure or mucin secretion, and the cells themselves will possess the stigmata of immaturity, particularly as regards the nuclear presentation.

Analogous to the mucin production of the well differentiated adenocarcinoma is the keratin formation of well differentiated squamous cell carcinomas. In a similar way, a fibrosarcoma if well differentiated will show a greater *fibrillar* content and a lessened *cellularity* compared to a poorly differentiated sarcoma, which will be more cellular and less fibrillar.

The more important organs and structures in the body are shown in Table 1.2 which relates to the more important histopathological conditions. It is not an exhaustive list, merely an attempt to highlight for the inexperienced worker the location of the more common lesions, i.e. those that are likely to be presented to the average histology laboratory.

Table 1.2 Some commonly received specimens in the surgical laboratory and their more common pathologies.

Tissue	Non-tumour pathology	Tumour pathology
Appendix	Appendicitis Mucocele	Carcinoid tumour Carcinoma, primary (rare) Carcinoma, secondary (uncommon)
Artery	Arteritis Atheroma Aneurysm	Chemodectoma (uncommon)
Bladder (biopsy or cystectomy)	Cystitis Diverticulae Fistulae Tuberculosis Shistosomiasis (uncommon)	Transitional cell carcinoma Squamous cell carcinoma Adenocarcinoma (rare)
Bone and bone marrow	Osteoporosis Osteomalacia Osteomyelitis Paget's disease	Osteochondroma Myeloma Metastatic tumour (e.g. breast, bronchus, thyroid, prostate, kidney) Leukaemia Osteosarcoma
Breast (biopsy or mastectomy)	Cysts Fibrocystic disease Abscess Fat necrosis	Adenoma Fibroadenoma Adenocarcinoma Paget's disease of nipple
Bronchial biopsy	Inflammation Squamous metaplasia	Squamous cell carcinoma Oat cell carcinoma
Cervix (cone biopsy or punch biopsy)	Inflammation Dysplasia (CIN)	Squamous carcinoma (in-situ (CIN) or invasive)
Colon and rectum (biopsy or colectomy)	Ulcerative colitis Crohn's disease Amyloidosis Fistulae Amoebiasis (uncommon) Diverticular disease	Adenomatous polyps Adenocarcinoma Lymphoma (uncommon) Polyps

Tissue	Non-tumour pathology	Tumour pathology
Endometrium (curettings)	Endometritis Abnormalities of cycle Hyperplasia	Adenocarcinoma Sarcomas (uncommon) Polyps
Epididymis	Cysts Inflammation Tuberculosis	Adenocarcinoma (rare)
Fallopian tubes	Salpingitis Ectopic pregnancy Endometriosis	
Gall bladder	Cholecystitis Calculi	Adenocarcinoma (uncommon)
Joints/tendons	Arthritis Crystal synovitis (e.g. gout)	Sarcoma (rare)
Kidney (biopsy or nephrectomy)	Amyloidosis Glomerulonephritis Pyelonephritis Cysts/calculi Tuberculosis	Adenocarcinoma Transitional cell carcinoma of pelvis
Larynx and vocal cords	Laryngeal nodules Inflammation Polyps	Squamous cell carcinoma
Liver (biopsy)	Hepatitis Cirrhosis Obstructive jaundice Sarcoidosis Amyloidosis Storage disorders	Hepatocellular carcinoma Secondary tumour, e.g. colon stomach, breast and pancreas Lymphoma
Lung (biopsy)	Pneumonia Alveolar fibrosis Pneumocystic carinii	Squamous carcinoma Oat cell carcinoma Adenocarcinoma Secondary tumours
Lymph node	Reaction to inflammation Tuberculosis Sarcoidosis	Hodgkin's and non-Hodgkin's lymphoma Secondary tumours, e.g. lung, breast, colon, testis
Muscle, voluntary (biopsy)	Myopathies Neuropathic atrophy	Rhabdomyosarcoma (rare)
Nasal mucosa	Polyps Inflammation	Muco-epidermoid carcinoma Squamous cell carcinoma
Oral cavity	Cysts (dental) Inflammation Polyps	Squamous cell carcinoma Salivary gland tumours
Oesophagus (biopsy)	Oesophagitis Strictures Ulceration (peptic)	Squamous cell carcinoma

Ovary	Cysts
	Endometriosis
		Both benign and malignant tumours of:
		    Epithelium, e.g. mucinous cystadenoma
		    Stroma, e.g. thecoma
		    Germ cells, e.g. dysgerminoma
		Metastatic tumours, e.g. stomach

Pancreas (biopsy)	Cysts Pancreatitis	Adenocarcinoma (exocrine elements) Apudomas (rare)
Parathyroid gland	Hyperplasia	Adenomas
Placenta and umbilical cord	Malformations Infarction	Hydatidiform mole Choriocarcinoma

Tissue	Non-tumour pathology	Tumour pathology
Pleural biopsy	Inflammations Tuberculosis	Mesothelioma Secondary tumour e.g. lungs, breast
Prostate gland	Hyperplasia Prostatitis	Adenocarcinoma
Salivary gland	Calculi Sialoadenitis	Pleomorphic adenoma Adenolymphoma (Warthins) Mucoepidermoid tumour
Skin (biopsy)	Cysts Dermatitis Reactive changes	Naevi Warts Skin appendage tumours Squamous cell carcinoma Basal cell carcinoma Malignant melanoma Carcinoma-in-situ (Bowen's disease)
Small intestine	Infarction Diverticulae Crohn's disease Coeliac disease	Carcinoid tumour Lymphoma Adenocarcinoma (uncommon)
Spleen	Traumatic rupture Thrombocytopenic purpura Hypersplenism syndromes Amyloidosis	Lymphoma Leukaemia
Stomach	Gastritis Peptic ulceration	Adenocarcinoma Lymphoma Leiomyoma
Testis	Infertility Orchitis Tuberculosis Hydrocele	Seminoma Teratoma Lymphoma (uncommon)
Thyroid	Nodular goitre Thyrotoxic hyperplasia Hashimoto's thyroiditis	Adenoma Adenocarcinoma Medullary carcinoma (amyloid associated)
Uterus (hysterectomy)	Abnormal cyclical bleeding Endometritis Adenomyosis Endometriosis	Leiomyoma (fibroid) Adenocarcinoma of endometrium
Vulva (biopsy or excision)	Leukoplakia Inflammation Dysplasia	Squamous carcinoma (in situ or invasive)

REFERENCES

Hudson R C B 1963 The human conducting-system and its
  examination. Journal of Clinical Pathology 16: 49
Robb-Smith A H T, Taylor C R 1981 Lymph node biopsy.
  Miller Heyden, London

2

Principles of tissue demonstration

In order to visualize detail and tissue structure at light microscope level it is usually necessary to impart colour to the element to be studied. When Zernicke in 1932 and later Kohler and Loos in 1941, introduced the phase contrast microscope it was hailed as the new means of examining tissue which, it was confidently forecast by many workers, would soon render conventional histological demonstration techniques obsolete. As we now know, phase contrast microscopy has indeed taken its place in the repertoire, particularly for studying fine detail in living material, but colouring of cells and tissues remains fundamental to the science of histology. The foregoing remarks apply to light microscopical examination only. When tissues are studied by electron microscopy colour definition is not involved, and 'staining' of cells is achieved by the application of salts of heavy metals such as those of lead and uranium. These build up a detailed image by varying the electron lucency or opacity, depending on the way they are bound to the tissue.

There are basically three ways in which we impart colour to tissue: staining with dyes, impregnation with metallic salts and the formation of coloured compounds in situ by means of chemical reactions and these are discussed below. It must be emphasized that this is a complex subject and we are only attempting to present the outlines of the principles of tissue demonstration. More detailed information is available (Horobin 1982, a, b).

STAINING WITH DYES

Fixed protein has approximately the same refractive index as glass, so that when one looks at a

12

stained section under the microscope which has been cleared and mounted in one of the standard media, it is not the tissue per se that is seen but dye particles attached to the (usually) protein molecules, so that the way in which we do this vitally affects the tissue picture that we see. The basic principle is as follows. When carrying out a staining method on tissue sections a dye is chosen which has a particular affinity for the element to be studied — this is the *primary* stain. In order to highlight the stained *primary* element it is common practice to counterstain the background: this *secondary* staining is carried out with dyes of a contrasting colour which have an affinity for the background tissues. How the dyes vary in colour and tissue affinity will now be described.

DYES AND THEIR DEVELOPMENT

Dyes of natural origin, i.e. those of animal and vegetable origin, have been in use for the study of tissue for a considerable period of time, possibly starting with Grew in 1682 who stained plant tissue with cochineal and certainly Leeuwenhoek who, in 1714, stained muscle fibres with saffron. These dyes were of animal (cochineal beetle) and plant (crocus) origin respectively.

Not, however, until Perkin successfully synthesized the dye aniline violet in 1856 did a visible dye industry emerge, from which sprang dyes for histological and bacteriological purposes. The impetus for a flourishing and successful dye industry came largely from German workers, as indeed did the staining of tissue in the laboratory. Prominent among these workers were household names such as Ehrlich, Weigert and Koch. Today, most dyes used in histology are synthetic ones but it is interesting to reflect that probably *the* most important early dye still in use today is a naturally derived one, namely haematoxylin which is extracted from the bark of a tropical logwood.

When dyes were first introduced their mode of action was ill understood and right up to the early 1950's many of the tissue – dye reactions remained empirical. These reactions are now better understood overall; also the dyes themselves are more completely classified and to some extent standardized. There is little room for complacency as even today there are staining reactions for which there is no accepted rationale, and the histologist is still too often plagued by variation in the quality and content of dye batches. Not infrequently there is variation, for example, in the proportion of substances such as dextrin or sodium chloride combined with the dye during manufacture. These are added to improve the solubility or flow properties of the dye, but as will be appreciated it is the percentage of dye actually present which is of most importance to the laboratory user. Most dyes were developed for use in the textile industry and the histologist's needs are, in consequence, secondary to those of the industrial users when one considers the enormous disparity in the quantities used. One means of establishing the uniformity of dye samples is to carry out simple paper chromatography. This will show whether or not there are secondary dye fractions present, and will also give some indication of dye particle size by the extent of travel in the paper in a given solvent and developing solution. A number 1 Whatman filter paper can be used for this exercise, and the procedure is clearly set out in an article by Rosenthal et al (1965) which should be consulted for full details.

Reference has been made to the importance of the natural dye haematoxylin in histology; this was introduced in 1863 by Waldeyer and still has a wide histological usage. Other natural dyes include carmine from the cochineal beetle, and orcein which is derived from a species of lichens; both dyes continue to have a significant, if small role in current histological practices.

In the last two decades comparatively few 'new' dyes have entered the repertoire (and more importantly remained there!). Examples of those that have are luxol fast blue, solochrome cyanine, sirius red, brilliant crystal scarlet, amido black, alcian blue and fluorescent dyes such as thioflavine T and fluoroscein isothiocyanate (FITC). Dye nomenclature is often descriptive and reflects either the colour of the product, e.g. *light green*, or occasionally, an association with a particular use, e.g. 'wool green' or even a particular event e.g. 'Congo red' whose introduction to the dye market coincided with the founding of the Congo Free State in 1885. Sometimes the dye name is followed by various letters or numbers, e.g. alcian blue GX and is allotted by the manufacturer to designate slight modifications in production.

THE CHEMISTRY OF DYES AND THEIR MODE OF ATTACHMENT TO TISSUE

Dyes

These are essentially aromatic benzene ring compounds (or derivatives) which possess the twin properties of colour and being able to bind to tissues. At one time most dyes were coal tar derivatives but an increasing number are now by-products of oil distillation.

Chromophores

The group on the benzene ring which confers colour is known as a chromophore and alters the light resonance properties of the compound, so that unequal absorption occurs when white light is passed through. As is well known, the colour *emission* of a given object depends on the colour spectrum *absorbed* when white light falls on it; so that a red rose is red because the arrangement of the rose fibre molecules is such that the blue-green component is absorbed out.

An important chromophore is the quinoid ring where two of the hydrogen atoms on the benzene ring have been replaced by oxygen atoms. The quinoid chromophore may occur alone, as in the triphenyl methane dyes (e.g. basic fuchsin), or together with chromophores such as the azo group (e.g. as in Congo red). Other important chromophoric groups are xanthene (e.g. eosin) and the quinone-imine group. The latter group is subdivided according to the element present in the interbenzene bonds, and includes the *oxazins* where an oxygen atom is incorporated (e.g. as in cresyl fast violet), and the thiazins where a sulphur atom is incorporated (e.g. as in toluidine blue).

It is important to appreciate that possession of colour alone does not itself constitute a dye; an auxochromic group is necessary (a substance possessing a chromophore is known as a chromogen, therefore; chromogen + auxochrome = a dye).

Auxochromes

In order for tissue to bind firmly to a given dye, it is necessary for the dye to possess auxochromic groups. These are groups on the benzene ring which can impart a net charge to the molecule by conferring the property of electrolytic dissociation. This electrical charge, as will be seen, is an important mechanism in the attachment of dyes to tissues.

The amino group is an important cationic auxochrome and the hydroxyl and carboxyl groups important anionic auxochromes.

DYE MODIFIERS

We have seen how the possession of a chromophore and auxochrome is integral to the formation of a dye, but there are other radicles which affect either the colour or properties of that dye; in other words they literally 'modify' the dye. Ethyl and methyl groups on the benzene ring have this effect and by increased methylation, for example, of methyl violet we can arrive at a bluer shade of dye namely crystal violet. Another type of dye modifier is the sulphonic acid radicle which can increase the water solubility of a dye and also confer anionic properties, even in the presence of a cationic auxochrome. Acid fuchsin for example, is virtually sulphonated basic fuchsin and as their names imply will have quite different staining properties.

Leuco dyes

Dyes that by a process of reduction lose their colour are termed 'leuco' dyes. A good example of this is the dye patent blue which becomes colourless on hydrogenation, but which may be restored to its original colour by a suitably catalysed oxidation process. Schiff's reagent is often referred to as

a 'leuocofuchsin', a term that is best avoided as strictly speaking it is a sulphurated fuchsin, rather than a reduced fuchsin. The use of Schiff's reagent is fundamental to the practice of histochemistry and is essentially a sulphurated pararosanilin dye which is capable of forming a magenta compound with tissue di-aldehydes. The precise nature of the magenta compound produced is still not unequivocally established, and is discussed in greater detail in the chapter on carbohydrates.

Fluorescent dyes

Fluorescence is emitted by certain substances when high energy, i.e. low wavelength light, is used to raise them to a higher energy level. Subsequently there is a fall to a lower energy level and because there is an energy loss, the energy they emit is of a higher wavelength. This is the basis of fluorescence microscopy, which is used as a means of identifying, or visualizing certain tissue entities. These fluorescent substances can be shown to increase the wavelength of the exciting light from the invisible (e.g. ultraviolet) to visible, or to increase the wavelength of visible exciting light and thus change the colour (e.g. blue to yellow).

Certain structures such as elastic fibres possess an inherent fluorescence property which is known as auto or primary fluorescence (more properly the latter). In addition there are compounds known as fluorochromes or fluorescent dyes which can bind to non-fluorescent tissue entities and thus demonstrate them by indirect fluorescence properties; this is termed secondary fluorescence. Examples of commonly employed fluorescent dyes are acridine orange, thioflavine T and fluorescein isothiocyanate (FITC). One particularly useful advantage of fluorescent over conventional dyes is that they are more sensitive and can aid the visualization of minute compounds or structures, but they are usually less selective.

DYE TO TISSUE MECHANISMS

Tissue will bind dyes by one of the following mechanisms:

1. *Electrostatic*. The majority of tissue-dye reactions involve some form of electrostatic mechanism, so that a cationic dye (e.g. neutral red) will bond to anionic tissue (e.g. nucleic acids). Conversely, anionic dyes (e.g. light green) will bond to cationic tissue (e.g. basic protein as in red cell envelopes). Amphoteric reactions also apply, an example being muscle protein which will behave as a base in the presence of an acid dye and bind that dye. Dyes too, may be amphoteric and behave as an acid or base when suitably buffered to below or above their isoelectric point.

2. *Hydrogen bonding*. Although relatively few staining effects are based on this type of reaction, it is important in view of the fact that one of the most useful and diagnostically significant techniques in the histological repertoire is involved; namely Congo red for amyloid. Other examples of hydrogen bond dye reactions are carmine for glycogen and the Weigert-type resorcinol dye methods for elastic fibres.

3. *Van der Waals forces and covalent bonding*. There has been in recent years, an increased awareness of the role played by the former mechanism in dye binding, and it has been shown that large dye-mordant complexes may bind to tissue by Van der Waals forces; an example of such binding is the staining of cell nuclei by alum haematoxylin solutions. Covalent bonding is also thought to be involved in dye-mordant-tissue reactions, but the precise nature of the binding is less clear.

4. *Physical staining*. The staining of lipids by a group of dyes known collectively as the Sudan dyes is the only noteworthy histological reaction where a purely physical mechanism pertains. These dyes (which are of the azo chromophoric group) possess the unique property of being more soluble in certain types of lipid than in their own solvent, so that diffusion, which is reversible, takes place from one medium to the other.

The Sudan dyes, with one exception, lack an auxochromic group so that they are not dyes in the true sense of the word. The exception is Sudan black which possesses an amino group auxochrome. In fact because of this, it has enhanced staining properties and a wider range of lipids can be stained compared to others of the Sudan group.

5. *Natural affinity*. There are a few examples where living material has an affinity for a particular dye the most noteworthy being that of Janus green for mitochondria in *Vital* dyeing.

FACTORS INFLUENCING DYE UPTAKE

These include *spatial relationships*, where the stereochemistry of the dye molecule and tissue results in a specific staining reaction, and *dye particle size related to tissue pore size* in controlled sequential staining by different coloured dyes having a similar electrical charge. Both of these factors will be further discussed in the chapters dealing with the demonstration of nucleic acids and connective tissue respectively, but it is important to appreciate that these merely *influence* the way in which dyes are bound to tissue by *conventional* (i.e. usually electrostatic) forces.

The third influencing factor in certain staining reactions is the use of *mordants*. These are double salts of metals such as lead, aluminium, copper, iron, molybdenum and tungsten and serve to enhance or make possible the binding of a particular dye to a particular tissue moiety. In a sense they act as a bridge between tissue and dye. Mordants can be incorporated into the stain solution, e.g. aluminium potassium sulphate in haematoxylin solutions, or as a separate step usually preceding the staining solution as in the Loyez technique for myelin.

EFFECTS OF FIXATION ON STAINING OF TISSUES

To discuss this in any detail is beyond the scope of this chapter, but it should be mentioned that certain fixatives either enhance or inhibit dye uptake by modifying the protein (usually) so that either dye diffusion is affected, or reactive radicals exposed or alternatively masked by protein rearrangement through denaturation. For example, formalin forms cross links with protein and tends to mask cationic tissue binding sites for anionic dyes so that acid dye uptake, e.g. eosin is suppressed.

Conversely, anionic binding sites are exposed so that basophilia of nuclei, for example, is enhanced.

IMPREGNATION WITH METALLIC SALTS

Only two metallic salts are of any importance as a means of demonstrating tissue morphology and of these it is really only silver nitrate that has a wide use. The other salt, gold chloride, was employed to a limited extent in an empirical manner by some of the early workers in the field of nerve fibre and nerve ending demonstration. The only technique employing a gold salt which is still widely used, is that of Cajal which incorporates an impregnating solution of gold chloride and mercuric chloride to demonstrate neuroglial astrocytes.

The use of silver nitrate in histological demonstration techniques is not new, a German worker von Recklinghausen having used it as long ago as 1862. It is one having many applications and can probably be best divided into three forms.

1. ARYGYROPHIL REACTIONS

There are many techniques to be found under this broad umbrella, quite often differing only in the length of the various steps or in the compostion of the silver solutions employed.

Essentially the reactions are those employed in black and white photography, although the precise rationale for many of these closely related methods is poorly understood. Certain tissue elements have a natural affinity (arygrophilia) for silver nitrate. This bound colourless silver salt (various complex solutions are actually employed) if subsequently reduced by substances such as hydroquinone or formalin will form a black reduced silver compound and show the particular elements to be demonstrated as black structures against (hopefully!) a colourless or pale yellow background. Examples of tissue elements demonstrated by an argyrophil technique are reticulin and nerve fibres, also calcium salts although this involves a somewhat different type of argyrophil reaction (q.v.).

2. ARGENTAFFIN REACTIONS

In this type of technique, use is made of the presence in structures of substances, often of the phenolic group, capable of reducing silver salts (and other metallic salts), i.e. they do not need an extraneous reducer as in the argyrophil method. One of the earliest applications of this principle in histology was by Gossett and Masson in 1914, who demonstrated carcinoid tumours (q.v.). Tissue granules, such as melanin and certain forms of enterochromaffin cells are good examples of argentaffin material.

3. ALDEHYDE REDUCTION

Certain carbohydrate-containing tissues when treated with suitable oxidants will form aldehydes, and these aldehydes are able to reduce a compound formed of hexamine (methenamine) and silver nitrate, under appropriate conditions of temperature and pH (q.v.).

We owe the popularity of this form of silver reduction in histology to that remarkable American histochemist Gomori, who in the mid 1940's introduced a method based on this principle which, with subsequent modifications by other workers, remains the standard technique for fungi and basement membranes (basal lamina).

FORMATION OF COLOURED COMPOUNDS BY MEANS OF A CHEMICAL REACTION

Rather like the silver techniques described above, the use of colour formation methodology has a firm place in the routine histological repertoire. In this type of technique the sections are treated with organic or inorganic salts which will react with the moiety to be demonstrated, and will either directly form a coloured reaction product in situ, or will form a colourless intermediate product which is capable of forming a coloured end-product when suitably treated in its turn. This is by no means new: as far back as 1849, Millon devised such a histochemical technique for tyrosine, also Perls introduced in 1867 his classical (and still widely used!) method for iron. Other techniques still in common use, and based upon colour formation by a chemical reaction, include the Schmorl method for melanin and the Fouchet method for bile which was adapted from its original use in biochemistry. These methods will be discussed in greater detail in the relevant chapters. There is another significant group of histochemical techniques which is the demonstration of enzymes; This received its impetus from the ubiquitous Gomori in 1939. He described a technique for the demonstration of alkaline phosphatase using a metallic substitution principle to produce a brown-black reaction product. Another later enzyme demonstration milestone, by Menten and co-workers in 1944 was the use of diazonium salts which react with enzyme-substrate reaction products to form an azo dye in situ. It is interesting that the whole field of enzyme histochemistry has taken on a new lease of life with the development of immunohistochemistry; one of the important techniques in this context being the DAB technique, which was introduced in 1966 by Graham and Karnovsky for the simple demonstration of the enzyme peroxidase in certain blood cells. How little could they have anticipated its eventual worldwide use in the immunoperoxidase method — currently the most exciting histochemical technique for which new applications are constantly being found.

SUMMARY OF COMMON TERMS USED IN TISSUE DEMONSTRATION

Argentaffin. Affinity of substances for silver salts and capable of reducing them to a black metallic silver without the need for an extraneous reducer, e.g. melanin pigment.

Argyrophil. Affinity of substances for silver salts which are subsequently reduced to a black metallic silver and consequently demonstrated, e.g. nerve fibres, using a reducing agent.

Auxochrome. A charged group present on dye molecules responsible for electrochemical binding of charged tissue molecules, e.g. OH, NH_2

Chromophore. An organic group, the presence of which confers colour to benzene ring compounds, e.g. quinoid group.

Diazonium salt. Organic compounds which have been nitrogenated ('diazotized') and which can combine with certain organic groups, such as naphthol, to form azo dyes. Used commonly in methods for tissue enzymes.

Fluorochrome. When tissues are stained with a fluorochrome, e.g. acridine orange, this confers the property of secondary fluorescence. In other words, a fluorochrome can increase the wavelength of high energy light passed through it and so can be used to confer secondary fluorescence.

Metachromasia. A metachromatic dye is one capable of staining certain negatively charged tissue moieties a colour which is not inherent in the dye itself, e.g. toluidine blue will stain cartilage metachromatically purple-red and the surrounding tissue blue. *Polychromasia*, by contrast, is when tissues are stained varying colours by a compound containing more than one dye fraction, e.g. Giemsa stain.

Mordant. Some dye-to-tissue reactions require the presence of an intermediate binding agent. This agent is termed a mordant and consists of the salts of various metals, e.g. aluminium potassium sulphate which will facilitate the binding of haematoxylin to cell nuclei.

REFERENCES

Horobin R 1982a Theory of staining. In: Bancroft J D, Stevens A (eds) Theory and practice of histological techniques, 2nd edn. Churchill Livingstone, Edinburgh

Horobin R 1982b Histochemistry. Butterworth, London

Lillie R D 1969 In: Conn H J (ed) Biological stains, 8th edn. chs I to IV. Williams and Wilkins, Baltimore

Rosenthal S I, Puchtler H, Sweat F 1965 Paper chromatography of dyes. Archives of Pathology 80: 190–6

3

Routine morphological staining

HAEMATOXYLIN AND EOSIN (H and E)

Notes

H and E staining usually denotes staining of nuclei by oxidized haematoxylin (haematein) through mordant (chelate) bonds of metals such as aluminium, followed by counterstaining by the xanthene dye eosin, which colours in varying shades the different tissue fibres and cytoplasms. A general tissue demonstration picture is produced and serves as the main diagnostic technique.

Haematoxylin, which is extracted from the bark of a tropical log wood, is not a dye as such, as it possesses neither tissue binding properties, nor indeed, colour to any marked degree. For nuclear staining it is necessary to oxidize the haematoxylin to haematein which is a weakly anionic purple dye. This oxidation or 'ripening' may be accomplished by a natural process of exposure to light and air over a long period of time, or by the addition of oxidizing agents. Examples of the latter are sodium iodate in Mayer's, Gill's or Carazzi's solutions, iodine in Cole's and mercuric oxide in Harris's haematoxylin.

Being anionic, the haematein will have no particular affinity for the nucleic acids of cell nuclei. Therefore it is also necessary to combine a metallic salt or 'mordant' with the haematoxylin which will confer a net positive charge to the dye compound by virtue of the metal cation present. Thus the cationic dye-metal complex will bind to the anionic nuclear chromatin. Haematoxylin solutions containing 'alums' formed of aluminium sulphate with either potassium or ammonium sulphate, are known as 'alum haematoxylins', and are suitable for routine nuclear staining with eosin as a counterstain. An alternative nuclear stain is provided by the 'iron haematoxylins'. These use mordants which combine ferric sulphate with ammonium sulphate and form a much stronger nucleic acid-dye bond. Consequently, these iron haematoxylins are employed when a particularly vigorous counterstain such as van Gieson is to be used, which might decolourize the weaker nuclear staining obtained with the alum haematoxylins.

Some haematoxylin solutions such as Harris's, tend to stain background tissue as well as nuclei, albeit to a lesser degree, and subsequent acid-alcohol differentiation will be required so that only the nuclei are stained. This is known as *regressive* staining and is the usual technique employed in routine morphological staining. Other haematoxylins, however, stain the background tissue to a much lesser extent, so that differentiation may not be necessary or need only be minimal. This is known as *progressive* staining and can be seen with haematoxylins such as those of Mayer and Carazzi.

The haematoxylin solutions are complex and will contain one or more of the following substances forming a composite solution bearing the originator's name.

An alum. This is the mordant of which the aluminium cation is the main reactant and is obtained as a combined salt with either potassium or ammonium sulphate.

An acid. This aims at making staining more precise ('accelerator').

An oxidizing agent gives speedy conversion of haematoxylin to haematein.

Glycerol. This slows the oxidation of naturally oxidizing haematoxylin and improves the keeping properties.

The choice of a haematoxylin solution is a personal decision as all the popular ones are capable of giving good results. There are minor attributes to be borne in mind. Mayer's and Carazzi's haematoxylin solutions have a shorter staining time and can be used progressively, whilst Harris's haematoxylin solution needs filtering before use and careful differentiation, but is regarded by many as giving the most intense and precise staining of all. Gill's haematoxylin seems to be quite popular, particularly amongst cytologists, for its avid staining allied to a short staining time and so may be used in the Papanicoloau technique for cervical smears. Ehrlich's haematoxylin solution, on the other hand, keeps well and stains certain of the mucins blue, but needs longer staining times.

Differentiation of haematoxylin is usually accomplished by an alcoholic solution of hydrochloric acid. It is thought the differentiation is achieved by the acid attacking and breaking the tissue to mordant bond, rather than the mordant to dye bond (Baker, 1962). Eosin was first used in 1875 (as 'Eosine') for the dyeing of silk and wool. There are various forms available commercially but the most commonly used is the water-soluble (ws) yellowish. Other variants are eosin B (a bluish form) and eosin ethyl and alcohol soluble form. Eosin is an anionic dye and combines electrostatically with tissue such as collagen and muscle, the latter in an amphoteric manner. By raising the pH of the solution, eosin will stain more intensely; this can be achieved either by the use of a suitable buffer or by dissolving the dye in tap water (the latter treatment will, of course, vary in its efficacy in different areas).

In the following procedures, dogmatic times of haematoxylin treatment will be omitted as these will depend very much on the preparation of the solutions and sections. For example, Ehrlich's haematoxylin staining time will vary according to the degree of oxidation obtained; also long formalin-fixed paraffin sections will stain more heavily with haematoxylin and more weakly with eosin, than sections of tissue fixed for a short time in, for example, Helly's solution. Frozen sections will stain more quickly than paraffin.

Solutions

Ehrlich's haematoxylin solution (Ehrlich, 1886)

Haematoxylin	16 g
Ethyl alcohol	480 ml
Potassium or ammonium alum	48 g
Distilled water	240 ml
Glycerol	240 ml
Glacial acetic acid	24 ml

Dissolve the haematoxylin in the alcohol with the aid of gentle heat (56° C oven or water bath). Dissolve the alum in the distilled water using heat (bunsen) and whilst warm add the glycerol. Allow to cool. Add the alcoholic haematoxylin solution in small volumes to the alum-glycerol solution, mixing well. Add the acetic acid and mix. Plug the container with cotton wool and allow to oxidize by exposure to light; this will take at least 6 weeks but ripening may be allowed to continue indefinitely beyond that period. Filter prior to use. Immediate oxidation may be achieved, if so desired by adding 0.1 g sodium iodate per 100 ml volume of prepared solution, then mixing and allowing to stand for at least 1 h before use.

Mayer's haematoxylin solution (Mayer, 1903)

Haematoxylin	1 g
Distilled water	1000 ml
Potassium or ammonium alum	50 g
Sodium iodate	0.2 g
Citric acid	1 g
Chloral hydrate	50 g

Dissolve the haematoxylin, alum and sodium iodate in the distilled water by standing the mixture overnight at room temperature. Add the chloral hydrate and citric acid, mix and boil for 5 min. Cool and filter. The solution is ready for use and should not need refiltering.

Harris's haematoxylin solution (Harris, 1900)

Haematoxylin	5 g
Ethyl alcohol	50 ml
Potassium or ammonium alum	100 g
Distilled water	950 ml
Mercuric oxide	2.5 g
Glacial acetic acid	40 ml

Dissolve the haematoxylin in the alcohol using gentle heat (56° C oven or water bath) and dissolve the alum in the distilled water using heat (bunsen) with frequent stirring. Whilst the aqueous alum solution is still hot, add the alcoholic haematoxylin solution and bring to the boil stirring frequently.

(Turn off the bunsen just before adding the mercuric oxide as the resultant effervescence may cause spillage.) Cool quickly by plunging the container into cold water, then add the acetic acid and filter. The solution is ready for immediate use but will need refiltering.

Cole's haematoxylin solution (Cole, 1943)

Haematoxylin	1.5 g
Saturated aqueous potassium or ammonium alum	700 ml
1% iodine in 95% alcohol	50 ml
Distilled water	250 ml

Dissolve the haematoxylin in the distilled water using gentle heat (56° C oven or water bath). Add to this the iodine solution and bring to the boil, then cool quickly. The solution is ready for immediate use but will need refiltering.

Carazzi's haematoxylin solution (Carazzi, 1911)

Haematoxylin	1 g
Glycerol	200 ml
Potassium or ammonium alum	50 g
Distilled water	800 ml
Potassium iodate	0.2 g

Dissolve the haematoxylin in the glycerol, and the alum in most (e.g. 750 ml) of the distilled water. The alum solution should be prepared at room temperature and is best left overnight for the alum crystals to dissolve. Mix the alum and haematoxylin solutions in small volumes shaking well. Dissolve the iodate salt in the remaining volume of distilled water (e.g. 50 ml) and add to the main solution with thorough mixing. Filter. The solution is ready for use.

Gill's haematoxylin solution (Gill, 1974)

Haematoxylin	2 g
Sodium iodate	0.2 g
Aluminium sulphate	17.6 g
Distilled water	750 ml
Ethylene glycol	250 ml
Glacial acetic acid	20 ml

Mix the distilled water and ethylene glycol and add the haematoxylin. Next add the sodium iodate

followed by the aluminium sulphate and mix. Finally add the acetic acid and stir for 1 h at room temperature using a magnetic stirrer. The solution is ready for immediate use and should be filtered when required.

Eosin 1% aqueous ws yellowish

Add a crystal of phenol or thymol to the prepared solution in order to inhibit mould formation. Filter prior to use.

Differentiator

1% hydrochloric acid in 70% alcohol.

Blueing agent

2% aqueous sodium bicarbonate.

Technique

1. Take sections to water, i.e. deparaffinize in xylene, wash in alcohol, then in water.
2. Stain with a haematoxylin solution for the requisite period, e.g. Carazzi's, Mayer's and Harris's up to 5 min; Cole's and Gill's up to 10 min; Ehrlich's up to 25 min. (Gill's solution will stain smears in 2 min.)
3. Wash briefly in water and differentiate in acid-alcohol.
4. Wash well in water and blue. At this stage check microscopically; the nuclei should be a deep blue colour with the vesicular nuclei showing a well marked chromatin pattern, whilst the background should show only weak residual haematoxylin colouration.
5. Wash in water and stain with the eosin solution for 5 min.
6. Wash fairly quickly in water, differentiate and dehydrate in alcohol. Clear and mount as desired.

Results

Keratohyalin, nuclei, cytoplasmic RNA, some calcium salts, urates, bacteria (weakly)	blue

Muscle, keratin, coarse elastic
fibres, fibrin, fibrinoid   bright red

Collagen, reticulin, myelinated
nerve fibres, amyloid   pink

Red blood cells   orange

In addition to the haematoxylin solutions detailed above there are others having a more specialized role (see Table 3.1) and include: Celestine blue — haematoxylin, Heidenhain, Weigert, Verhoeff, Loyez, PTAH, Solcia lead haematoxylin and Thomas molybdenum.

Table 3.1 Specialized (non-nuclear) uses of haematoxylin/haematein

Technique	Mordant	Demonstration
Baker	Potassium dichromate	Phospholipids
Heidenhain	Iron alum	Mitochondria, striated muscle
Kultschitsky	Potassium dichromate/chromic fluoride	Normal myelin
Loyez	Iron alum	Normal myelin
Mallory	Phosphotungstic acid	Fibrin, glial fibres Striated muscle
Mallory	None	Lead, copper
Mayer	Aluminium chloride	Mucins
Solcia	Lead nitrate	APUD cells
Thomas	Molybdenum	APUD cells, collagen etc.
Verhoeff	Ferric chloride	Elastic fibres
Weigert	Ferric chloride	Normal myelin
Weil	Iron alum	Normal myelin

CARMALUM STAIN FOR NUCLEI (Mayer, 1892)

This can conveniently be used when a red nuclear stain is required. Unlike neutral red it is stable even if the section is mounted in an aqueous mountant. It is valuable as a nuclear counterstain to the Sudan black stain for lipid. However, it must be said that it is not a particularly avid stain and a lengthy (30 min) staining time is required. Note that formalin fixed material gives in general poor results; mercuric chloride-containing solutions are preferred.

Solution

Carminic acid   2 g
5% aqueous ammonium alum   100 ml
Salicylic acid or thymol   0.2 g

Add the carminic acid to the ammonium alum solution and dissolve by boiling for 1 h. Cool and restore to original volume with distilled water. Add the fungicidal agent and mix thoroughly. Filter and use. The solution keeps quite well if stored at 4° C.

RAPID STAINING FOR URGENT FROZEN SECTIONS

HAEMATOXYLIN AND EOSIN TECHNIQUE FOR FRESH CRYOSTAT SECTIONS

Notes

Whilst fixation prior to staining is not essential, brief (1–2 min) immersion of the slide in 10% formalin will enhance the nuclear basophilia. Sections of certain material, e.g. mucoid tumours, may lift off the slides when placed in the formalin and this step should, therefore, be avoided and a dry section celloidinized instead.

Solutions

Harris's haematoxylin (prefiltered).

1% acid alcohol.

2% aqueous sodium bicarbonate.

1% aqueous ws yellowish eosin.

Technique

1. Wash sections in water for 10–20 s.
2. Stain with haematoxylin for 1 min.
3. Wash briefly in water, differentiate in acid-alcohol for 1–2 s.
4. Wash briefly in water and 'blue' in sodium bicarbonate.
5. Wash in water 10–20 s and, if time permits, check nuclear staining microscopically.
6. Stain with eosin for 30 s.
7. Wash briefly, dehydrate, clear and mount as desired.

Results

Nuclei	blue
Background	shades of pink to red

H AND E TECHNIQUE FOR FORMALIN-FIXED FROZEN SECTIONS

Notes

The essential differences in technique when staining fixed — as opposed to — unfixed frozen sections are based upon the former's tendency to come away from the slide very much more easily during staining, and also the fact that eosin staining is depressed and nuclear staining enhanced. Providing that a celloidin film is applied which is reasonably thin and even, there should be no need to remove it at the conclusion of staining.

Solutions

As for the fresh cryostat section staining technique with the exception of the eosin solution which is as follows:

2% ws yellowish eosin in tap water, see notes on page 20.

Technique

1. Mount the frozen sections on a slide and blot dry.
2. Rinse in equal parts ether-alcohol and then cover with 0.5% celloidin in ether-alcohol.
3. Drain slide, *allow to air dry*, before washing in water for ½–1 min to complete the process of hardening the celloidin film.
4. Stain with haematoxylin for 40–50 s.
5. Wash briefly in water and differentiate in acid-alcohol for up to 5 s.
6. Wash briefly in water and 'blue' in sodium bicarbonate solution.
7. Wash in water and if time permits check nuclear staining microscopically.
8. Stain with eosin for 1 min.
9. Wash briefly in water, dehydrate thoroughly because of the celloidin film, clear and mount as desired.

Results

Nuclei	blue
Background	shades of pink to red

POLYCHROME METHYLENE BLUE TECHNIQUE (Morris, 1947)

Notes

The use of polychrome methylene blue for rapid frozen sections was quite popular at one time, either in place of the H and E stain, or as a preceding stain so that the pathologist could study the methylene blue stained section whilst the comparatively slower H and E stained section was completed. Touch or imprint smears of unfixed tumours, e.g. breast lumps or lymph nodes, may also be stained to advantage with polychrome methylene blue. Polychroming of methylene blue is achieved by potassium carbonate when various azures are formed. This process is accentuated by ageing of the solution.

Solution

Methylene blue	1 g
Potassium carbonate	1 g
Glacial acetic acid	3 ml
Distilled water	300 ml

Place the distilled water in a large (1 litre) flask and add, with mixing, the methylene blue and potassium carbonate. Boil for 10–15 min. Whilst still hot add the glacial acetic acid drop by drop shaking vigorously, until the formed precipitate is dissolved. Continue boiling until the volume of fluid is reduced to 100 ml. Cool and filter. Allow to stand 4 weeks prior to use.

Technique

1. Rinse frozen sections and imprint smears in water.
2. Filter on the polychrome methylene blue for ½–1 min.
3. Wash in water and blot dry.
4. Dehydrate in tertiary butyl alcohol, clear in xylene and mount in a DPX-type mountant, (conventional ethanol dehydration will diminish the polychromasia).

Results

Nuclei   blue
Background   various shades of red-purple.

ROUTINE STAINING FOR THIN PLASTIC RESIN SECTIONS

Staining resin sections for light microscopy presents problems that are absent when dealing with paraffin or frozen material. This is often the result of the inability of dye molecules to penetrate the plastic resin, so that it is necessary to dissolve the resin from the section prior to staining. This is a variable. In general the acrylics will permit staining without the need for resin extraction, and usually it is the epoxy resin sections that require treatment. Whether or not it is necessary to carry out section resin extraction, it may be necessary to modify the normal staining times or precede staining by permanganate oxidation to intensify the reaction. A case in point is the H and E technique. Whilst haematoxylin stains nuclei effectively in thin resin sections, eosin does not stain the cytoplasm to the same degree. It is common practice to use a related dye, phloxine, instead. Also described below is toluidine blue staining, which is the standard morphological technique for general oversight staining of tissue. This gives nuclear detail not readily obtained in toluidine blue staining of paraffin or frozen sections.

RESIN EXTRACTION OF SECTIONS PRIOR TO STAINING

1. Dissolve 2 g sodium hydroxide in 100 ml absolute ethanol and allow to stand overnight.
2. Place sections in the solution for 1 h at room temperature. Wash well in water (at least 15 min).

TOLUIDINE TECHNIQUE FOR THIN RESIN SECTIONS

Notes

Epoxy resins are more difficult to stain, even after sodium ethoxide extraction, and will necessitate a heated toluidine blue solution. Other resins such as L. R. White and glycol methacrylate are adequately stained using the room temperature solution. At the conclusion of staining it is better to air dry and mount, as the usual alcohol-xylene treatment may cause cracking or lifting of the section.

Solution

1% toluidine blue in 1% aqueous borax (sodium tetraborate). Filter, the solution has a pH of approximately 11.0.

Technique

1. Rinse sections in distilled water.
2. Stain with refiltered toluidine blue, either (see notes) at room temperature for 15 s or, for $1\frac{1}{2}$–2 min on a hot plate (temperature in the region 60–65°C).
3. Blot and allow to thoroughly air dry.
4. Mount as desired.

Results

Nuclei   deep blue
Background   pale blue

HAEMATOXYLIN-PHLOXINE TECHNIQUE FOR THIN RESIN SECTIONS

Notes

The nuclei of resin sections will usually stain perfectly well but less readily than non-plastic resin sections, so that it is important to use an avid alum haematoxylin. Harris's haematoxylin is commonly employed. It will be noted that somewhat longer times of staining are necessary with fairly brief subsequent acid-alcohol differentiation.

Solutions

Harris's haematoxylin, see page 19.

1% acid-alcohol.

2% aqueous sodium bicarbonate.

1% aqueous phloxine (add a few crystals of thymol after filtering to prevent fungal growth).

Technique

1. Rinse sections in water.
2. Stain with haematoxylin for 10 min.
3. Rinse in water.
4. Differentiate in acid-alcohol for 1–2 s.
5. Wash in water and blue in sodium bicarbonate.
6. Wash in water.
7. Stain with phloxine for 5 min.
8. Blot and allow to thoroughly air dry. Mount as desired.

Results

Nuclei	blue
Background	pale pink

Having considered some of the staining techniques in general use it would be profitable to consider two practical aspects of staining sections on slides. These concern keeping the section on the slide during treatment with reagents, and the measures to be adopted when a slide is broken which (inevitably!) carries an all-important section and for a variety of reasons is impossible to replace.

SECTION ADHESION

Most *well-processed*, *well-cut* paraffin sections if adequately dried on the slide, present few problems during staining. Badly prepared and dried sections are more likely to become detached, as are well-prepared sections of tissues such as brain, bone, keratinous skin lesions and material containing tuberculous caseation. In addition to the above, techniques involving high temperatures or exposure to strongly alkaline solutions will produce conditions where even the hardiest of sections will float quietly off the slide.

Recommended procedures in cases of difficulty

1. Mount the section on a microscope slide washed in 1% acid-alcohol (as per the standard H and E technique) for 10 min, wash in water and then wipe dry. When the section has been mounted on the slide it is often worthwhile drying at a lower-than-usual temperature but for a longer period, e.g. 3–4 h at 56° C or overnight at 37° C.

2. Should the above procedures fail, it will be necessary to coat the slide with a section adhesive. For the occasional section it is effective if the slide is smeared with a thin layer or *normal* plasma (Cook, 1965). The mounted section is then heat dried in the usual way. Note that too thick a layer of plasma will take up counterstains such as eosin. From a health and safety aspect it is important to check that the plasma has been obtained from patients in whom there is no risk of serum hepatitis. For larger numbers of sections we would recommend the following procedure in which slides are prepared in advance and en masse.

  a. Prepare a 0.2% aqueous solution of gelatin to which a few crystals of thymol have been added to discourage bacterial growth. Allow to dissolve at 56° C (30 min will usually suffice). The volume of solution to be prepared will depend on the number of slides to be coated, and the size of container.

  b. Dip clean microscope slides into the gelatin solution *when cool*, agitating for several seconds. Take out the slides, drain thoroughly and allow to dry on edge (for maximum drainage) at room temperature. It may be found useful, if slide racks are being used, to place these on clean cloth to obviate the collection of gelatin solution at the bottom edge of the slides.

  c. Dry the coated slides for 1 h at 56° C.

  d. Allow to cool and store until required in suitable containers.

Sections may be subsequently mounted in the usual way from the floating-out bath, followed by conventional drying treatment.

TRANSFERENCE OF SECTIONS (Clayden, 1955 slightly modified)

Notes

The transfer of a section from one glass slide to another is effectively achieved by covering the section with a plastic resin film, which when hardened can be soaked off together with the section.

For a successful result, it is important that the solution be of the right consistency and that the hardening of the film be complete. Too thin a film and it will fail to attach to the section; too thick and problems will be encountered when finally coverslipping.

Solution

D.P.X. or Styrolite mountant	1 part
Butyl acetate	6 parts

This is conveniently done in a glass test-tube and will require thorough mixing by repeated inversion.

Technique

1. Remove the coverslip from the section to be transferred and completely remove the existing mountant in xylene.

2. Cover the whole slide with the resin solution and leave for up to 30 min at 56° C until a hard film is formed. (This is conveniently done by resting the slide on glass rods in a Petri dish.)
3. Using a sharp scalpel blade make a firm cut in the resin film around the section.
4. Place the slide in distilled water until the film plus section starts to lift; this may take several minutes and can be expedited by levering one corner of the film with the scalpel blade.
5. When the section has completely floated off, take up on a clean slide, wipe off the excess water and place in a rack in the 56° C incubator until completely dry.
6. Wash carefully with several changes of butyl acetate, then in xylene and finally mount as desired.

REFERENCES

Baker J R 1962 Experiments on the action of mordants: 2, aluminium-haematin. Quarterly Journal of Microscopic Science 103: 493

Carazzi D 1911 Eine neue Hamatoxylinosung. Zeitschrift für wissenschaftliche Mikroskopie und für mikroskopische Technik 28: 275

Clayden E C 1955 Practical section cutting and staining. Churchill, London

Cole E C 1943 Studies in haematoxylin stains. Stain Technology 18: 125

Cook H C 1965 A comparative survey of section adhesives and of factors affecting adhesion. Stain Technology 40: 321–8

Ehrlich P 1886 Frageskasten. Zeitschrift für wissenschaftliche Mikroskopie und für mikroskopische Technik 3: 150

Gill G W, Frost J K, Miller K A 1974 A new formula for a half-oxidised haematoxylin solution that neither overstains or requires differentiation. Acta Cytologica 18: 300–11

Harris H F 1900 On the rapid conversion of haematoxylin into haematein in staining reactions. Journal of Applied Microscopic Laboratory Methods 3: 777

Mayer P 1892 Uber das Farben mit Carmin, Cochenille und Hamatein-Tonerde. Mitt. zool. Stat. Neapel 10: 480

Mayer P 1903 Notiz über Haematein und Hamalaum. Zeitschrift für wissenschaftliche Mikroskopie und für mikroskopische Technik 20: 409

Morris A A 1947 The histological use of the smear technique in the rapid histological diagnosis of tumours of the central nervous system. Journal of Neurosurgery 4: 497

4

Clinical (exfoliative) cytology

INTRODUCTION

Under the heading of 'exfoliative cytology' are grouped many cells from widely differing environments. The presentation of material is variable due to the different circumstances surrounding a given fluid when concentrating the contained cells. For example, where there are few cells in abundant fluid such as cerebrospinal fluid (c.s.f.), or urine it is useful to be able to filter off the contained cells by passing the fluid through one of the membrane filters such as the millipore filter. These filters can be chosen to have a pore size of 5 μm so that only particles of a greater diameter will be retained, i.e. most cells. Another useful method is the use of the Shandon Cytospin centrifuge, where cells in fluid are deposited directly on the slide surface by centrifugal force. Concentration of cells in sputum presents special problems due to the viscous nature of the mucous material. This high viscosity prevents membrane filtration and normal centrifugation methods; therefore we need to have recourse to mucolytic pretreatments such as the use of various enzymes or chemical reagents, with or without ultrasonic disintegration, followed by centrifugation. It is most important that all specimen preparation be carried out in an approved safety cabinet and that appropriate protective clothing be worn. In particular, handling of tuberculous, or possibly tuberculous material needs careful handling and all safety measures observed relating to this as prescribed by the 'Code of Practice for the prevention of infection in clinical laboratories and post-mortem rooms' (Howie Report, 1978). The materials most likely to carry this risk are sputum and serous effusions.

In recent years aspiration techniques have proved of increasing value in this field. Cells from a wide variety of tissues such as breast lumps and palpable lymph nodes can be aspirated using fine bore needles. The aspirated material may be put in fixative for subsequent concentration or placed directly on slides for fixation and staining. Other material which may be profitably examined in a clinical cytology laboratory, include seminal fluids (for infertility and vasectomy cases), breast fluids (discharges and cysts) and gastric brushings.

Choice of fixative is important and most cytological fixatives are based on the use of alcohol. There are three good reasons for this. (1) Alcohol is a protein coagulant and smears of predominantly protein material will remain better attached to the slide during staining. There are problems associated with non-protein fluids such as urine, and to help keep these smears on the slide one should mix the centrifuged deposit with Carbowax fixative (aqueous wax in alcohol), and use an adhesive on the slide. Other coagulant fixatives may be used such as mercuric chloride; non-coagulant fixatives such as formal-saline are not suitable. (2) Alcohol gives good chromatin preservation and delineation. (3) Alcohol in whatever form is easily dispensed to clinics and will store without undue deterioration. It must not be sent through the post.

There are several popular alcoholic-type fixatives. These include butanol-ethanol, ethanol-acetic and Carnoy's solution. In our experience 95% alcohol (95 parts 74 O.P. industrial methylated spirit (I.M.S.), 5 parts distilled water) or undiluted 74 O.P. I.M.S. give perfectly satisfactory results.

As a general rule, if smears are made they should be wet-fixed, i.e. the slide should be placed in the fixing solution before the smear dries. If the smear is allowed to dry various artefacts may occur; the most common of these are enlarged nuclei exhibiting ill-defined weakly staining chromatin and indistinct cell outlines. It is important also, to fix material as rapidly as possible. This applies particularly to serous effusions, as storage of the specimen even at 4°C will cause some cellular changes. Bulk urine specimens should have the fixing solution added if a delay in laboratory preparation is anticipated.

In the following pages will be presented techniques in common use in clinical cytology laboratories, but it is important to bear in mind that most histological demonstration techniques can also be used for cytological purposes, including those of immunohistochemistry. The difference is that dye uptake or reagent reaction times will tend to be shorter when dealing with smears.

Joint fluids which involve crystal identification, will be dealt with in the 'Miscellany' section which covers crystal identification in general.

The question is sometimes asked 'What is the value of exfoliative cytology in diagnostic pathology?'. The essential advantages are; (1) earlier indications of a symptomless lesion may be given by exfoliated cells, e.g. as in a cervical lesion; (2) there may be information given over a wider area than is likely to be the case with a single surgical biopsy, e.g. sputum examination for carcinoma of the lung. Added to these two important advantages are accessibility of most exfoliated material and simplicity of technique (no processing, sectioning or time-consuming surgical procedures).

Against these advantages must be set the paucity of useful cellular material often gained, and the relatively limited information provided by exfoliated material when compared to a histological preparation. For example, a section of a cervical carcinoma will indicate the degree of invasion, cell differentiation, and so on as an aid to prognosis. Another point to be considered is that whilst a cytological preparation showing a positive result (such as malignant change or inflammation) is of definite value, a 'negative' result is of considerably less value. For example, a sputum smear showing malignant cells is conclusive whilst a benign smear pattern in a patient suspected of having lung

cancer is inconclusive, as the failure to demonstrate malignant cells may be due to sampling error or simply failure to expectorate 'positive' material. Lastly, one must always bear in mind that exfoliative cytology is, of necessity, limited to tissues which exfoliate cells in reasonably accessible sites.

In conclusion, it may be said that, providing one keeps the aims of exfoliative cytological examination in perspective, it is a facet of laboratory work which has taken its place as a useful member of the pathology community.

GENERAL STAINING OF SMEARS

PAPANICOLAOU TECHNIQUE
(Papanicolaou, 1942)

Notes

This method is popular for the cytological examination of smears of the female reproductive tract. This is partly due to the variegated colour staining which is helpful with hormonal studies and with the detection of Candida and Trichomonas infestation (immunohistochemistry can be used to advantage, particularly for the latter organism) and partly due to the fact that the type of picture produced results in less eye-fatigue. This latter point is not unimportant when one considers the continuous microscopy involved in screening.

The nuclei are stained with Harris's haematoxylin which seems to give the most precise staining of exfoliated cells. There is considerable division of opinion as to the advisablity of incorporating acetic acid in the solution, some workers feeling that better results are given by using unacidified Harris's haematoxylin.

Following haematoxylin staining, the smears are stained with 'OG6'. This solution contains the yellow dye orange G, and is probably concerned with keratin staining, as for example in smears of vulval carcinoma. The final stage is where the cytoplasm of the cells are stained with solutions variously termed 'EA 36' or 'EA 50'. Different staining results may be given by solutions from different commercial firms bearing the same EA number, so that it is advisable to select the solutions giving the most acceptable results. These

EA solutions contain eosin, light green and Bismarck brown. Intermediate (non-cornified) vaginal cells usually stain green and superficial (cornified) cells stain pink. The principle by which this differential staining occurs is not clear, neither is the role of the Bismarck brown. The pink or green staining is affected by various conditions, such as inflammation, so that distinction between cornified and noncornified cells is more reliably made using nuclear criteria, i.e. pyknotic nuclei for cornified and vesicular nuclei for noncornified cells.

The staining schedule to be given is that for the automatic (Shandon) staining machine; when staining by hand one should increase the staining times of the OG and EA stains by about 50%. Different sources of stain will vary slightly and the staining times should be adjusted to suit the particular solutions. The times given are those using acidified Harris's haematoxylin and OG6 and EA 36 modified solutions available from Raymond A. Lamb*.

Solutions

Orange G

Orange G	0.5 g
Phosphotungstic acid	0.015 g
95% ethanol	100 ml

EA 50

0.1% light green SF in 95% ethanol	45 ml
0.5% eosin ws yellowish in 95% ethanol	45 ml
0.5% Bismarck brown in 95% ethanol	45 ml
Phosphotungstic acid	0.2 g
Saturated aqueous lithium carbonate	1 drop

Technique

The following is a 30 min schedule for the standard timing disc on the double-stage Shandon staining machine and utilizes 22 containers.

*Raymond A. Lamb, 6 Sunbeam Road, London N. W. 10.

1. Treat with 95% alcohol for 1 min.
2. Treat with 70% alcohol for 2 min.
3. Rinse with distilled water for 3 min.
4. Treat with Harris's haematoxylin solution for $2\frac{1}{2}$ min.
5. Rinse in tap water for 1 min.
6. Treat with 1% acid-alcohol for 3 s.
7. Rinse in tap water for 2 min.
8. Treat with ammoniated water (distilled water to which are added a few drops of concentrated ammonia) for 1 min.
9. Rinse in tap water for 3 min.
10. Treat 70% alcohol for 2 min.
11. Treat with 95% alcohol for 2 min.
12. Stain with OG6 solution for 1 min.
13. Treat with 95% alcohol for $\frac{1}{2}$ min.
14. Treat with 95% alcohol for $\frac{1}{2}$ min.
15. Stain with EA 36 solution for $1\frac{1}{2}$ min.
16. Treat with 95% alcohol for $\frac{1}{2}$ min.
17. Treat with absolute alcohol (74 O.P. industrial methylated spirit) for 1 min.
18. Treat with absolute alcohol for 1 min.
19. Treat with absolute alcohol for 1 min.
20. Treat with xylene for 2 min.
21. Treat with xylene for 2 min.
22. Treat with xylene and mount as desired.

Results

Nuclei	blue
Superficial (cornified) cells	pink
Intermediate (non-cornified) cells	green
Candida (monilia)	red
Trichomonads	grey-green
Parabasal cell cytoplasms	deep green
Red blood cells	orange

HAEMATOXYLIN AND EOSIN TECHNIQUE

Notes

H and E staining of smears follows the same broad pattern as when staining paraffin sections. The principal difference is that smears take up dyes more readily, and therefore staining times are shortened. There is no need to take smears down through xylene prior to staining. The following technique utilizes Harris's haematoxylin which we find gives good results for general smear staining including imprint preparations. It is important that the Harris's haematoxylin be filtered before use.

Solutions

Harris's haematoxylin, see page 19.

1% hydrochloric acid in 70% alcohol.

2% aqueous sodium bicarbonate.

0.5% aqueous eosin (ws yellowish).

Technique

1. Alcohol-fixed smears are washed well in water.
2. Stain with haematoxylin for 1 min.
3. Wash in water and differentiate in acid-alcohol until the nuclei are sharply stained blue and the background is relative unstained. The length of this step will depend on the type of material being stained, the fixative used and, more importantly, the avidity of the particular haematoxylin solution employed. An average differentiation time is from 2–6 s.
4. Wash in water and blue in the bicarbonate solution for 10–20 s.
5. Wash well in water.
6. Stain with eosin for 10–20 s.
7. Wash in water, dehydrate, clear and mount as desired.

Results

Nuclei	blue
Cytoplasm	pink
Red blood cells	orange

SHORR TECHNIQUE (Shorr, 1941)

Notes

This technique gives results similar to the Papanicolaou method. The staining results are probably a little brighter although it should be appreciated

that nuclear detail is inferior to those techniques which employ an alum haematoxylin step.

Solution

Biebrich scarlet ws	0.5 g
Orange G	0.25 g
Fast green FCF	0.075 g
Phosphotungstic acid	0.5 g
Phosphomolybdic acid	0.5 g
Acetic acid	1 ml
50% ethanol	100 ml

Technique

1. Stain smears for approximately 1 min.
2. Rinse in 70% alcohol then absolute alcohol for approximately 10 s.
3. Rinse well in xylene and mount as desired.

Results

Nuclei	red
Superficial (cornified) cells	orange-red
Intermediate (non-cornified) cells	green

MODIFIED MAY-GRUNWALD-GIEMSA TECHNIQUE

Notes

Some workers prefer one of the Romanowsky-type stains for examination of sputum and serous fluid smears. Certainly it is true that nuclear detail, particularly that of nucleoli, is well delineated but experience is still needed for accurate cell determination. Used on cervical or vaginal smears the staining effect seems to show *Trichomonas vaginalis* parasites clearly. With serous fluid, adenocarcinoma cells are well picked out, especially if any intracytoplasmic vacuolation is present.

Solutions

May-Grunwald stock solution

Grind 0.3 g of the powdered May-Grunwald dye in a little methanol, decant, add more methanol and grind. Continue until the dye is in solution and make up to a final volume of 100 ml. Filter.

Working solution May-Grunwald

Dilute 20 parts of May-Grunwald solution with 30 parts of pH 6.8 buffer.

Giemsa stock solution

See page 63.

Working solution Giemsa

Dilute 10 parts Giemsa with 40 parts of pH 6.8 buffer. (pH 6.8 phosphate buffer see Buffer Tables, Appendix 3).

Technique

1. Stain fixed smears in the diluted May-Grunwald solution for 10 min.
2. Rinse in tap water.
3. Stain in the diluted Giemsa solution for 30 min.
4. Wash and differentiate in buffer for 5–20 min until the desired colour balance is achieved.
5. Allow smears to dry and mount in a DPX-type mountant.

Results

Nuclei	purple
Cell cytoplasms	blue to mauve
Red blood cells	pink

ACRIDINE ORANGE TECHNIQUE
(von Bertalanffy et al, 1956; 1958)

Notes

Fluorescent staining of exfoliated material, particularly that of the female reproductive tract, has enjoyed some popularity owing to the clarity with which the fluorescence of RNA is seen. Rapidly growing cells such as malignant cells, have an increased cytoplasmic RNA content and this has afforded a means by which malignant cells may

be detected. The early popularity of the technique has tended to wane somewhat due to the impermanence of the preparations and the fact that interpretation, particularly of squamous carcinoma cells, still requires expertise and experience on a level with other techniques (Lowhagen, 1966). The technique requires a pH of 6.0 for the differential staining of RNA and DNA. Formalin-fixed material such as tissue sections does not stain satisfactorily, neither does tissue fixed in Bouin's solution; alcohol is the fixative of choice.

Solutions

Acridine orange solution

0.1% aqueous acridine orange. Before use dilute one part stain with 10 parts of pH 6.0 0.06 M phosphate buffer to give a 0.01% solution.

Buffer

pH 6.0 phosphate buffer (see Buffer Tables, Appendix 3).

Differentiator

0.1 M calcium chloride (11.099 g calcium chloride in 100 ml distilled water).

Technique

1. Take alcohol-fixed smears to distilled water.
2. Rinse in 1% acetic acid for a few seconds and in two changes of distilled water over 1 min.
3. Stain in the diluted acridine orange solution at pH 6.0 for 3 min.
4. Rinse in pH 6.0 buffer for 1 min.
5. Differentiate in the 0.1 M calcium chloride solution for $\frac{1}{2}$–1 min.
6. Wash in phosphate buffer and mount in same.

Results (with fluorescence microscope)

DNA	yellow-green
RNA, some mucins	red

NILE BLUE SULPHATE TECHNIQUE FOR FETAL CELLS (Brosens & Gordon, 1965, 1966)

Notes

This technique makes use of the fact that when material containing fetal cells is stained with Nile blue sulphate, the fetal sebaceous cells containing lipid will stain red as against the non-lipid cells which stain blue. There are two possible uses for the method. First, for detecting leaking fetal membrances near term; vaginal fornix aspiration is done and the fluid stained to detect fetal cells deposited by leaking amniotic fluid. Second, it sometimes happens that a pregnant patient appears to be past full term according to the menstrual history, and it is helpful to the obstetrician to know the precise fetal age before a decision as to initiation of parturition can be made. A sample of amniotic fluid is drawn off and the ratio of fetal lipid to non-lipid cells determined using the Nile blue sulphate technique. According to Brosens the stage of pregnancy can be determined as in Table 4.1 (counting at least 200 cells of all types).

Table 4.1

Fetal lipid-containing cells as percentage of total cells	Pregnancy development (weeks)
1	Up to 34
1–10	34–38
10–50	38–40
Over 50	Over 40

A number of workers (Sharp, 1968; Droege-mueller et al, 1969; Lind & Cheyne, 1969) have criticized not only the accuracy of such figures but the origin of the fat-containing cells. It seems fairly certain that whatever type of cell stains red in the method, reliance may only be placed on the cell count at the upper end of the scale. The technique is not permanent and the smear should be examined within an hour or so, as the fat globules tend to disperse. A guide to the identification of the cells if the staining is equivocal, is that the lipid-containing cells are usually anucleate compared to the nucleated non-lipid cells.

Solution

1% aqueous Nile blue sulphate. Test for high oxazone content before use (see p. 133). Better results are given if the solution is relatively fresh (less than 1 month old).

Technique

1. If amniotic fluid is received, centrifuge at low speed (1500 r/min) for 5 min.
2. Decant supernatant and resuspend the deposit in the remaining fluid.
3. Place one or two loop-fulls on a clean slide, add 1 or 2 drops of filtered Nile blue sulphate and apply a cover slip.

Results

Lipid-containing cells	red
Non-lipid-containing cells	blue

SPERMATOZOA IN SEMINAL FLUID

Notes

The following technique enables examination of spermatozoa in fixed, stained preparations. Initial fixation is in osmium tetroxide vapour followed by Schaudinn fixation which, being a coagulant fixative, serves to prevent loss of material during staining. Haematoxylin staining of spermatozoon heads is followed by counterstaining with Rose Bengal, a homologue of eosin which gives superior staining of spermatozoon tails.

When making the smears it is important not to make them too thick, as they have a tendency to flake off during staining. Even though Schauddin's solution contains mercuric chloride, it is not usually necessary to subsequently treat for mercuric precipitates, as they are rarely formed.

Solutions

1% osmium tetroxide.

Schaudinn's solution
Saturated aqueous mercuric chloride	2 parts
Absolute alcohol	1 part

0.5% aqueous rose bengal

Technique

1. Make thin smears and wet-fix in osmium tetroxide vapour for 3 min (a Coplin jar painted black containing a few ml of fixative usually suffices).
2. Transfer direct to Schaudinn's solution for 10 min.
3. Wash in water for 5 min.
4. Stain with Mayer's haematoxylin solution for 5 min. Wash in water. Differentiate in acid-alcohol and blue.
5. Stain with rose Bengal solution for 3 min.
6. Wash in water. Dehydrate, clear and mount as desired.

Results

Spermatozoon heads	blue
Spermatozoon tails	bright pink
Background	pale pink

SEX CHROMATIN

The sex chromatin mass was first shown to be peculiar to female cells by Barr & Bertram (1949) and is popularly known as the 'Barr body'. It is thought to be the genetically inactive X chromosome, the active X chromosome in the female not being seen in interphase nuclei. These Barr bodies are present on the nuclear membrane only (the reason for this is not clear), are approximately 1 μm in diameter and typically crescentic in shape. Normal males with XY sex chromosomes do not show the Barr body but those with a cytogenetic abnormality such as Klinefelter's syndrome with XXY sex chromosomes will show a sex chromatin mass. Those patients who are XXXY will show two Barr bodies and so on. Similarly, female subjects may show an increase in sex chromatin masses above the normal. Figure 1 illustrates the association of sex chromatin masses and sex chromosome complement. It should be noted that absence of the sex chromatin or inactive X can be present in disease. A good example of this is Turner's syndrome where the female patient is sex

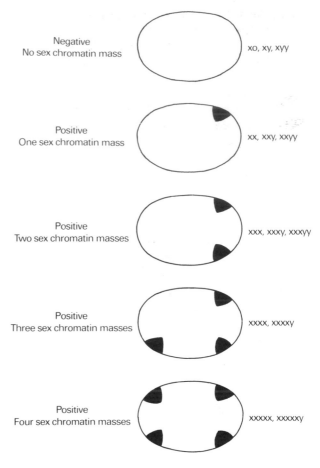

Fig. 4.1 Correlation of number of Barr bodies and sex chromosome complement.

chromatin negative, i.e. XO, instead of the normal XX.

In the routine laboratory the demonstration of the sex chromatin mass usually revolves around those patients suspected of suffering from Klinefelter's or Turner's syndromes (sex chromatin positive males and sex chromatin negative females, respectively). For this purpose the most convenient site for taking smears is from the buccal cavity. To obtain a successful smear there are several points to be observed:

1. It is important to scrape firmly as otherwise only the superficial and less well preserved cells will be gained.

2. Take at least four smears but avoid scraping an area previously scraped.
3. The slides should be covered with an adhesive, e.g. plasma to prevent subsequent loss of material during staining.
4. Smears should be wet-fixed; ether-alcohol (equal parts) or 95% alcohol serve equally well for this purpose. Slides should be fixed for at least 30 min but may be safely left in the fixative for several days.
5. Smears should also be taken from normal male and female subjects to serve as control material for the particular technique adopted.

In addition to the techniques described one may use either carefully differentiated Harris's haematoxylin method or the Feulgen technique. Staining of bacteria with the former method can be suppressed by using a Feulgen-type hydrolysis (Klinger & Ludwig, 1957). This will depolymerize the haematoxylin-positive bacterial RNA and thus prevent salt linkage with the component phosphate groups.

CRESYL FAST VIOLET TECHNIQUE (Moore, 1962)

Notes

This is a popular technique and one that is simple to do. Differentiation of the dye, however, requires some experience before really good results are obtained.

Solution

1% aqueous cresyl fast (echt) violet.

Technique

1. Celloidinize both test and control smears (previously fixed) with 0.5% celloidin in ether-alcohol. Rinse in alcohol then harden in water for several minutes.
2. Stain with the cresyl fast violet solution for 15 min.
3. Wash in water and differentiate in 95% alcohol until the chromatin of cell nuclei is clearly seen.
4. Rinse in absolute alcohol, remove celloidin film, clear and mount as desired.

Results

Sex chromatin	purple body lying on the nuclear membrane
Background	pale blue purple

ACETO-ORCEIN TECHNIQUE (Sanderson & Stewart, 1961)

Notes

Highly satisfactory results can be given by this method but, unfortunately, it tends to be inconsistent. This variability is almost certainly due to non-uniformity of dye batches. The technique itself is simple and involves simultaneous fixing and staining with the acetic acid–orcein mixture. Squash preparations are subsequently made and it is important to squash firmly, in order to be able to render the cells flat and, therefore, easily seen.

Solution

Dissolve 1 g of synthetic orcein in 45 ml of hot (80–85° C) acetic acid, cool to room temperature and add 55 ml distilled water. Filter. Fresh solutions give better results.

Technique

1. Make a buccal smear on a clean slide and add one or two drops of aceto-orcein solution. Place on a coverslip and make a squash preparation as follows.
   Squash preparation:
   Place several sheets of blotting paper on the slide to absorb excess stain and, holding one corner of the coverslip down with one hand, make several firm strokes with the other hand on the blotting paper.
2. Examine microscopically and if satisfactory make a permanent preparation as follows.
   a. Freeze the slide on solid carbon dioxide or by using the chuck of a freezing-microtome. When frozen remove the coverslip.
   b. Dehydrate in alcohol and clear by treating with two changes of Cellosolve (2-ethoxyethanol) for 5 min each time.

3. Finally mount. The method originally called for treatment with Euparal essence for 5 min and mounting in Euparal vert. This is almost certainly not essential and the routine mountants should be satisfactory.

Results

Nuclear chromatin, particularly
   the sex chromatin body   dark brown
Cytoplasm   light brown

BIEBRICH SCARLET-FAST GREEN TECHNIQUE (Guard, 1959, slightly modified)

Notes

In our experience this is undoubtedly the method of choice for sex chromatin demonstration. It is not a short technique in terms of time nor is it particularly simple to do but it has the over-riding advantage of consistency of results even with inexperienced personnel.

The principle of the technique seems to be that following short staining in diluted alum haematoxylin (the function of this is obscure), nuclear chromatin is stained red with acidified Biebrich scarlet. Subsequent replacement staining is carried out using acidified fast green until only pyknotic nuclei and the sex chromatin of vesicular nuclei are stained red, all other structures being stained green.

In practice this differential staining effect is difficult to achieve consistently and requires freshly prepared Biebrich scarlet solution. We have found it better to overstain with the fast green solution with the result that the sex chromatin, although also stained green, is a darker colour and seems to stand out against the nuclear membrane. In this way it is possible to obtain consistent, easily achieved results.

Solutions

Mayer's haematoxylin diluted one part with five parts distilled water.

Biebrich scarlet
  Biebrich scarlet ws   1 g

Phosphotungstic acid	0.3 g
Acetic acid	0.5 ml
50% ethanol	100 ml

Fast green
Fast green FCF	0.5 g
Phosphomolybdic acid	0.3 g
Phosphotungstic acid	0.3 g
Acetic acid	5 ml
50% ethanol	100 ml

Technique

1. Celloidinize smears, as for the cresyl fast violet technique, and take to water.
2. Treat with the diluted Mayer's haematoxylin solution for 15s.
3. Drain and transfer direct to the Biebrich scarlet solution for 2 min.
4. Rinse in 50% alcohol.
5. Place in a Coplin jar of fast green solution for 3–4 h.
6. Rinse in water. Dehydrate (removing celloidin film), clear and mount as desired.

Results

Nuclear chromatin,
  particularly the sex
  chromatin body   dark green
Cell cytoplasm   light green

DEMONSTRATION OF Y CHROMOSOMES

Notes

As a corollary to Barr body X chromosome demonstration in the nuclei of female subjects it is possible to demonstrate the Y chromosome in males, using the following fluorescence technique on buccal smears.

In our limited experience the demonstration and visualization of the Y chromosome by this method is not an easy one. The chromosome appears a small structure (when compared to the female Barr body) and differentiating it from the adjacent chromatin particles requires experience. A good fluorescence microscope is important preferably of the epi-illumination type. It is essential to stain in parallel with the test smears a buccal smear from a normal male and a normal female as a positive and negative control respectively.

Solutions

0.5% aqueous quinacrine hydrochloride (prepare fresh).

1% aqueous potassium chloride.

Technique

1. Buccal smears are conventionally fixed in an alcohol-based fixative.
2. Wash in distilled water.
3. Stain with the quinacrine solution for 5 min.
4. Wash in distilled water.
5. Differentiate in potassium chloride for approximately 1 min.
6. Wash in distilled water and 'mount' in same.

Results

Using a BG 12 exciter filter and K530 barrier filter with ultraviolet light excitation — Y chromosome small yellow intranuclear body.

G-BANDING FOR CHROMOSOME IDENTIFICATION (Seabright, 1971; mod. Coban p. comm)

Notes

In order to more precisely identify the different human chromosomes, a technique has been devised in which following partial digestion by the enzyme trypsin, the chromosomes of, for example, tissue culture preparations are stained by Giemsa. This so-called G-banding technique reveals typical banding of the denatured DNA, in which the heterochromatin areas stain purple in contrast to the relatively unstained euchromatin.

A fluorescent dye quinacrine may be used in a similar way to differentiate human chromosomes and is termed, appropriately, Q-banding. The former method is more commonly used and is given below. When diluting the Hanks solution it is important to use deionized water for standard results. When preparing the Trypsin-Hanks' stock solution aliquots use aseptic conditions.

Solutions

Trypsin in Hanks' solution

Stock solution
2.5% trypsin solution*	80 ml
1 × Hanks' solution*	22.5 ml

Aliquot in 5 ml amounts and store at −20°C.

Working solution
Stock solution	5 ml
1 × Hanks' solution	45 ml

Hanks' solution
10 × Hanks' solution*	15 ml
Deionized water	135 ml

5% Giemsa in pH 6.8 buffer

Technique

1. Test and control slides are washed in Hanks' solution adjusted to pH 6.8 with 0.1M sodium bicarbonate for 1 min.
2. Treat with the trypsin-Hanks' solution adjusted to pH 6.6 with 0.1 M sodium bicarbonate for 40–60 s.
3. Give slides one quick dip in Hanks' solution adjusted to pH 6.0 with 0.1 M hydrochloric acid.
4. Stain with Giemsa solution for 4 min.
5. Give slides one quick dip in deionized water, blot dry, and remove last traces of water under a lamp. Examine slides using the oil-immersion (×100) objective.

Results

Typical chromosomal patterns as shown in purple bands of varying width.

SPUTUM SPECIMENS

INTRODUCTION

A smear technique and a concentration technique are described. The latter method uses hydrochloric

---

*Obtainable from Flow Laboratories Ltd, Irvine, Ayrshire, Scotland.

acid as a mucolytic agent and has the advantage of allowing subsequent cell concentration. Cell morphology, including that of squamous carcinoma cells, is surprisingly well-preserved and where these are suspected, the smear technique should also be carried out. Carnoy's fixative is recommended for sputa, although 95% alcohol gives results almost as good. With the Carnoy fixation red blood cells are lysed and with very haemorrhagic specimens will give a clearer background. Ehrlich's haematoxylin solution should not be used for sputum smears as the component mucins will also stain blue.

SMEAR TECHNIQUE

Solutions

Carnoy's fixative, see page 256.

Mayer's haematoxylin solution, see page 19.

0.5% aqueous eosin was yellowish.

Technique

1. Using a safety cabinet, select suitable material from the sputum specimen displayed in a Petri dish and make smears on two or three slides using either wooden applicator sticks or wire loops.
2. Wet-fix the smears in Coplin jars filled with Carnoy's fixative.
   Leave for a minimum of 20 min but not longer than 24 h.
3. Rinse smears in water for several minutes.
4. Stain with Mayer's haematoxylin solution for 10 min. Wash in water.
5. Differentiate in 1% acid-alcohol for 5–8 s depending on the avidity of the particular haematoxylin batch in use at the time. Wash in water and blue in 2% aqueous sodium bicarbonate. Wash again in water.
6. Treat with the eosin solution for 20–30 s.
7. Wash in water, dehydrate, clear and mount as desired. For thick specimens which do not

clear easily, leave in one part alcohol to three parts xylene overnight. Rinse in xylene and mount.

Results

Nuclei	blue
Background	pink

CONCENTRATION TECHNIQUE (TAPLIN, 1966)

Notes

The principle of the technique is that the component mucins (particularly sialomucins) are hydrolysed by hydrochloric acid. Thus the sputum viscosity is lowered, enabling concentration by centrifugation. Normally the sputum is treated with the acid overnight at a concentration of 8%. Should it be necessary, on occasion, to leave the specimen more than 24 h in acid, then a 4% solution of hydrochloric acid should be employed. When the smears are eventually prepared they may be safely air-dried without, seemingly, producing the usual artefacts.

In our hands atypical squamous cells are well preserved, but adenocarcinoma cells less so.

Solutions

8% hydrochloric acid v/v.

Scott's tap water substitute

Sodium bicarbonate	3.5 g
Magnesium sulphate	20 g
Distilled water	1 litre

(By using distilled water, moulds occur less often.)

Mayer's haematoxylin solution.

1% eosin ws yellowish.

Technique

1. Add approximately 15 ml of hydrochloric acid to the specimen in the container. Mix well and leave overnight at room temperature.
2. Pour the now liquid contents into a centrifuge

tube and spin at 3000 r/min for 5 min.

3. Pour off the supernatant. Add approximately 15 ml of the Scott's tap water substitute and re-spin for 5 min at 3000 r/min.
4. Pour off the supernatant and re-suspend the cells in Scott's tap water substitute, using just enough solution to give a 'thin cream' consistency. Make smears on clean slides using wooden applicators. Allow to air dry.
5. Stain with H and E preparation in the same way used for sputum smears but giving rather less acid-alcohol differentiation.

Results

Cell nuclei	blue
Background	bright pink

SEROUS FLUIDS

CONCENTRATION TECHNIQUE

Notes

The method described is particularly useful for highly cellular fluids such as effusions of the peritoneum ('ascitic' fluid) and pleura.

Heavy effusions are often the result of nonspecific inflammation or infections such as peritonitis or empyema but occasionally are due to serous membrane involvement in malignant growth. This may be due to direct spread from adjacent organs such as that from carcinoma of the colon or lung, or to secondary 'seedlings' from tumours elsewhere. For example, ovarian adenocarcinomas not infrequently involve the pleural membranes causing a heavy effusion. In addition, a rather uncommon tumour of mesothelial cells lining the serous membranes may occur (mesothelioma). A non-malignant inflammatory effusion will contain a mixed cell population comprising neutrophils, lymphocytes, etc. and usually varying numbers of mesothelial cells.

Whilst our experience has been mainly concerned with H and E staining of this type of material, there is no reason why the other popular cytological stains (see below) should not be used. The principle of the concentration technique is the

centrifuged deposit of the fluid is mixed with plasma to which thrombin is added. The cells are enmeshed in the resultant clot which is fixed in formalin, and subsequently paraffin processed and sectioned as for a tissue block.

Solutions

Plasma

The most useful source of plasma will be a haematology/blood transfusion laboratory. It should be stored at 4°C.

Thrombin

Thrombin is available in ampoules,* each containing 50 units of topical thrombin. The contents of each ampoule are mixed with 1 ml of normal saline diluent, which is also supplied in ampoules of 1 ml amounts.

Technique

1. The serous fluid, which is preferably citrated to prevent spontaneous clotting, is centrifuged for 5–10 min at 3000 r/min.
2. Pour off the supernatant and if the centrifuged deposit is scanty make smears and fix and stain as for sputum smears. If the deposit is reasonably substantial proceed as follows.
3. Add approximately twice the volume of plasma to the centrifuged deposit and remaining fluid. Mix thoroughly and add one drop of thrombin. Mix well. A thrombin clot will form, usually within 1 min. If this does not occur it may be due to an insufficiency of plasma; therefore add a little more plasma and remix.
4. When the clot has formed, fill the tube with 10% formalin and allow to fix overnight.
5. Place the clot in suitable thin wrapping paper and paraffin process. Cut thin (5 μm) sections at three levels in the block.
6. H and E staining is preferred and should be

*Available from S. Maw Son & Sons Ltd., Aldersgate House, Barnet, Herts.

according to the conventional schedule used for paraffin tissue sections.

Results

Cell nuclei	blue
Cytoplasms, plasma clots	pink

DEMONSTRATION OF METACHROMATIC LEUCODYSTROPHY USING URINE SPECIMENS

Notes

We are indebted to Francis (p. comm) for the following technique in which urine cell deposits are smeared on slides and stained with Toluidine blue. In cases of the lipid storage disorder metachromatic leucodystrophy, cells may be discerned containing metachromatic granules.

Solution

0.1% Toluidine blue in pH 5.0 acetic-acetate buffer (see Appendix 3).

Technique

1. The urine sample is centrifuged and the spun deposit washed thoroughly in pH 5.0 buffer.
2. Recentrifuge the buffer-urine deposit and make smears on slides coated with an adhesive such as gelatin or plasma.
3. Fix the smears in formalin vapour for 30 min. This may conveniently be done by placing them in a Coplin jar containing a small (0.5–1 ml) amount of concentrated formalin.
4. Allow the smears to thoroughly dry at room temperature (30 min or so).
5. Stain with Toluidine blue overnight at room temperature.
6. Rinse slides in pH 5.0 buffer, blot dry and mount in a DPX-type mountant.

Results

Positive cells will show purple-red stained granules. All other cellular material will stain blue.

REFERENCES

Brosens I, Gordon H 1965 Cytological diagnosis of ruptured membranes usine Nile blue sulphate staining. Journal of Obstetrics and Gynaecology of the British Commonwealth 72: 342

Brosens I, Gordon H 1966 The estimation of maturity by cytological examination of the liquor amnii. Journal of Obstetrics and Gynaecology of the British Commonwealth 73: 88

Francis R 1982 Personal communication

Guard H R 1959 A new technic for differential staining of the sex chromatin, and the determination of its incidence in exfoliated vaginal epithelial cells. American Journal of Clinical Pathology 32: 145

Klinger H P, Kurt S L 1957 A universal stain for the sex chromatin body. Stain Technology 32: 235

Moore K L 1962 The sex chromatin: its discovery and variations in the animal kingdom. Acta Cytologica 6: 1

Moore K L, Barr M L 1955 Smears from the oral mucosa in the detection of chromosomal sex. Lancet 2: 57

Papanicolaou G N 1942 A new procedure for the staining of vaginal smears. Science NY 95: 438

Sanderson A R, Stewart J S 1961 Nuclear sexine with aceto-orcein. British Medical Journal 2: 1065

Seabright M 1971 Rapid banding technique for human chromosomes. Lancet 2: 971

Shorr E 1941 A new technic for staining vaginal smears: III, a single differential stain. Science NY 94: 545

Taplin D J 1966 Malignant cells in sputum: a simple method of liquefying sputum. Journal of Medical Laboratory Technology 23: 252–5

von Bertalanffy L, Masin F, Masin M 1956 Use of acridine orange fluorescence technique inexfoliative cytology. Science N Y 124: 1024

von Bertalanffy L, Masin M, Masin F 1958 A new and rapid method for diagnosis of vaginal and cervical cancer by fluorescence microscopy. Cancer NY 11: 873

5

The connective tissues

This term is used in its widest connotation to include not only the fibrillar connective tissue, but also the tissues which are histologically associated with them such as muscle and basement membranes (basal lamina).

The types of technique to fall within this group are those which involve many of the more colourful dyes, whose roots are firmly set in the earlier more empirical years of histological staining. Their role has changed comparatively little over the decades as has their value to the histologist, for these methods comprise some of the most often-requested in the repertoire of the routine diagnostic laboratory.

Whilst the chief components of connective tissue are dealt with in this chapter, there are other entities which because of their specialized chemical constituents are dealt with separately. For example, cartilage, owing to its high mucin content, will be dealt with under 'Carbohydrates' and adipose tissue under 'Lipids'. Bone is a somewhat specialized area of histology and will be dealt with under 'Miscellany'.

Demonstration of the different forms of muscle is largely achieved by the use of a trichrome-type technique. These will distinguish muscle from connective tissue in a tinctorial manner, although it should be appreciated that the different types of striated muscle fibre (Types I, 2a, 2b, 2c) can only be reliably distinguished by means of enzyme histochemistry. This will be dealt with in the appropriate chapter.

COLLAGEN

These fibres are formed by fibroblasts and may be fine or coarse, and quite dense, as in dermis or tendons, or relatively scanty as in lymphoid tissue. At least four types (I–IV) can be identified based on variation in alpha helix protein content.

Collagen is also found in the widely occuring areolar tissue together with reticulin and elastin fibres. Different types of cells are found normally in loose connective tissues and include histiocytes, mast cells, fibroblasts, neutrophils and lymphocytes.

Van Gieson's technique which follows together with the methyl blue variant, is the most widely used technique along with the trichromes for the demonstration of collagen. Pathologically, this is done usually either to show the extent of fibrosis in a given tissue, or to identify collagenous tumours such as the benign fibromas or malignant fibrosarcomas.

VAN GIESON'S TECHNIQUE (van Gieson, 1889)

Notes

Van Gieson's technique is probably the most successful single histological technique ever devised; 95 years or so after its inception it is still in use in histological laboratories in most countries in the world.

Its success is due to the remarkably specific staining of collagen in clearly seen colour distinction to tissues such as muscle. Unfortunately one rather serious drawback is the nonstaining of young collagen fibres; to demonstrate these fibres use one of the trichrome stains (see p. 42). Apart from its role as a specific indicator of collagen, van Gieson stain makes for a useful counterstain in a number of techniques e.g. in the Fouchet technique for bile (p. 147) and the von Kossa method for calcium (p. 244). In the latter instance the van Gieson stain demonstrates very effectively the osteoid material in bone (red) against the mineralized bone (black). The rationale seems to be that when using combined solutions of picric acid and acid fuchsin the small molecules of picric acid penetrate all tissues rapidly, but are only firmly retained in the close-textured red blood cells and muscle. The larger molecules of the acid fuchsin are able to enter the larger pores of the collagen fibres when they are able to displace the picric acid particles (Seki, 1932).

Hydrochloric or nitric acid can be added to the van Gieson's solution (0.25 ml) and this sometimes results in brighter staining. However, the acid has a tendency to cause further differentiation of haematoxylins and elastin stains and therefore must be used cautiously.

Other dyes can be used in combination with picric acid in place of acid fuschsin and will give similar results; these include methyl blue, aniline blue, amido black 10B and violamine.

Due to the tendency for the picric acid moiety to differentiate haematoxylin it is customary to stain the nuclei with iron salt-mordant haematoxylin solutions such as Weigert's iron haematoxylin, or a celestine blue/Mayer's haematoxylin sequence. If using the latter sequence, it should be borne in mind that celloidin often strongly retains celestine blue and therefore avoid celloidinization of sections prior to staining. On the whole, Weigert's stain is to be preferred. A ferrous sulphate iron haematoxylin is included and will give a very intense, dark nuclear stain suitable for use with the van Gieson and trichrome techniques. For the brightest staining results avoid tap water rinsing before and after van Gieson staining; use distilled water instead. Dehydrate fairly quickly at the conclusion of the technique lest the highly alcohol-soluble picric acid be extracted. Differentiation of the haematoxylin with the acid alcohol should be minimal as during staining with van Gieson's solution some further differentiation will occur.

Solutions

Weigert's iron haematoxylin (Weigert, 1904)

This is normally stored as two separate solutions and mixed in equal proportions immediately prior to use. However, it has been shown (Ibeachum, 1971) that the working solution retains its staining avidity for up to 60 days if stored at 4° C. The alcoholic haematoxylin solution gives better results when young; in older solutions overoxidation results when the ferric chloride is added. The hydrochloric acid probably acts as an accentuator.

Solution A

Haematoxylin	1 g
Ethyl alcohol	100 ml
Dissolve with gentle heat.	

Solution B

30% aqueous ferric chloride	4 ml
Conc. hydrochloric acid	1 ml
Distilled water	100 ml

Add together equal volumes of A and B prior to use.

Celestine blue (Gray et al, 1956)

Celestine blue B or R	1 g
Conc. sulphuric acid	0.5 ml
2.5% aqueous ferric ammonium sulphate (iron alum) solution	86 ml
Glycerol	14 ml

Grind the celestine blue to a paste with the sulphuric acid and then gradually add the iron alum solution with frequent mixing. Add the glycerol, mix and place in the 56°C oven to dissolve. Cool and filter. It is advisable to filter again prior to use. We find this variant gives particularly intense staining.

Ferrous sulphate iron haematoxylin (Slidders, 1968)

In the following solution the ferrous salt is used in place of a ferric salt mordant as is customary with iron haematoxylins. This is intended to give a more stable and vigorous solution as it will not overoxidize the haematoxylin. Aluminium is incorporated as a stabilizing salt. A staining time of 5–10 min is recommended and may be followed by the usual counterstains including van Gieson. Nuclei are stained a very dark almost black colour.

Iron haematoxylin

Haematoxylin	1 g
Aluminium chloride	10 g
Ferrous sulphate	10 g
Conc. hydrochloric acid	2 ml
95% ethanol	100 ml
Saturated (9%) aqueous sodium iodate	2 ml
Distilled water	100 ml

Dissolve the haematoxylin in the 95% ethanol. Next add the aluminium chloride and ferrous sulphate to the distilled water. Mix the two solutions together then add the hydrochloric acid and sodium iodate solutions. Mix, stand for 48 h and filter before use.

Van Gieson stain

Saturated aqueous picric acid	100 ml
1% aqueous acid fuchsin	10 ml

Boil for 3 min, cool and filter.

Curtis's stain (1905)

An acceptable modification of van Gieson's stain is that of Curtis which undoubtedly seems to give brighter results and is claimed to fade less easily than the conventional stain.

Saturated aqueous picric acid	90 ml
1% aqueous Ponceau S	10 ml
Glacial acetic acid	1 ml

Technique

1. Take sections to water.
2. Stain nuclei with either Weigert's haematoxylin solution for 15–30 min, or with celestine blue then Mayer's haematoxylin solution for 5 min each.
3. Wash in water, differentiate with acid-alcohol. Wash and blue.
4. Check microscopically; the nuclei should be a dark blue-black and the background a paler blue-black colour.
5. Rinse well in distilled water.
6. Stain with van Gieson's solution for 5 min.
7. Rinse in distilled water or drain, then rinse in alcohol. Dehydrate and clear in xylene.

Mount, preferably in either acid balsam or a DPX-type mountant.

Results

Nuclei	brown-black
Mature collagen	red
Other tissue, e.g. muscle and red blood cells	yellow
Some bile pigments	green

METHYL BLUE-VAN GIESON TECHNIQUE FOR YOUNG AND MATURE COLLAGEN (Herovici, 1963)

Notes

The method depends on the affinity of young collagen (and reticulin) for methyl blue and the mature fibres for acid fuchsin, and is of possible use in the demonstration of recent fibrosis as in healing processes in tissue. This variable affinity is presumably due to variation in particle size in the two dyes, and in the structure of the fibres; i.e. the maturer having larger intermicellar spaces and the younger fibres smaller spaces. The recommended fixative is formal-acetic-alcohol (10 : 5 : 85) and good results may be obtained although, on occasion capricious results can occur. We have noticed that fibrin may also stain blue. The original method used a final metanil yellow step to stain cytoplasms but we usually omit this.

Solutions

Modified van Gieson's stain

0.05% aqueous methyl blue	50 ml
0.1% acid fuchsin in saturated aqueous picric acid	50 ml
Mix, then add glycerol	10 ml
Saturated aqueous lithium carbonate	0.5 ml

Technique

1. Take sections to water.
2. Stain nuclei with an iron haematoxylin solution. Differentiate and blue.

3. Stain with modified van Gieson's solution for 2 min.
4. Wash in 1% acetic acid solution for 2 min.
5. Dehydrate, clear and mount as for the conventional van Gieson technique.

Results

Nuclei	brown black
Reticulin, young collagen and (?) fibrin	blue
Mature collagen	red
Red blood cells, muscle, etc.	yellow

TRICHROMES

Under this heading may be grouped a number of multi-stage techniques which aim at differentiating tissue structures such as collagen from muscle, in contrasting colours: A potential use for example, being the differentiation of myosarcomas from fibrosarcomas, or their benign counterparts the leiomyoma and fibroma.

The rationale underlying most of these methods is while the firm attachment of dye to tissue is probably electrostatic in nature, the means by which selective sequential staining with a number of anionic dyes is achieved is almost certainly bound up with physical structure of dye and tissue. To take an example, the red blood cells may be stained first with a small particle of dye such as orange G, which is more firmly retained in the small intermicellar spaces of the red cell than in the looser texture of structures such as collagen or muscle. If this is then followed by acid fuchsin staining, which has a larger particle size, the dye molecules will not be able to enter the red cells pores, but will enter those of muscle and collagen. Should the tissue be treated with phosphomolybdic or phosphotungstic acid solutions there will be displacement of the acid fuchsin particles from collagen, where they are insecurely held in the large intermicellar spaces. Finally, a dye of large particle size, such as aniline blue, is used which is able to enter collagen.

The trichrome stains are of primary value for demonstrating fibrin or young collagen fibres and for differentiating muscle from connective tissue. The method used is largely immaterial, as with all of them good results are possible; it is a matter of experience. Mercuric chloride, potassium dichromate and picric acid fixation give best results. Formalin fixation can lead to indifferent results which may be partly overcome by premordanting sections in Helly's fixative (see Appendix 1) for at least 5 h.

A useful tip, when dealing with a section in which there are few normal tissue structures to act as a guide to staining, is to select a reasonably sized artery to act as a control, relying on the fact that the tunica media should be red and the tunica adventitia blue or green. When staining voluntary (striated muscle) it will be found that type I fibres stain a deeper red colour than type II. This effect is heightened if formalin fixation only was used and less easily seen if the normally recommended fixation was carried out. So it would appear that the formaldehyde cross-linking masking effect on amino group acidophilia is less pronounced with type I muscle protein.

MALLORY'S TECHNIQUE (Mallory, 1905)

Notes

This, one of the earliest and most popular of the trichrome methods, is no longer widely used in Britain. Mallory himself slightly modified the method in later years but the following technique is his original one. We see no reason why nuclei may not be stained first with haematoxylin.

Solutions

0.5% aqueous acid fuchsin.

Orange G-aniline blue stain

Orange G	2 g
Aniline blue	0.5 g
Phosphomolybdic acid	1 g
Distilled water	100 ml

Dissolve the phosphomolybdic acid in the water, then add the two dyes and mix. Filter before use.

Technique

1. Take sections to water.
2. Stain with the acid fuchsin solution for 5 min.
3. Drain and stain with the orange G-aniline blue solution for 20 min.
4. Differentiate in 95% alcohol, dehydrate, clear and mount as desired.

Results

Nuclei	blue or red depending on whether or not a haematoxylin step was introduced
Muscle, fibrin	red
Collagen, reticulin	blue
Red blood cells	yellow

Note that elastin tends to stain a weak red colour.

PICRO-MALLORY TECHNIQUE (McFarlane, 1944)

Notes

When differentiating the picro-orange solution, it is wise to leave a little in the background as it will tend to be masked by the subsequent dyes. Differentiation of the acid fuchsin is usually more prolonged than that of the collagen stain, and one should be prepared to treat as long as necessary in order to obtain the desired effect, a maxim that can safely be applied to all histological methods.

Acid mucins can be stained a different colour by introducing an alcian green step (Cook, unpublished data). The brightest mucin staining is achieved by staining both before and after haematoxylin staining.

Solutions

1% alcian green 2 GX in 3% acetic acid.

0.2% orange G in saturated alcoholic picric acid.

Ponceau-acid fuchsin solution
Equal volumes of 0.5% Ponceau 2 R in 1% acetic acid and 0.5% acid fuchsin in 1% acetic acid.

Aniline blue solution

Boil 97.5 ml of distilled water and add 2 g aniline blue ws. While still hot, add 2.5 ml glacial acetic acid. Cool and filter.

Differentiators

Stock solution	
Phosphotungstic acid	25 g
Picric acid	2.5 g
95% alcohol	100 ml

'Red' differentiator	
Stock solution	40 ml
95% alcohol	40 ml
Distilled water	20 ml

'Blue' differentiator	
Stock solution	20 ml
Distilled water	80 ml

Technique

1. Take sections to water.
2. Stain with the alcian green solution for 3 min (optional).
3. Wash, and stain nuclei with an iron haematoxylin solution. Differentiate well and blue.
4. Wash, then stain again with the alcian green solution for 3 min (optional).
5. Wash and stain with the picro-orange solution for 7 min.
6. Differentiate in water for approximately 5 s until red blood cells are yellow and background is faint yellow.
7. Treat with the ponceau-acid fuchsin solution for 2–3 min.
8. Rinse in 2% acetic acid then differentiate in red differentiator until the muscle is red and connective tissues are almost colourless, this may take several minutes. In order to check microscopically, rinse in 2% acetic acid, this will stop further differentiation.
9. Finally, rinse in 2% acetic acid then in tap water for 10 s or so to remove the acetic acid.
10 Stain with the aniline blue solution for 10 min.

11. Rinse in 2% acetic acid and differentiate in the blue differentiator until excess blue staining is removed (usually 10–20 s).
12. Rinse in 2% acetic acid. Dehydrate, clear and mount as desired.

Results

Nuclei	blue-black (may be coloured red)
Acid mucins	green (optional step)
Fibrin, muscle	red
Reticulin, collagen	blue
Red blood cells, colloid	yellow

HEIDENHAIN'S 'AZAN' (Heidenhain, 1915)

Notes

This is one of the less widely used trichrome methods. To obtain good results, stain strongly with the azocarmine and then slightly underdifferentiate with the aniline-alcohol, otherwise the counterstain will tend to mask the staining of muscle, etc. It should be noted that although orange G is incorporated into the counterstain, very little yellow colouration is in fact imparted to such structures as red blood cells. Although this is, perhaps, one of the less successful trichromes, we have found it to be useful when examining renal tissue.

Solutions

Azocarmine

Add 0.1 g azocarmine GX or 1 g azocarmine B to 100 ml distilled water and bring to the boil. Cool and add 1 ml acetic acid. Filter.

Orange G-aniline blue

Dissolve 0.5 g aniline blue ws and 2 g orange G in 100 ml of 8% aqueous acetic acid solution. Dissolve with the aid of gentle heat (56° C oven). Cool and filter. Dilute 1:3 with distilled water prior to use.

Technique

1. Take sections to water.
2. Stain with the azocarmine solution for 45–60 min at 56°C in a Coplin jar.
3. Cool to room temperature for approximately 10 min before removing the slide and washing.
4. Differentiate in 0.1% aniline in 95% alcohol so that the muscle is red and the collagen a paler red colour (usually 10–30 s).
5. Rinse in 2% acetic acid to stop differentiation. Wash.
6. Complete differentiation in 5% phosphotungstic acid in 25% methanol (30–60 min).
7. Wash, and counterstain in the orange G-aniline blue solution for 15 min.
8. Wash, dehydrate and differentiate in alcohol, clear and mount as desired.

Results

Nuclei, red blood cells, fibrin	red
Muscle	orange-red
Collagen	blue

MASSON'S TECHNIQUE (Masson, 1929)

Notes

The success of this method largely devolves on the degree of differentiation of the ponceau-acid fuchsin by the phosphomolybdic acid. It is important to prolong differentiation until the connective tissue is almost unstained. This differentiation may be expedited by carrying it out at 56°C if necessary. (Phosphotungstic acid may be used equally well.)

Whether one uses aniline blue or light green for the fibre stain is a matter of choice. We prefer the latter stain if only because it makes for more striking photomicrographs.

Solutions

Ponceau-acid fuchsin solution, see p. 43.

1% aqueous phosphomolybdic acid.

Either *aniline blue solution* (see p. 43) or 2% light green in 2% acetic acid diluted 1:10 with distilled water prior to use.

Technique

1. Take sections to water.
2. Stain nuclei with an iron haematoxylin solution. Differentiate and blue. Wash in water.
3. Treat with the ponceau-acid fuchsin solution for 2–3 min.
4. Wash in water and differentiate in the phosphomolybdic acid solution (usually for between 5 and 15 min at room temperature).
5. Wash well in water.
6. Counterstain either with the aniline blue solution for 5 min, or the light green solution for 1 min.
7. Wash, dehydrate, clear and mount as desired.

Results

Nuclei	blue-black
Muscle, red blood cells, fibrin	red
Connective tissue	blue or green according to the counterstain used

GOMORI RAPID ONE STEP TRICHROME
(Gomori, 1950A)

Notes

The main advantage of this method is its simplicity, in that unlike other trichrome techniques the inexperienced worker can easily obtain good results. A useful if rarely called for variant of this solution is for demonstrating nemaline rods in nemaline rod myopathy. For this the traditional formula is used but at a slightly higher pH; also frozen sections should be used, not paraffin (Francis, 1982).

Solutions

Stain solution
Chromotrope 2 R   0.6 g

Fast green FCF	0.3 g
Phosphotungstic acid	0.6 g
Glacial acetic acid	1 ml
Distilled water	100 ml

The solution keeps well. For demonstrating nemaline rods adjust the pH of the solution to 3.4 using 1 M sodium hydroxide (Dubowitz & Brooke, 1973).

0.2% glacial acetic acid.

Technique

1. Take paraffin sections to water.
2. Stain nuclei with an alum haematoxylin.
3. Differentiate in acid alcohol and blue as per the standard technique.
4. Wash well in tap water, then in distilled water.
5. Stain in the Gomori solution 5–20 min.
6. Rinse well in the acetic acid solution.
7. Blot dry, dehydrate, clear and mount in a DPX-type mountant.

Results

Nuclei	grey-blue
Collagen	green
Muscle, cytoplasm, red blood cells, fibrin	red

Using the higher pH solution:	
Nemaline rods	red
Background	blue-green

MALLORY'S PHOSPHOTUNGSTIC ACID-HAEMATOXYLIN (PTAH)

Notes

This is a good example of a 'standard' method which is anything but in its application, as no two laboratories seem to carry it out in an identical manner. It is a popular method, demonstrating as it does a wide range of fibrillar elements clearly and in a progressive manner. The results are less subjective than the usual regressive type of technique.

In diagnostic work it is of value in demonstrating gliosis in central nervous system (CNS) tissue and tumours of voluntary muscle such as the rhabdomyosarcoma, also fibrin deposits in a wide variety of lesions.

The mechanism by which two-colour staining is achieved from a mixture of haematein and phosphotungstic acid is obscure. Terner et al (1964) carried out an investigation and concluded that the blue colour produced was a metachromatic-type staining effect.

The technique can be capricious and this may well be the result of variation in batches of dye. Fixation in a mercuric chloride-containing solution gives the brightest staining, although perfectly satisfactory results may be obtained with most routine fixatives, providing that fixation times are not prolonged. An effective means of improving staining is by immersing sections in Helly's fluid for several hours prior to staining.

Some of the more important modifications of the PTAH technique are Mallory (1900), Lieb (1948), Bohacek (1966). We prefer the method of Shum & Hon (1969) which follows.

According to the authors (Shum & Hon, 1969) the proportion of phosphotungstic acid to haematein is important for good results (0.9%: 0.08%). They also state that premordanting is unnecessary and that long room-temperature staining gives slightly more precise results than shorter staining at 56°C. We concur with the latter statement. The solution may be used repeatedly and should be filtered after use.

Solution

Take 0.08 g haematein and grind to a chocolate-brown paste with 1 ml distilled water (an unsatisfactory batch of haematein will appear lighter, more straw coloured and should be discarded). Dissolve 0.9 g phosphotungstic acid in 99 ml distilled water and mix with the ground haematein solution. Bring to the boil, cool and filter.

Technique

1. Take sections to water.
2. Treat with 0.25% aqueous potassium permanganate solution for 5 min.
3. Wash, then bleach with 5% aqueous oxalic acid solution.
4. Wash well, then stain in the PTAH solution for 12–24 h at room temperature.
5. Wash in distilled water. Dehydrate, clear and mount in a DPX-type mountant.

Results

The following have variously been reported as staining blue: Keratin, red blood cells, nuclei, some fibrin, intercellular bridges of squamous cells, muscle, bile canaliculi, cilia, Paneth cells, neuroglia fibres, coarse elastin, alpha pancreatic cells, myelin, oncocytes.

Collagen, reticulin, mucins   brick red

LISSAMINE FAST RED TECHNIQUE
(Lendrum, 1947a)

Notes

Although not strictly speaking a trichrome, this method gives clear-cut differentiation of muscle from collagen. Its main attribute is the striking demonstration of myofibrils; it should be noted that cross-striations of muscle are not particularly well-shown. It may be used to advantage in the demonstration of leiomyosarcoma providing it is a reasonably well differentiated tumour. Differentiation of the lissamine fast red by phophomolybdic acid should stop when there is still a little excess dye in the collagen, as the final tartrazine counterstain tends to remove some of the red dye. Should differentiation be found too rapid at 56°C carry out the procedure at room temperature. The lissamine fast red solution does not keep well and should be discarded after 3 weeks or so. Like all trichrome-type techniques mercuric chloride/potassium dichromate fixation seems to give improved results. This may be achieved by secondary fixation of either tissue or section, if they were initially formalin fixed. As a guiding rule, large tumours fixed in formalin for several days will give indifferent staining with lissamine fast red unless secondarily fixed as indicated.

Solutions

1% lissamine fast red in 1% acetic acid.

1.5% tartrazine in 1.5% acetic acid.

1% aqueous phosphomolybdic acid.

Technique

1. Take sections to water.
2. Stain nuclei with an iron haematoxylin solution. Differentiate well and blue.
3. Stain with the lissamine fast red solution for 5 min.
4. Wash briefly in water, then differentiate in the phosphomolybdic acid solution at 56°C until the connective tissue is destained (5 min will usually suffice).
5. Wash briefly in water.
6. Counterstain with the tartrazine solution for 5 min.
7. Wash briefly in 90% alcohol.
8. Dehydrate, clear and mount as desired.

Results

Nuclei	blue-black
Muscle and red blood cells	red
Connective tissue, etc.	yellow

ACID FUCHSIN TECHNIQUE FOR EARLY MYOCARDIAL INFARCTION (Poley, et al, 1964)

Notes

This is a method for detecting ischaemic and degenerating myocardium before changes are evident in conventional (e.g. H and E) histological methods. It is based on the greater affinity of degenerating myocardium for dyes such as acid fuchsin, compared to normal myocardium which is counterstained a contrasting blue-green colour. The practical utilization of such a concept was introduced by Selye (1958) and is incorporated by the stain later devised by Poley et al (1964).

The rationale is not fully understood, but it has been suggested that a pH change or electrolyte shift may be responsible for the increased affinity for acid stains of damaged myocardium (Lie, 1968). The latter worker examined the usefulness of the acid fuchsin technique for detecting early myocardial infarction, and found it to be a sensitive technique. When carrying out the method, it is important to take through a set of control slides i.e. (if possible) a normal myocardium, one showing minimal infarction, and a myocardium showing well-marked infarction changes. The times of staining should be regarded as somewhat variable and will need to be altered according to the results obtained with the control material.

In our limited experience with this technique, we have found that practice is necessary to achieve consistent results, for like most trichrome-type techniques, the results tend to be subjective. Mechanical mixing during the acid fuchsin staining has been found to increase reproducibility (Berry, 1967).

An alternative method for demonstrating early myocardial infarction is that of Carle (1981). This worker utilized the enhanced acidophilia of necrotic myocardium by examining conventional H and E preparations with a fluorescence microscope. Necrotic muscle fibres give a bright yellow secondary fluorescence compared to the dull green fluorescence of normal myocardium. The effects result from the fact (not always appreciated!) that eosin is a fluorochrome.

Solutions

Stain A:

Stock solution

Cresyl fast violet	0.2 g
Distilled water	100 ml
Allow to stand 1 h and filter.	

Working solution (prepare on day of use)

Stock solution	10 ml
Distilled water	40 ml
1% aqueous oxalic acid	0.2 ml

Stain B

0.01% aqueous acid fuchsin	20 ml
0.01% aqueous orange G	15 ml
0.01% methyl green	0.1 ml
1% aqueous oxalic acid	0.2 ml

1% aqueous phosphotungstic acid

0.05% glacial acetic acid.

Technique

1. Take sections to water.

2. Place in stain A for 15 min.
3. Wash in running water for 10 min.
4. Mordant in the phosphotungstic acid for 15 min.
5. Wash in running water for 3 min.
6. Place in stain B for 30 min at 60°C (if possible using a mechanical stirrer).
7. Rinse in the weak acetic acid.
8. Dehydrate, clear and mount as desired.

Results

Myocardial fibres are stained progressively red in proportion to the degree of myocardial infarction.

Normal myocardium   blue green

COLLAGENASE DIGESTION

Notes

Collagenase derived from the Clostridia group of organisms, was described by Green (1960) as an enzyme for the digestion of collagen and reticulin fibres in tissue sections. This, used in conjunction with suitable connective tissue methods, would enable presumptive identification of these fibres. Another later variant (Vice, 1968) gives, in our opinion better results and will be described below. The rationale is collagen and reticulin are depolymerized into randomized peptides.

Fixation should be preferably in Carnoy's fluid or alcohol and after thorough washing in water, frozen sections should be prepared. We have found it necessary to extend digestion time in order to achieve full digestion of the fibres. Even so, complete digestion of all collagen and reticulin fibres is not invariable.

Solution

1 mg high-purity collagenase, 800–1600 units/mg dissolved in 1 ml pH 7.0 buffer (see Buffer Tables, Appendix 3.)

Technique

1. Take two test and two positive control sections to distilled water.
2. Treat one test and one control section with collagenase for at least 5 h, and if necessary up to 24 h at 37° C. Treat the remaining test and control sections with buffer only at 37° C for a similar period of time.
3. Wash all sections well in running tap water. Carry out a suitable demonstration technique, e.g. trichrome or van Gieson for collagen, and a silver method for reticulin.

Results

Collagen and reticulin fibres will fail to stain and will not, therefore, be apparent when the digested sections are compared to the undigested control sections. Young collagen is reported to be more susceptible to digestion that mature fibres (Montford & Perez-Tanyayo, 1975). When silver techniques for reticulin are carried out following collagenase digestion, an increase in background argyrophilia will be seen.

RETICULIN

Reticulin fibres (collagen type III) are fine branching fibres which are difficult to see in H and E preparations and need special stains to be visualized. The fibres are normally seen to best advantage in lymphoid tissue and liver.

The demonstration of reticulin fibres can be of assistance in diagnosis in certain instances; e.g. myelosclerosis in bone biopsies, where there is an excess of reticulin fibres; also in differentiating poorly differentiated carcinomas from certain of the lymphomas, the carcinoma showing a poorly marked reticulin pattern compared to the lymphoma where there is likely to be a profuse reticulin network. Reticulin demonstration is often useful in liver biopsies to show alterations to the normal architecture in certain types of cirrhosis.

To show these fibres one may carry out a trichrome-type technique where they stain blue or green; the PAS technique where they are positive or, more popularly, one may take advantage of their argyrophilia. There are many silver techniques for reticulin in common use, the more important of which will be described. Whilst we prefer to use the Gordon and Sweets' technique, all the methods described in this chapter are capable of yielding good results given the necessary expertise.

The rationale for the various silver methods for reticulin is they are modifications of the Bielschowsky techniques for nerve fibres in which, by means of various metallic sensitizers, silver from silver oxides is selectively deposited on the fibres. This is subsequently converted to reduced (black) silver by suitable reducing agents allowing visualization of the fibres.

Most silver techniques for reticulin are preceded by a permanganate oxidation step; this is thought to prevent the normal argyrophilia of such structures as nerve fibres.

As in any silver method, toning in gold chloride is optional and if used will give a clearer background and render collagen a purple-grey colour instead of a yellow-brown. We prefer not to tone and thus retain the colour distinction between collagen and reticulin (brown/black respectively).

The final step in all silver methods is to remove any remaining unreduced silver by treating with sodium thiosulphate ('hypo'). This prevents subsequent background precipitation due to light reduction and does not appear to be strictly necessary in reticulin methods.

Formalin is probably the best fixative in this instance, but most fixatives are satisfactory with the exception of Helly's.

Decalcified material often gives poor results with silver techniques for reticulin. For example, needle biopsies may exhibit argyrophilia of the red blood cells in the marrow. There is no clear cut answer to this problem but the result may be improved if non-acidic decalcification is used e.g. EDTA at 48°C.

GORDON AND SWEETS' TECHNIQUE
(Gordon & Sweets, 1936)

Notes

This is a popular and reliable method. The ammoniacal silver solution may be kept without deterioration for many weeks, even when stored at room temperature in a clear container. The formalin is best diluted with tap water which gives a better and more even reduction; this is probably due as much to the dissolved chlorides giving more intense reduction as to the higher pH of tap water.

Solutions

5% aqueous oxalic acid.

2% aqueous ferric ammonium sulphate (iron alum).

Acidified potassium permanganate solution

0.25% aqueous potassium permanganate	47.5 ml
3% aqueous sulphuric acid	2.5 ml

(These may conveniently be kept as stock solutions; the composite solution will normally keep for several weeks).

Ammoniacal silver solution

10% aqueous silver nitrate	5 ml

Add concentrated ammonia drop by drop with frequent mixing until the formed precipitate just redissolves. Then add 5 ml of 3.1% aqueous sodium hydroxide and mix. A precipitate will form which gradually dissolves upon the addition of ammonia, drop by drop as before. Stop when there are only a few precipitate granules remaining. Make up the final volume to 50 ml with water.

Technique

1. Take sections to water.
2. Treat with acidified potassium permanganate solution for 5 min.
3. Wash off, and bleach with oxalic acid solution for approximately 1 min. Wash well in water.
4. Rinse in distilled water then treat with the iron alum solution for 5 min.
5. Wash well in several changes of distilled water.
6. Treat with the ammoniacal silver solution for 4–5 s with agitation.
7. Wash well in several changes of distilled water.

8. Reduce in 10% formalin in tap water for ½–1 min with agitation.
9. Wash and tone if desired in 0.1% aqueous yellow gold chloride for 2 min.
10. Wash, treat with 5% hypo for 5 min.
11. Wash, counterstain if desired in 1% aqueous neutral red for 5 min. Wash, dehydrate, clear and mount as desired.

Note that neutral red may diffuse from the section in Canada balsam.

Results

Reticulin	black (some pigments such as lipofuscins and melanin are also weakly impregnated)
Collagen	yellow-brown if untoned
Background	clear if not counterstained, red if counterstained.

WILDER'S TECHNIQUE (Wilder, 1935)

Notes

This is a rapid method but one which has a tendency to give background silver deposition.

Solutions

0.25% aqueous potassium permanganate.

5% aqueous oxalic acid.

1% aqueous uranyl nitrate.

Ammoniacal silver solution
As for Gordon and Sweets' method.

Reducer

1.5% aqueous uranyl nitrate	1.5 ml
Formalin	0.5 ml
Distilled water	50 ml

Technique

1. Take sections to water.
2. Treat with the potassium permanganate solution for 1 min.

3. Wash off and bleach with the oxalic acid solution for approximately 1 min.
4. Wash well in water, then in distilled water.
5. Treat with the 1% uranyl nitrate solution for 3–5 s.
6. Wash well in distilled water.
7. Treat with the ammoniacal silver solution for 1 min.
8. Dip quickly into 95% alcohol.
9. Reduce for 1 min. Wash and tone if desired in 0.2% aqueous gold chloride.
10. Wash, treat with 5% hypo for 5 min.
11. Wash and counterstain in 1% aqueous neutral red if desired.
12. Wash, dehydrate, clear and mount as desired.

Results

Reticulin (and some pigments)	black
Collagen	yellow-brown if untoned
Background	light brown if not counterstained, red if counterstained

LAIDLAW'S TECHNIQUE (Laidlaw, 1929)

Notes

This method is a little more time-consuming than some, but gives good results.

Solutions

1% iodine in 95% alcohol.

0.25% aqueous potassium permanganate.

5% aqueous oxalic acid.

Ammoniacal lithium-silver solution

To 230 ml saturated aqueous lithium carbonate add 20 ml 60% aqueous silver nitrate, in a 250 ml measuring cylinder. Mix and allow the formed precipitate to settle to a 70 ml volume. Decant the supernatant and replace with distilled water. Mix well then repeat this washing of the precipitate twice more. Finally, having decanted the supernatant for the third time, add concentrated ammonia, with mixing, until the precipitate is almost dissolved. Make up the final volume to 120 ml with distilled water and filter.

Technique

1. Take sections to water.
2. Treat with the alcoholic-iodine solution for 5 min.
3. Wash and treat with 5% hypo to bleach the iodine colouration.
4. Wash, then treat with the potassium permanganate solution for 3 min.
5. Wash, bleach with the oxalic acid solution for approximately 1 min.
6. Wash well in water, then in several changes of distilled water.
7. Treat with the ammoniacal lithium-silver solution for 5 min at 56° C (preheated).
8. Rinse well in distilled water.
9. Reduce in 1% formalin in a Coplin jar until satisfactory reduction is obtained; this may take from 3–60 min.
10. Wash, tone if desired, treat with 5% hypo. Counterstain if wished in 1% aqueous neutral red.
11. Dehydrate, clear and mount as desired.

Results

Reticulin (and some pigments)	black
Collagen	yellow-brown if untoned
Background	clear if not counterstained, red if counterstained

ROBB-SMITH'S TECHNIQUE (Robb-Smith, 1937)

Notes

This is a flotation method which is rather laborious but it can give crisp reticulin demonstration. A convenient method is to float the paraffin sections onto the appropriate reagent in a glass Petri dish at the end of the treatment time then to take off the solution using a suction pump. Finally, pour in the new solution with care. With practice it will be found fairly easy to take off the solution in the dish without losing or damaging the section.

Solutions

10% aqueous ammonia (conc. ammonia diluted 1:10).

0.25% aqueous potassium permanganate.

1.5% aqueous oxalic acid.

5% aqueous silver nitrate.

Ammoniacal silver
  Add 6 drops of 10% aqueous sodium hydroxide to 8 ml 10% aqueous silver nitrate. Mix, and add conc. ammonia with mixing until the resultant precipitate is almost redissolved. Make up to 28 ml volume with distilled water.

Technique

1. Cut paraffin sections and float them onto distilled water at room temperature.
2. Transfer to the ammonia solution for 5 min.
3. Wash in three changes of distilled water.
4. Treat with the potassium permanganate solution for 10 min.
5. Wash with one change of distilled water, then bleach in the oxalic acid solution for 1–2 min.
6. Give four changes of distilled water then treat with the aqueous silver nitrate solution for 1 h.
7. Give three changes of distilled water.
8. Treat with the ammoniacal silver solution for 15 min.
9. Wash with three changes of distilled water.
10. Reduce in 30% formalin for 3 min.
11. Wash, tone if desired in 0.2% aqueous gold chloride and fix in 5% hypo. Wash.
12. Float onto warm water to flatten the section, pick up on a clean slide and dry in a 56°C oven for 30 min.
13. Dewax in xylene, rinse in clean xylene and mount as desired.

Results

Reticulin (and some pigments)	black
Collagen	yellow-brown if untoned
Background	pale yellow

GOMORI'S TECHNIQUE (Gomori, 1937)

Notes

This is a popular method which is comparable to Gordon and Sweets' not only in technique detail, but also as regards consistency of result. Gomori indicated a second reducing step following gold chloride toning.

Solutions

1% aqueous potassium permanganate.

3% aqueous potassium metabisuliphite.

2% aqueous ferric ammonium sulphate (iron alum).

Ammoniacal silver
To 20 ml of 10% aqueous silver nitrate add 4 ml of 10% aqueous potassium hydroxide. Add conc. ammonia with repeated mixing until the formed precipitate is just dissolved. Then add 10% aqueous silver nitrate slowly with frequent mixing, until only a faint opalescence remains. Dilute with an equal volume of distilled water.

Technique

1. Take sections to water.
2. Treat with potassium permanganate solution for 1–2 min.
3. Wash in water, then bleach with the potassium metabisulphite solution. Wash well in water.
4. Treat with iron alum solution for 1 min. Wash well in tap, then distilled water.
5. Treat with ammoniacal silver solution for 1 min.
6. Wash briefly in distilled water and reduce in 10% formalin for 3 min.
7. Wash, then tone in 0.2% gold chloride for up to 10 min.
8. Rinse in distilled water, then treat with the potassium metabisulphite solution for 1 min.
9. Rinse with distilled water and fix with 5% hypo for 1–2 mins.
10. Wash, dehydrate, clear and mount as desired.

Results

Reticulin (and some pigments)	black
Nuclei	grey
Collagen	grey-purple

JAMES TECHNIQUE (James, 1967)

Notes

Good results may be obtained with this technique for reticulin fibres, which has the added advantage of a standard treatment time for each step.

Solutions

Acidified potassium permanganate
0.3% aqueous potassium permanganate.
3% sulphuric acid.
Mix equal parts immediately prior to use.

5% aqueous oxalic acid.

5% aqueous silver nitrate.

Ammoniacal silver solution
To 20 ml of 10% aqueous silver nitrate add concentrated ammonia drop by drop with frequent mixing until the formed precipitate just redissolves. Add one drop of 10% aqueous silver nitrate and 20 ml distilled water. Filter and store in the dark.

5% formalin.

5% aqueous sodium thiosulphate ('hypo').

Technique

1. Take sections to water.
2. Treat with acidified permanganate for 5 min.
3. Rinse three times in distilled water.
4. Treat with the oxalic acid for 5 min.
5. Rinse three times in distilled water.

6. Treat with the 5% silver nitrate for 5 min.
7. Rinse three times in distilled water.
8. Treat with the ammoniacal silver for 5 min.
9. Rinse three times in distilled water.
10. Reduce in formalin for 5 min.
11. Rinse three times in distilled water.
12. Fix in hypo for 5 min.
13. Wash well in water.
14. Dehydrate, clear and mount as desired.

Results

Reticulin fibres	black
Collagen	yellow to brown

ELASTIC FIBRES

Elastic fibres are branching fibres of varying size and diameter which are particularly well seen in tissue sites such as dermis of skin, lung, heart and blood vessel walls. The demonstration of elastin has a firm place in diagnostic pathology. In conditions such as arteriosclerosis and temporal arteritis, for example, the elastic laminae of the affected blood vessels may be disorganized or absent, or one may encounter an excess of elastic tissue ('elastosis') in certain conditions of the heart and bladder neck, also in skin from some elderly subjects ('senile elastosis').

The finer elastic fibres are not easily delineated in an H and E preparation and one normally makes use of special stains. The fibres are weakly PAS positive, exhibit a green-yellow primary fluorescence and stain with Congo red and related dyes. It is said that prior methylation will block the reactivity of elastin (Fullmer, 1958).

Fixation is not, on the whole, critical although Heidenhain's 'Susa' may give inferior staining results. Celloidinization of sections prior to staining, particularly of skin and blood vessels, is often desirable as they may detach from the slide.

WEIGERT-TYPE TECHNIQUES

Notes

There are several variations of the original Weigert technique resulting in a choice of final colour product. The rationale of these methods is obscure, but it has been stated (Baker, 1966) that resorcinol fuchsin stains elastin by a hydrogen bonding mechanism; the same mechanism probably underlies the staining of elastin by Congo red.

Most of the Weigert-type methods evince a remarkable demonstration selectivity for elastic fibres and give what is, in our opinion, the best demonstration of fine fibres. The techniques tend to be slow and the solutions are rather time-consuming to prepare. If the solution fails to stain satisfactorily the likely cause is a poor batch of either the dye or the ferric chloride. An avid staining solution may be used repeatedly, it being merely necessary to filter the solution after use.

The main variants are as follows:

Weigert's resorcinol fuchsin (1898)	elastic fibres, dark blue-black
Hart's modification (1908)	elastic fibres, dark blue-black
French's modification (1929)	elastic fibres, dark blue-green
Sheridan's modification (1929)	elastic fibres, green.

All of these solutions stain well at room temperature and may be used repeatedly. Some variation in staining avidity will be found with different batches so that variation in staining times will occur. By and large, it will be found that staining at room temperature for longer periods gives better results that a shorter time in the 56° C oven. Pretreatment with acidified permanganate/oxalic acid solution sequence gives a clearer background.

Solutions

Weigert's resorcinol fuchsin solution

Basic fuchsin	2 g
Resorcin	4 g
Distilled water	200 ml
30% aqueous anhydrous ferric chloride	25 ml
95% alcohol	200 ml
Conc. hydrochloric acid	4 ml

Dissolve the basic fuchsin and resorcin in the distilled water bringing to the boil in a porcelain evaporating dish. Whilst still boiling, slowly add the aqueous anhydrous ferric chloride solution with continuous stirring. Continue this boiling and stirring for approximately 5 min. Cool and filter into a conical flask taking care that all available precipitate is collected. Discard the filtrate, then dry the flask into which is now put the dried filter paper containing the precipitate. Add the alcohol and heat gently on a hotplate until the precipitate is dissolved. Remove the filter paper, add the conc. hydrochloric acid, cool and filter. Make up the final volume to 200 ml by pouring fresh 95% alcohol through the used filter paper. The purified basic fuchsin commonly used for Schiff's reagent gives inferior results.

Hart's modification

This is Weigert's solution diluted with 1% acid-alcohol. The proportions will vary according to the avidity of the particular batch of stain prepared and should be calculated using a trial run. The usual proportions are Weigert's solution 5–20 ml acid alcohol 30–40 ml.

French's modification

The solution is that of Weigert excepting that in place of basic fuchsin 2 g, use 1 g each of basic fuchsin and crystal violet.

Sheridan's modification

The solution is that of Weigert excepting that in place of the basic fuchsin 2 g, use 2 g each of crystal violet and dextrin.

Technique

1. Take sections to water.
2. Treat with the acidified potassium permanganate solution for 5 min. Wash and bleach with oxalic acid for approximately 1 min.
3. Having washed well in water, rinse in alcohol.
4. Stain in the elastin solution. The time will vary according to the batch and type of solution, e.g. Weigert's elastin solution will usually stain sufficiently well in 1–3 h at room temperature whilst the other three elastin solutions may require overnight staining at room temperature.
5. Wash in water and differentiate in acid-alcohol until the background is clear of stain. Wash well in water. Note that with Sheridan's solution the green colouration of the elastin is enhanced by increased acid-alcohol differentiation.
6. Counterstain as required, e.g. neutral red, eosin or van Gieson.
7. Dehydrate, clear and mount as desired.

Results

| Elasticfibres | dark blue-black (Weigert and Hart), dark blue-green (French), green (Sheridan) |
| Background | according to counterstain used |

MODIFIED WEIGERT ELASTIN TECHNIQUE (MILLER, 1971)

Notes

The following stain for elastic fibres is a fairly rapid one and is used progressively i.e., no differentiation is required.

Solutions

0.5% aqueous potassium permanganate.

1% aqueous oxalic acid.

Stain solution
Victoria blue 4 R	1 g
New fuchsin	1 g
Crystal violet	1 g

Dissolve in 200 ml of hot distilled water and add in the following order:
Resorcin	4 g
Dextrin	1 g
Freshly prepared 30% aqueous ferric chloride	50 ml

Boil for 5 min and filter whilst still hot. Transfer the precipitate plus filter paper to the original flask and redissolve in 200 ml of 95% alcohol. Boil for 15–20 min. Cool, filter, and make up to a 200 ml volume with 95% alcohol. Finally add 2 ml of conc. hydrochloric acid.

Technique

1. Take sections to water.
2. Treat with potassium permanganate for 5 min.
3. Wash in water and bleach with oxalic acid for 2–3 min.
4. Wash well in water, then in 95% alcohol.
5. Place in either (a) undiluted stain for 1–3 h or (b) diluted stain (equal parts with 95% alcohol) overnight.
6. Wash in 95% alcohol then in water.
7. Counterstain as desired, e.g. van Gieson's stain in the usual manner (see p. 41).
8. Dehydrate, clear and mount as desired.

Results

Elastic fibres and mast cell granules	black
Background	according to counterstain used

ORCEIN TECHNIQUE (Unna, 1891)

Notes

This method shares with the Weigert-type techniques a remarkable selectivity for elastic tissue. Occasionally it may fail to give good results and this can nearly always be traced to a faulty batch of the dye. The fact that it stains elastin a brown colour makes it less suitable than the Weigert methods for use in conjunction with a van Gieson counterstain.

The precise rationale of orcein binding by elastin is not clear, although van der Waals forces are considered to be involved. As will be discussed in the Shikata technique for viral hepatitis antigen (p. 215), following suitable pre-oxidation of tissue, orcein has a firm affinity for sulphur-containing compounds.

Solution

Dissolve orcein (preferably synthetic) 1 g in 100 ml of 70% alcohol with the aid of gentle heat. Cool, filter and add 1 ml of conc. hydrochloric acid.

Technique

1. Take sections to 70% alcohol.
2. Stain with the orcein solution for 1–2 h at 37° C.
3. Rinse in 70% alcohol, differentiate in 1% acid-alcohol if necessary then wash well in water.
4. Counterstain as required. Suitable counterstains are haematoxylin, 0.1% aqueous azure A or methylene blue for 1–2 min.
5. Finally, dehydrate, clear and mount as desired.

Results

Elastin	dark brown
Background	according to counterstain used

ALDEHYDE-FUCHSIN TECHNIQUE (Gomori, 1950B)

Notes

This is quite a popular method for elastin as it stains both coarse and fine fibres strongly. However, it is less selective than other elastin methods as it demonstrates a number of tissue entities a similar colour. The rationale is obscure, although it has been stated the combination of aldehyde and basic fuchsin demonstrates organically bound sulphur, e.g. sulphated mucins, also insulin as in beta cells of pancreas (Rhinehart, 1952–53). Whether or not elastin contains such a sulphur moiety has yet to be firmly established.

Strictly speaking no pre-oxidation is necessary in order to stain either elastin or sulphated mucins, for without pre-oxidation only these two materials will stain. Staining is speeded up by pre-oxidation and will increase the number of tissue entities demonstrated, e.g. beta cells of pancreas. If periodic or peracetic acid is used as the oxidant, glycogen and neutral mucin will be stained by Schiff's base formation.

The solution can be capricious and there are a number of factors to be observed in its preparation. The basic fuchsin should be of the finer granule size (as for PAS); if in doubt use pararosanilin. It has been stated that the paraldehyde is prone to decomposition and that one should use only freshly opened samples (Moment, 1969). Following preparation the solution must be allowed to 'blue' for at least 2 days at room temperature, preferably longer. This blueing has been attributed to the formation of acetaldehyde from the acidic paraldehyde, which condenses with the amino groups of basic fuchsin moving the absorption spectrum to the longer wavelengths (Summer, 1965). Older aldehyde fuchsin solutions will need filtering prior to use and one may need to extend times of staining by 100%.

Various counterstains have been proposed for aldehyde fuchsin. Providing that a suitably contrasting one is used the final choice is not important. Obviously, van Gieson's solution is not the most suitable owing to the close colour similarity of the collagen fibres and elastin.

Solutions

Acidified potassium permanganate solution see page 49.

5% aqueous oxalic acid.

Aldehyde fuchsin
  Dissolve basic fuchsin 1 g in 100 ml of 60% alcohol. Add conc. hydrochloric acid 1 ml and paraldehyde 2 ml. Allow to blue at room temperature for at least 2 days before using. Store at 4°C. The solution should keep for 1–2 months. Deterioration will be evidenced by increased background staining.

Technique

1. Take sections to water.
2. Treat with the acid potassium permanganate solution for 1 min. Wash, bleach with the oxalic acid solution then wash well in water.
3. Rinse in 70% alcohol.
4. Stain with the aldehyde fuchsin solution for 4 min.
5. Rinse well in 70% alcohol, then in water.
6. Counterstain suitably, e.g. 0.1% aqueous methylene blue, 0.2% light green in 0.2% acetic acid or saturated tartrazine in

Cellosolve (rinse in Cellosolve not water) for $\frac{1}{2}$–1 minute.
7. Dehydrate, clear and mount in a DPX-type mountant.

Results

Elastin, sulphated mucins (includes mast cells), beta cells of pancreas and pituitary, some lipofuscins, gastric chief cells, hypothalamic neurosecretory cells, HBS antigen — purple.

Background   according to counterstain used

VERHOEFF'S TECHNIQUE (Verhoeff, 1908)

Notes

This is a popular, quick method, staining elastic fibres a strong black colour. A major disadvantage is the fact that some expertise is necessary in order to stain the finer elastic fibres, and at the same time obtain a well differentiated background.

It will be found that the elastin staining is extracted by the van Gieson counterstain to a certain extent. Consequently, to obtain good results one should aim at slightly underdifferentiating the Verhoeff stain in the ferric chloride solution.

The rationale of the technique like most other elastin stains, is rather obscure. Both iodine and ferric chloride with which the haematoxylin is combined, are oxidizing agents and it is this property which probably accounts for the production of a black dye with cationic properties (nuclei are also stained), rather than a simple dye-mordant-tissue mechanism.

Solutions

Verhoeff's stain
5% alcoholic haematoxylin (freshly
prepared solutions give stronger
staining results)   20 ml
10% aqueous ferric chloride   8 ml
Lugol's iodine (see below)   8 ml
2 g potassium iodide are dissolved in a few ml of distilled water; dissolve in this 1 g of iodine and

finally make up to 100 ml volume with distilled water.

2% aqueous ferric chloride.

Technique

1. Take sections to alcohol.
2. Stain with Verhoeff's solution for 15 min (make up prior to use).
3. Wash in water and differentiate in the ferric chloride solution until the nuclei and elastic fibres are black and the background is still weakly stained.
4. Wash in water then in alcohol for approximately 5 min to remove iodine colouration of the background.
5. Wash in water and counterstain as desired; with solutions such as van Gieson or neutral red for standard times.
6. Dehydrate, clear and mount as desired.

Results

Nuclei and elastic fibres	black
Background	according to the counterstain used

ELASTASE DIGESTION (Fullmer, 1958)

Notes

It may be desirable on occasion to confirm that the particular material reacting with the elastin methods is elastin and the use of this enzyme will be of assistance. It should be noted that elastase is an expensive enzyme. It is derived commercially from pig pancreas.

We have found the following technique to work well although the time of digestion may need to be increased with certain material up to 18 h. Unlike collagenase, formalin fixation does not seem to inhibit the enzyme action. Elastin molecules are made soluble by fission of peptide linkages.

Solution

Dissolve 15 mg elastase (15–20 units/mg elastase) in 100 ml pH 8.8 buffer (see Buffer Tables).

Technique

1. Take two test sections plus suitable positive control sections to distilled water.
2. Treat one of the test and one of the positive control sections with the preheated enzyme for 6 h at 37°C. Duplicate sections are treated with pH 8.8 buffer only for the same time and temperature.
3. Wash all sections in water for several minutes.
4. Finally stain all sections with one of the preceding methods for elastic fibres.
5. Dehydrate, clear and mount as desired (if the aldehyde fuchsin technique is used mount in one of the DPX-type mountants).

Results

Sections treated with the enzyme should show loss of elastic fibre staining, when compared with the section treated with buffer only.

OXYTALAN FIBRES

First recognized by Fullmer (1958), oxytalan fibres are connective tissue in type with a morphology and (modified) histochemistry similar to that of elastic fibres. They are found in close association with tendons and ligaments and are particularly well seen in periodontal ligaments, where they insert into the cementum layers of teeth.

Oxytalan fibres have also been reported in the blood vessels of pregnant uteri (Manning, 1974), and in pathological cornea (Alexander et al, 1981).

OXYTALAN FIBRE DEMONSTRATION

Notes

An important feature of oxytalan histochemistry is that the fibres react with some, but not all, elastic fibre techniques and only after pre-oxidation with certain substances. Similarly, elastase will not digest oxytalan fibres unless pre-oxidation is carried out. The most satisfactory dye for demonstration purposes would seem to be aldehyde fuchsin using as a pre-oxidant either peracetic acid or peroxymonosulphate (Alexander et al, 1981). Potassium permanganate can also be used but is less effective.

The need for pre-oxidation in oxytalan fibre demonstration presumably denotes the presence of masking ethylene groups, which when oxidized either make available reactive sulphate radicals capable of ionic linkage or hydrogen bonding with appropriate dyes. It has also been considered that it is a mucopolysaccharide present in the fibres which requires oxidation to open reactive bonds (Fullmer, 1965). Table 5.1 is taken from Fullmer (1964), and Fullmer & Lillie (1958). It illustrates the reactions to various stains by oxytalan and elastic fibres using peracetic pre-oxidation.

Table 5.1 Staining reactions of oxytalan and elastic fibres

Peracetic oxidized	Oxytalan fibres	Elastic fibres
Orcein	Brown (some)	Brown
Aldehyde fuchsin	Purple	Purple
Resorcin fuchsin	Purple-black (some)	Purple-black
Verhoeff's stain	Negative	Black
PAS	Negative	Magenta
Elastase digestion	Digested	Digested

Solutions

Peracetic acid

Glacial acetic acid	95.6 ml
30% (100 volumes) hydrogen peroxide	259 ml
Conc. sulphuric acid	2.2 ml

Add disodium hydrogen orthophosphate 0.04 g as a stabilizer, and allow to stand 1–3 days before use. The solution will keep for several months at 4°C.

10% aqueous potassium peroxymonosulphate
Obtainable as 'Caroat' from: Bayley Degusse Ltd., Stanley Green Trading Estate, Cheadle Hulme, Cheadle, Cheshire.

Technique

1. Take duplicate paraffin sections of test material to distilled water.

2. Treat one section only with either peracetic acid for 30 min or potassium peroxymonosulphate for 60 min.
3. Wash well in water.
4. Carry out the aldehyde fuchsin stain for elastic fibres (p. 55) on both sections as per standard technique.
5. Dehydrate, clear and mount as desired.

Results

An increase in fibre staining in the oxidized section when compared to the unoxidized section, will denote the presence of oxytalan fibres.

BASEMENT MEMBRANES (BASAL LAMINA)

Basement membranes (basal lamina) are composed of mucoprotein and are associated with specialized reticulin fibres (collagen type IV). They normally underlie epithelial surfaces and are particularly pronounced around hair follicles and epididymal tubules. It is occasionally of some importance to be able to demonstrate basement membranes; for example, they may be greatly thickened in renal glomeruli in diseases such as lupus erythematosus and membranous glomerulonephritis, also in bronchial vessels in asthma. They may be demonstrated by the trichrome methods, in which they take up the fibre stain; by the periodic acid-Schiff (PAS) technique and a variant of this, the Allochrome method; or by a modification of Gomori's hexamine-silver technique. Undoubtedly, the latter method gives the most precise demonstration of basement membranes. Thinner than usual sections should be employed. The PAS technique will be fully dealt with in the chapter dealing with carbohydrates, and although the PAS method for basement membranes (basal lamina) is essentially the same in principle, it is important to extend the times of oxidation and Schiff treatment by upto half as much again.

A point to bear in mind is that the proportions of fibres to mucoprotein varies in different tissues with a consequent variation in staining reactions. For example, the basement membrane (basal lamina) of the renal tubules is well shown by PAS (for the mucoprotein content), whereas in the intestine the basement membrane (basal lamina) is poorly outlined by PAS but well shown by techniques for reticulin fibres. It has been shown (Laurie et al, 1981) that two types of glycoprotein may be found in basement membrane, fibronectin and laminin.

MODIFIED HEXAMINE-SILVER TECHNIQUE (Gomori, 1946; Jones, 1957)

Notes

Periodate-formed aldehydes from certain carbo-hydrate-containing material (in this case, basement membranes) will selectively reduce an alkaline hexamine-silver salt mixture. The technique, whilst a rather laborious one, demonstrates the finer basement membranes such as those of the renal glomerulus probably better than any other method. Connective tissue fibres are also demonstrated to a variable degree. When demonstrating the basement membranes (basal lamina) of renal glomeruli, it is important to slightly overimpregnate with the hexamine-silver solution. Take through a control section to test the efficacy of the solution. When dealing with renal tissue it is important to examine the glomeruli *not* the tubules to determine the end-point of the reaction. This is because the glomerular basement membrane (basal lamina) consists only of structural proteins. The tubular basement membrane, on the other hand, also contain a reticulin element and will more readily stain.

Fixation may be important. Bouin fixation leads to the best results as impregnation times will be shorter. Formalin is satisfactory but following long-standing fixation sections will need prolonged impregnation in the hexamine-silver. Formal sublimate fixation of tissue will result in relatively poor results, and in general terms it is better to avoid mercuric chloride-containing fixatives when intending to carry out this technique.

Solutions

1% aqueous periodic acid.

Stock hexamine-silver solution

Mix 5 ml of 5% aqueous silver nitrate and 100 ml of 3% aqueous hexamine (synonyms: methenamine or hexamethylenetetramine). A white precipitate will form which dissolves on shaking. This solution will keep for a limited time (1–2 months) if stored in a dark container at 4°C.

Working solution

Dilute 2 ml of a 5% aqueous sodium borate solution with 25 ml of distilled water. Mix and add 25 ml of the stock hexamine-silver solution.

Technique

1. Take sections to distilled water.
2. Treat with the periodic acid solution for 10 min.
3. Wash well in several changes of distilled water.
4. Place in preheated hexamine-silver solution in a 56° C water bath. Examine after 20 min and subsequently at frequent intervals until the basement membranes are blackened; this will take from 25–40 min.
5. Wash well in several changes of distilled water.
6. Tone in 0.1% aqueous yellow gold chloride for 2–5 min.
7. Wash in water and treat with 5% hypo for 5 min.
8. Wash, counterstain in 0.2% light green in 0.2% acetic acid for ½–1 min.
9. Wash, dehydrate, clear and mount as desired.

Results

Basement membranes (basal lamina)   black
Background   green

ALLOCHROME TECHNIQUE (Lillie, 1951)

Notes

This method is the PAS technique followed by a picro-methyl blue counterstain to give combined staining of basement membranes and connective tissue fibres in contrasting colours. We see little value in this method but it seems to enjoy some popularity.

Solutions

PAS solutions, see page 102.

0.04% methyl blue in saturated aqueous picric acid.

Technique

1. Take sections to distilled water and treat with periodic acid and Schiff's reagent as for the PAS technique.

2. Stain nuclei with an iron haematoxylin solution. Differentiate and blue.
3. Counterstain with the picro-methyl blue solution for 6 min.
4. Differentiate briefly in 95% alcohol. Dehydrate, clear and mount as desired.

Results

Nuclei	brown-black
Collagen and reticulin	blue
Cytoplasm and muscle	greenish-yellow
Basement membranes (basal lamina) and other periodate-reactive material	magenta

Table 5.2 Connective tissue staining results

Technique	Collagen	Reticulin	Elastin	Oxytalan	Basement memb.	Muscle
Van Gieson	Red	—	—	—	—	Yellow
Trichromes	Blue	Blue	Red/Blue	—	Blue	Red
PTAH	Red	Red	Blue	—	—	Blue
Silver (untoned)	Brown	Black		—	—	—
Weigerts elastin	—	—	Blue-black	Blue-black	—	—
Weigerts with preoxid.	—	—	Blue-black	Blue-black	—	—
Sheridan's elastin	—	—	Green	—	—	—
Sheridan's with preoxid.	—	—	Green	Green	—	—
Orcein	—	—	Brown	Variable brown	—	—
Aldehyde fuchsin	—	—	Purple		—	—
Aldehyde fuchsin with preoxid.	—	—	Purple	Purple	—	—
PAS	Weak magenta	Magenta	Weak magenta	—	Magenta	Volunt. and cardiac magenta
Hexamine silver (Jones mod.)	—	—	—	—	Black	—

REFERENCES

Abul-Haj S K, Rinehart J F 1952/53 Fuchsin-aldehyde staining of sulfated mucopolysaccharides and related substances. Journal of the National Cancer Institute 13: 232–3

Alexander R A, Clayton D C, Howes R C, Garner A 1981 Effect of oxidation upon demonstration of corneal oxytalan fibres: a light and electron microscopical study. Medical Laboratory Sciences 38: 91–101

Baker J R 1966 Cytological technique, 5th edn. Methuen, London

Berry C L 1967 Myocardial ischaemia in infancy and childhood. Journal of Clinical Pathology 20: 38–41

Bohacek L G 1966 Acceleration of Mallory's phosphotungstic acid-haematoxylin staining for skeletal muscle fixed in formalin. Stain Technology 41: 101–3

Carle B N 1981 Autofluorescence in the identification of myocardial infarcts. Human Pathology 12: 643–6

Cooper J H 1969 The evaluation of current methods for the diagnostic histochemistry of amyloid. Journal of Clinical Pathology 22: 410

Disbrey B D, Rack J H 1970 Histological Laboratory Methods. Livingstone, Edinburgh

Drury R A B, Wallington E A 1980 Carleton's histological technique. Oxford University Press, Oxford

Dubowitz V. Brooke M H 1973 Muscle biopsy: a modern approach. W B Saunders, London

Francis R 1982 Personal communication

French R W 1929 Elastic tissue staining. Stain Technology 4: 11

Fullmer H M 1958 Differential staining of connective tissue fibres in areas of stress. Science (New York) 127: 1240

Fullmer H N 1964 In: Provenza DV (ed) Oral histology inheritance and development. Pitman Medical, London

Fullmer H M, Lillie R D 1958 The oxytalan fibre: a previously undescribed connective tissue fibre. Journal of Histochemistry and Cytochemistry 6: 425–30

Gitlin D, Craig J M 1957 Variations in the staining characteristics of human fibrin. American Journal of Pathology 33: 267

Glynn G E, Loewi G 1952 Fibrinoid necrosis in rheumatic fever. Journal of Pathology and Bacteriology 64: 329

Gomori G 1937 Silver impregnation of reticulum in paraffin sections. American Journal of Pathology 13: 993

Gomori G 1946 A new histochemical test for glycogen and mucin. American Journal of Clinical Pathology 16: 177

Gomori G 1950A A rapid one-step trichrome stain. American Journal of Clinical Pathology 20: 661

Gomori G 1950B Aldehyde fuchsin a new stain for elastic tissues. American Journal of Clinical Pathology 20: 665

Gordon H, Sweets H H 1936 A simple method for the silver impregnation of reticulum. American Journal of Pathology 12: 545

Gray P, Pickle F M, Muser M D, Hayweiser J 1958 Oxazine dyes. I. Celestine blue with iron as a mordant. Stain Technology 31: 141

Green J 1960 Digestion of collagen and reticulin in paraffin sections by collagenase. Stain Technology 35: 273–6

Hart K 1908 Die Farbung der elastischen Fasern mit dem von Weigert angegebenen Farbstoff. Zentralblatt für Allegemaine Pathologie und Pathologische Anatomie 19: 1

Heidenhain M 1915 Zeitschrift fur wissenschaftliche Mikroskopie und fur mikroskopische Technik 21: 1

Herovici C 1963 A polychrome stain for differentiating pre-collagen, from collagen. Stain Technology 38: 204–6

Ibeachum G I 1971 The storage of Weigert's iron haematoxylin. Medical Laboratory Technology 28: 117–20

James K R 1967 A simple silver method for the demonstration of reticulin fibres. Journal of Medical Laboratory Technology 24: 49–51

Jones D B 1957 Nephrotic glomerulonephritis. American Journal of Pathology 33: 313

Laidlaw G F 1929 Silver staining of skin and of its tumours. American Journal of Pathology 5: 239

Laurie G W, Lebold C P, Cournil I, Martin G R 1981 Immunohistochemical evidence for the intracellular formation of basement membranes collagen (type IV) in developing tissues. Journal of Histochemistry and Cytochemistry 28: 1267

Lendrum A C 1947A The phloxine-tartrazine method as a general histological stain and for the demonstration of inclusion bodies. Journal of Pathology and Bacteriology 59: 399

Lendrum A C 1947B Routine diagnostic technique of the general morbid anatomist. In: Dyke S C (ed) Recent Advances in Clinical Pathology. Churchill, London

Lendrum A C, Fraser D S, Slidders W, Henderson R 1962 Studies on the character and staining of fibrin. Journal of Clinical Pathology 15: 401

Lie J T 1968 Detection of early myocardial infarction by the acid fuchsin staining technic. American Journal of Clinical Pathology 50: 317–9

Lieb E 1948 Modified phosphotungstic acid-haematoxylin stain. Archives of Pathology 45: 559

Lillie R D 1951 The allochrome procedure: a differential method segregating the connective tissues, collagen, reticulin and basement membranes into two groups. American Journal of Clinical Pathology 21: 484

Lillie R D 1965 Histopathologic technic and practical histochemistry 3rd edn. McGraw-Hill, New York

McFarlane D 1944 Picro-Mallory. An easily controlled regressive trichromic staining method. Stain Technology 19: 29

McManus J F A 1946 Histological demonstration of mucin after periodic acid. Nature, London 158: 202

Mallory F B 1900 A contribution to staining methods. Journal of Experimental Medicine 5: 15

Mallory F B 1905 A contribution to the classification of tumours. Journal of Medical Research, Boston 13: 113–36

Manning P J 1974 The staining of elastic tissue and related fibres in uterine blood vessels. Medical Laboratory Technology 31: 115–25

Masson P 1929 Some histological methods. Trichrome stainings and their preliminary technique. Bulletin of the International Association of Medicine 12: 75

Miller P J 1971 An elastin stain. Medical Laboratory Technology 28: 148–9

Moe N, Abilgaard U 1969 Histological staining properties of in vitro formed fibrin clots and precipitated fibrinogen. Acta Pathologica Microbiologica Scandinavica 76: 61–73

Moment G B 1969 Deteriorated paraldehyde: an insidious cause of failure in aldehyde fuchsin staining. Stain Technology 44: 52–3

Montford P, Perez-Tanyayo R 1975 The distribution of collagenase in normal rat tissues. Journal of Histochemistry and Cytochemistry 22: 910–20

Muirhead E E, Booth E, Montgomery P O B 1957 Derivation of certain forms of 'fibrinoid' from smooth muscle. Archives of Pathology 63: 213–28

Poley R W Fobes C D, Hall M J 1964 Fuchsinophilia in early myocardial infarction: a method for the demonstration of early myocardial infarction using acid fuchsin staining. Archives of Pathology 77: 325–9

Robb-Smith A H T 1937 Device to facilitate impregnation of reticulin fibrils in paraffin sections. Journal of Pathology and Bacteriology 45: 312–3

Schiff H 1866 Eine neue Reihe organischer Diamine. Justus Liebigs Annin Chem 140: 92

Seki M 1932 Folia anat Jap. 10: 635

Selye H 1958 Chemical prevention of cardiac necroses. Ronald Press, New York

Sheridan W F 1929 Journal of Technical Methods Bulletin of International Association of Medical Museums 12: 123

Shum M W K, Hon J K Y 1969 A modified phosphotungstic acid-haematoxylin stain for formalin fixed tissues. Journal of Medical Laboratory Technology 26: 38–42

Singer M, Wislocki C B 1948 Affinity of syncytium, fibrin and fibrinoid of human placenta for acid and basic dyes under controlled conditions of staining. Anatomical Record 102: 175–93

Slidders W 1961 The fuchsin-Miller method. Journal of Medical Laboratory Technology 18: 36–7

Slidders W 1968 A stable iron-haematoxylin solution for staining the chromatin of cell nuclei. Journal of Microscopy 90: Pt 1, 61–5

Summer B E H 1965 Experiments to determine the composition of aldehyde fuchsin solutions. Journal of the Royal Microscopical Society 84: 181–7

Terner J Y, Gurland J, Gaer S 1964 Phosphotungstic acid-haematoxylin: spectrophotometry of the lake in solution and in stained tissue. Stain Technology 39: 141–153

Unna P G 1891 Ueber 'Ichthyolfirnisse' Monatsh f. prakt. Dermat Hamb. XII: 49–56

van Gieson I 1889 Laboratory notes of technical methods for the nervous system. New York Medical Journal 50: 57

Verhoeff F H 1908 Some new staining methods of wide applicability, including a rapid differential stain for elastic tissue. Journal of American Medical Association 50: 876

Vice P 1968 Collagenase digestion for distinguishing neural from reticular fibres in silver stains. Stain Technology 43: 183–6

Wiegert C 1898 Ueber eine Methode zur Farbung elastischer Fasern. Zentralblatt Für Allgemeine Pathologie und Pathologische Anatomie 9: 289

Weigert C 1904 Eine kleine Verbesserung der Hamatoxylin-van Gieson Methode. Zeitschrift fur wissenschaftliche Mikroskopie und Fur mikroskopische Technik 21: 1

Wilder H C 1935 Improved technique for silver impregnation of reticulin fibres. American Journal of Pathology 11: 817–9

6

Intracellular granules

EOSINOPHIL CELLS

The granules of eosinophil cells are intensely acidophilic and stain perfectly well in an H and E preparation. They also stain with Congo red, the DMAB-nitrite reaction and amido black. Eosinophils are of some significance pathologically in that they may be present in excessive numbers in such diverse conditions as parasitic infestations, chronic inflammations, eosinophil granuloma and in certain forms of Hodgkin's disease.

The two methods below give good selective staining of the granules.

CARBOL CHROMOTROPE TECHNIQUE
(Lendrum, 1944)

Notes

This is an empirical, but remarkably selective technique for eosinophils. It is simple to do and reliable. The presence of the phenol presumably lowers the pH of the stain solution and increases selectivity for the granules.

Solution

Melt 1 g phenol in a flask under hot water and add 0.5 g chromotrope 2R. Mix, then dissolve the resultant sludge in 100 ml distilled water. The solution should keep for up to 3 months.

Technique

1. Take sections to water.
2. Stain the nuclei with one of the alum haematoxylin solutions. Differentiate and blue.

3. Stain with the carbol chromotrope solution for 30 min.
4. Wash, dehydrate, clear and mount as desired.

Results

Nuclei	blue
Eosinophil granules	red
Red blood cells	pale red
Paneth cell granules	rust-coloured
Enterochromaffin granules	weak brown

GIEMSA TECHNIQUE (Giemsa, 1902)

Notes

This is a slightly modified version of the original Giemsa technique which will give good results for sections. It will be appreciated that most acidophil cells as well as eosinophils will be stained a similar colour. To achieve a good colour balance it is necessary to initially overstain with the Giemsa stain, and then slightly overdifferentiate in weak acetic acid until there is an overall pink cast to the cells. This is done to offset the loss of eosinophilia and gain in basophilia which results upon eventual alcohol dehydration. Decalcification of tissue using strong acids should be avoided, as it results in a poor colour balance.

Solution

A standard Giemsa staining solution is readily available from most commercial firms dealing in dyes for laboratories, but for those wishing to prepare their own batch, the following formula may be used.

Mix 7.36 g Giemsa dry stain in 500 ml glycerol

which is heated to 50° C in a water bath. Leave for 30 min at 50° C with periodic mixing. Allow to cool and add 500 ml methanol (the acetone content is immaterial). Mix and filter.

Technique

1. Take sections to distilled water.
2. Filter enough Giemsa stain into a Coplin jar filled with distilled water to render the solution a dark blue colour (0.5–1 ml). Stain with the solution for at least 20 min at 56° C until the section is an overall dark blue.
3. Rinse in distilled water and differentiate in a very weak acetic acid solution (approximately 1:10 000 v/v) until the section is predominantly pink in colour.
4. Rinse in distilled water, dehydrate, clear and mount as desired.

Results

Nuclei	purple
Azurophilic granules	blue
Eosinophil granules, red blood cells and other acidophil structures	pink

PANETH CELLS

It is a curious fact that while there is a legion of special stains for these cells, their demonstration is rarely called for in diagnostic histopathology. The cells were first described by Schwalbe and later by Paneth whose name they acquired. Paneth cells are situated in the bases of the crypts of Lieberkühn in the small bowel. Less often they can be seen in the appendix and proximal colon. In pathological conditions they can occur in the stomach and large bowel. There appears to be a decrease of the cells in coeliac disease, and an increase in ulcerative colitis. The granules are similar to the zymogen granules of the pancreas in appearance and their staining reactions are not dissimilar. The function of Paneth cells has not been resolved but it is well known that they contain zinc (Ham, 1969). For the best results

with Paneth cells prompt fixation is necessary to preserve the granules. Acid fixation will destroy the reactive elements so neutral formal saline or formal calcium fixation is recommended. Acidic fixatives can be used as secondary solutions if required. The cells are strongly acidophilic and can be seen in routine H and E sections. Two techniques are given below and their reactions to other staining methods in Table 6.1.

Table 6.1 Staining reactions of Paneth cells

Method	Colour
Phloxine tartrazine	Red to orange
Fuchsin Miller	Red
DMAB-nitrite	Blue
MSB	Red
Giemsa	Red
Gram	Positive
PAS	Variable positive
PTAH	Blue
Amido black	Dark blue

PHLOXINE-TARTRAZINE TECHNIQUE (Lendrum, 1947)

Notes

This popular technique for Paneth cells, relies on overstaining with phloxine and then progressive substitution by tartrazine. The method is not specific for the granules as number of other substances may also be demonstrated, e.g. fibrin and virus inclusion bodies. Muscle also tends to retain the phloxine, albeit weakly.

Solutions

0.5% phloxine in 0.5% aqueous calcium chloride.

Saturated tartrazine in Cellosolve (2-ethoxyethanol).

Technique

1. Take sections to water.
2. Stain the nuclei with one of the haematoxylin solutions (e.g. Mayer's). Differentiate and blue. Wash.
3. Stain with the phloxine solution for 10–15 min.
4. Wash in water, then in Cellosolve.

5. Treat with the tartrazine solution. At intervals, wash off in water and note remaining phloxine staining; repeat until only red blood cells and Paneth cell granules are strongly stained red. Finally, treat with the tartrazine solution for 3–4 s, sufficient to restain the background yellow.
6. Wash in Cellosolve, then xylene. Mount as desired.

Results

Nuclei	blue
Red blood cells and Paneth cell granules	red-orange
Muscle and keratin	pale red
Other tissues	yellow

AMIDO BLACK TECHNIQUE (Bower & Chadwin, 1968)

Notes

Like most other methods for Paneth cell granules this does not give specific staining. It is highly selective however, and easy to carry out.

Solution

0.5% amido black 10B (syn. naphthalene black) in equal parts of propylene glycol and distilled water.

Technique

1. Take sections to water.
2. Stain with the amido black solution for 30 min.
3. Wash, then differentiate in 0.01% aqueous lithium carbonate until excess stain is removed.
4. Wash and counterstain with neutral red for 5 min. Wash.
5. Dehydrate, clear and mount as desired.

Results

Paneth cell granules, red blood cells, eosinophil granules	dark blue
Nuclei	red

GASTRIC GLAND CELLS

The cells we are concerned with are those of the gastric fundus and body, and comprise epithelial lining cells, gastric neck cells, parietal (syn. oxyntic) cells and peptic (syn. chief, central or zymogen) cells. The demonstration of secretory cells of the stomach may be of use in highlighting, for example, gastric metaplasia in a Meckel's diverticulum (a congenital diverticulum of the ileum), but in the main these techniques are intended to show the normal histological structure of the gastric mucosa. They are useful for teaching purposes. The following two techniques are representative of the sparse literature on the subject.

PAS-TOLUIDINE BLUE-AURANTIA TECHNIQUE (Cook, 1962)

Notes

The rationale of the method depends partly on the PAS reactivity of the epithelial lining and mucous neck cells, and on the RNA content of the peptic cells having a strong affinity for contrasting cationic dyes such as toluidine blue. The parietal cells take up the yellow counterstain aurantia. The dye aurantia is considered by some to be potentially explosive and the safety-conscious worker may prefer to use a more innocuous dye such as Milling yellow. When differentiating the toluidine blue in 70% alcohol one should aim at underdifferentiation to avoid masking by the subsequent yellow dye.

Dehydration is in t-butanol to avoid extraction of the toluidine blue.

Solutions

1% aqueous periodic acid.

Schiff's reagent, see page 102.

0.5% aqueous toluidine blue.

0.25% aurantia in 50% alcohol, or 2.5% Milling yellow 3G in Cellosolve. See Slidder's technique for fibrin, page 249.

Technique

1. Take sections to distilled water.
2. Carry out the PAS technique giving 5 min periodic acid and 15 min Schiff treatment. Wash well.
3. Stain the nuclei with an iron haematoxylin solution (a celestine blue/Mayer's haematoxylin sequence gives good results). Differentiate and blue so that the cell cytoplasms are left unstained. Wash.
4. Stain in the toluidine blue solution for 1 min.
5. Wash in water, then differentiate in 70% alcohol for up to 1 min until the peptic cells are blue and the background relatively clear.
6. Wash in water to stop the differentiation, and stain in the aurantia solution for 10 s, or wash in water then Cellosolve, stain with the Milling yellow solution for 3–5 min (a gradual replacement of toluidine blue will occur with prolonged treatment).
7. Wash, blot dry, dehydrate in tertiary butanol or cellosolve. Clear in xylene and mount as desired.

Results

Nuclei	blue-black
Epithelial and mucous neck cells	magenta
Peptic cells	blue
Parietal cells and red blood cells	yellow

METHASOL FAST BLUE-ALCIAN YELLOW TECHNIQUE (Maxwell, 1963)

Notes

This particular technique gives useful staining of the gastric cells. The mucin-containing cells are stained with alcian yellow, having first introduced acidic groups on to the component neutral mucin. This enables good colour contrast to be achieved using a blue dye and a red dye to stain the parietal and peptic cells respectively.

Solutions

0.5% aqueous periodic acid.

0.1% alcoholic methasol fast blue.

10% aqueous sodium metabisulphite 100 ml acidified with molar hydrochloric acid 10 ml.

1% aqueous alcian yellow.

0.01% aqueous lithium carbonate.

2% aqueous pyronin.

Technique

1. Take sections to alcohol.
2. Stain with the methanol fast blue solution for 8–16 h at 60° C.
3. Wash in water, then differentiate in the lithium carbonate solution until the parietal cells are prominently shown against the background.
4. Wash in distilled water well, then treat with the periodic acid solution for 5 min.
5. Wash briefly in distilled water then treat with the acidified metabisulphite solution for 5 min.
6. Transfer direct to the alcian yellow solution for 10 min.
7. Wash and counterstain with the pyronin solution. (The time for this was not specified; we suggest 5 min.)
8. Wash, dehydrate, clear and mount as desired.

Results

Epithelial lining cells and mucous neck cells	yellow
Parietal cells	blue
Peptic cells	red

ANTERIOR PITUITARY CELLS

The adenohypophysis which is the anterior lobe of the pituitary is composed of epithelial cells. They are divided into three groups on the basis of their staining reactions:

1. *Chromophobe cells* are the largest population, approximately 50% of the total. They have small nuclei and a scanty non-granular cytoplasm. At the electron microscope level a few secretory granules can be seen and it is thought that some of the cells secrete adrenocorticotrophic hormone (ACTH).

2. *Acidophils* (α) account for 40% of the cell number, they are usually clumped together in the lateral wings of the anterior lobe. The acidophils have many cytoplasmic granules, some of the cells secrete growth hormone, these are termed somatotrophs. Other cells, mammotrophs, secrete prolactin.

3. *Basophils* (β). These cells are about 10% of the total. They are usually larger than acidophils, and are divided into two groups on the basis of their staining reactions. Basophil-S-cells are so-called because alcian blue demonstrates sulphur containing amino acids; basophil-R-cells are for their resistance to oxidation and subsequent alcian blue staining. The secretions of the two types of cell are different, the S cell is thought to produce adenocorticotrophic hormone (ACTH) while the R cell secretes thyrotrophic hormone (TSH), luteinizing hormone (LH) and follicle stimulating hormone (FSH).

Most fixatives give acceptable staining results, although some people prefer mercuric, we have noticed little difference. What is important is to have thin sections between 3–4 μm, especially for H and E. The staining reactions are shown in Table 6.2

KERENYI & TAYLOR'S (1961) PONTAMINE SKY BLUE METHOD

Notes

A simple method that demonstrates acidophils well.

Solutions

1% aqueous pontamine sky blue.

Mayers haematoxylin, see page 19.

1% acid alcohol.

0.5% ws eosin.

Technique

1. Take sections to water.
2. Stain in 1% aqueous pontamine sky blue 5BX for 2 min.
3. Wash in running water for 1 min.
4. Stain nuclei in Mayer's haematoxylin.
5. Rinse in tap water and differentiate nuclei in 1% acid alcohol.
6. '*Blue*' nuclei in running tap water for at least 5 min.
7. Stain in 0.5% aqueous eosin for 2 min.
8. Differentiate eosin in water, dehydrate in alcohol, clear in xylene and mount in a synthetic resin medium.

Results

Nuclei	blue to blue-black
Basophils	bluish-purple
Acidophils	bright red
Chromophobes	pale pink

PAS-ORANGE G METHOD FOR ANTERIOR PITUITARY CELLS (Pearse, 1953)

Notes

This method is an extension of the PAS reaction. Whilst the basophils are stained by the Schiff's reagent, the acidophils by the orange G and the chromophobes are stained by haematoxylin. Other PAS positive structures will also stain.

Technique

Steps 1–7 as in standard PAS method (p. 102).
8. Stain in 2% orange G in 5% phosphotungstic acid for 20 s.

Table 6.2 Staining reactions of anterior pituitary cells

Cell type	MSB	Sky blue eosin	PAS-OG	OFG	BR.AB. OFG
Chromophobes	—	Pale pink	Blue-grey	Pale blue-grey	Grey-green
Acidophils	Red	Red	Yellow	Yellow	Yellow
Basophil-R-cell	Blue	Blue-purple	Magenta	Magenta	Magenta
Basophil-S-cell	Blue	Blue-purple	Magenta	Magenta	Green-blue

9. Differentiate in tap water until macroscopically the section is pale yellow. Check microscopically that only the RBC's and acidophil cells are yellow.
10. Dehydrate, clear and mount in DPX.

Results

Basophils	magenta
Acidophils	yellow
Red blood cells	yellow
Nuclei	blue-black
Chromophobes	pale blue-grey

ONE-STEP MSB FOR ANTERIOR PITUITARY CELLS (Lendrum et al, 1962; Dawes & Hillier, 1964)

Notes

This is a modification of the MSB method. It is an easy and reliable method that requires no differentiation. It separates acidophils and basophils well.

Solutions

Yellow solution

Martius yellow	100 mg
Absolute alcohol	95 ml
Distilled water	5 ml
Phosphotungstic acid	2 g

Red solution

1% brilliant crystal scarlet in 2.5% acetic acid.

Blue solution

0.5% aniline blue in 1% acetic acid.

Staining solution

Yellow solution	45 ml
Red solution	30 ml
Blue solution	45 ml

The three solutions are filtered through separate filter papers in the order above. The solution is allowed to stand for 3 days before use.

Technique

1. Sections to water.
2. Stain nuclei with celestine blue-haematoxylin (see p. 40).
3. Differentiate in acid-alcohol.
4. Blue in tap water.
5. Place in staining solution for 8 min.
6. Rinse rapidly in tap water and blot dry.
7. Dehydrate in absolute alcohol, clear in xylene.
8. Mount in DPX.

Results

Acidophils	red
Basophils	blue
Red blood cells	yellow
Nuclei	blue-black

ORANGE G-ACID FUCHSIN-GREEN (OFG) TECHNIQUE (Slidders, 1961a)

Notes

A certain amount of expertise is needed to obtain good results but colourful and clear-cut cell demonstration is possible. The staining of the basophils by acid fuchsin is progressive and one should stain until the cells, but not the background, are a well-defined red-purple.

Solutions

Saturated orange G in 2% phosphotungstic acid in 95% alcohol.

0.5% acid fuchsin in 0.5% acetic acid.

1.5% light green in 1.5% acetic acid.

Technique

1. Take sections to water and stain the nuclei in an iron haematoxylin solution. Differentiate and blue. Wash in water, then in 95% alcohol.
2. Stain with the orange G solution for 2 min.
3. Rinse in distilled water and stain in the acid fuchsin solution for 2–5 min.
4. Rinse in distilled water, then treat with 1%

aqueous phosphotungstic acid for 5 min.
5. Rinse in distilled water and stain in the light green solution for 1–2 min.
6. Wash in distilled water and blot dry.
7. Dehydrate, clear and mount as desired.

Results

Nuclei	blue-black
Basophils	red-purple
Red blood cells, acidophils	yellow
Chromophobes	pale blue-grey
Connective tissue	green

BR.AB-OFG METHOD FOR CELLS OF THE ANTERIOR PITUITARY (Slidders, 1961b)

Notes

This method is a development of performic acid-alcian blue PAS-orange G. It separates the two types of basophil cell. Bromine is used in this method instead of performic acid as in the performic acid alcian blue-orange G method.

Solutions

Bromine water
10% hydrobromic acid (aqueous)	45 ml
2.5% potassium permanganate (aqueous)	5 ml

Alcian blue
Alcian blue	100 mg
Sulphuric acid (conc.)	1 ml
Glacial acetic acid	9 ml
Distilled water	90 ml

Carefully mix the dye and the sulphuric acid, stir with a glass rod. Slowly add the glacial acetic acid. Stir again. Make up to 100 ml with the distilled water and filter.

Technique

1. Sections to water.
2. Treat with bromine water for 5 min.
3. Wash in running tap water for 5 min.
4. Rinse in distilled water.

5. Stain in alcian blue solution for 1 h.
6. Wash well in tap water.
7. Proceed with the OFG method (p. 68).

Results

Acidophils	orange-yellow
Basophils (S)	dark green-blue
Basophils (R)	magenta-red
Chromophobe cells	pale blue-grey
Nuclei	grey-blue
Red blood cells	yellow

CARMOISINE-ORANGE G-WOOL GREEN TECHNIQUE FOR DIFFERENTIATING ACIDOPHIL CELLS (Brookes, 1968)

Notes

The following technique is capable of giving good results but requires some degree of expertise in order to obtain clear-cut colour differentiation of somatotrophic from lactotrophic pituitary acidophil cells.

Solutions

1% carmoisine L in 1% acetic acid.

Saturated orange G in 2% phosphotungstic acid in 95% ethanol.

0.5% wool green S in 0.5% acetic acid.

Technique

1. Take sections to water and mordant in 10% aqueous copper sulphate for 2 h at 44° C.
2. Wash well in tap water for 10–20 min then in distilled water.
3. Stain with the carmoisine solution for 30 min.
4. Wash in distilled water, then in 95% alcohol.
5. Stain with the orange G solution for 5–30 min. Replacement of the carmoisine by the orange G in the somatotrophic cells will take place; this should be controlled by washing the slide at intervals in 2% phosphotungstic acid in 95% ethanol and examining microscopically.
6. Rinse well in distilled water.

7. Restain in the carmoisine solution for 5 min.
8. Rinse in distilled water and counterstain in the wool green solution for 10 min.
9. Rinse in distilled water, then treat with 1% acetic acid for 2 min to remove excess wool green.
10. Dehydrate, clear and mount in a DPX-type mountant.

Results

Somatotropes	yellow
Red blood cells, lactotropes	red
Basophils	green

METHYL BLUE-EOSIN TECHNIQUE (Mann, 1894)

Notes

Colourful staining can be obtained with this method, but unbalanced results sometimes occur; this is almost certainly due to variation in dye batches. In such cases it is worthwhile experimenting with the proportions of methyl blue to eosin; for example 5% aqueous eosin instead of the 1% solution sometimes gives better results.

Solution

Methyl blue-eosin solution

1% aqueous methyl blue (this solution should be freshly prepared)	35 ml
1% aqueous eosin ws yellowish	45 ml
Distilled water	100 ml

Differentiator

Add 5 drops of saturated potassium hydroxide in ethanol to 30 ml ethanol.

Technique

1. Take sections to water.
2. Stain with the solution overnight at room temperature.
3. Rinse in distilled water.

4. Drain slide, and differentiate sections in the alcoholic potassium hydroxide solution until a lighter, more precise result is obtained.
5. Rinse and dehydrate in alcohol, clear and mount as desired.

Results

Nuclei and basophil cell granules	blue
Red blood cells and acidophil cell granules	red
Chromophobes	colourless

BASIC FUCHSIN-ALCIAN BLUE TECHNIQUE (Monroe & Frommer, 1966)

Notes

The rationale is tannic acid forms a mordant-dye complex with dyes having free amine radicals, in this case basic fuchsin, leading to strong staining of acidophil cells and weaker staining of delta basophil cells. Following phosphomolybdic acid treatment the beta basophils stain a blue-green colour.

This is the type of technique where good results are possible, providing one is willing to persevere until the necessary expertise is acquired.

Solutions

10% aqueous tannic acid.

1% basic fuchsin in 20% alcohol.

1% aqueous alcian blue.

1% aniline in 90% alcohol.

1% aqueous phosphomolybdic acid.

Technique

1. Take sections to water.
2. Treat with the tannic acid solution for 15 min.
3. Wash well in water for 5 min.
4. Dilute the basic fuchsin solution with equal parts of distilled water and treat for several seconds, agitating the slide.
5. Wash in water.
6. Differentiate in the alcoholic aniline solution

until the acidophil cells are red and the delta basophil cells pink.

7. Place in the phosphomolybdic acid solution for 30 s.
8. Wash, then stain in filtered alcian blue solution for 30 s.
9. Wash, dehydrate, clear and mount as desired.

Results

Acidophils	red
Beta basophils	blue-green
Delta basophils	purple
Chromophobes	colourless
Collagen	blue-green

THE PANCREAS

The organ is divided into two parts, the larger portion of the gland is exocrine. The exocrine cells are acidophilic and contain zymogen granules in the cytoplasm. These granules are involved in the production of digestive enzymes. Cells of the exocrine component are not difficult to demonstrate as they are easy to see in a conventional H and E as well as in trichrome stains and phloxine-tartrazine. Zymogen granules are particularly well shown with freeze dried sections. Fixation for the pancreas is important: all specimens should be freshly fixed avoiding acidic solutions.

The smaller portion of this organ is endocrine, the components of which are the islets of Langerhans. These are groups of endocrine cells surrounded by exocrine glands. The endocrine function of the pancreas is performed by the cells within the islets. The distribution of the islets of Langerhans is throughout the organ but are found in greater number in the pancreatic tail. The cells that make up the islets are of different types and each produce a different hormone. At the present time four separate cells have been identified and it is clear which specific hormone two of them secrete. The A (α_2) cells produce glucagon, the B (β) cells secrete insulin. The D cells (α_1) are thought to produce different hormones, mainly a somatostatin-like one, and the C cells are considered to be precursors of the alpha and beta cells. The further development and elucidation of the endocrine role of the pancreas awaits the results of the specific immunohistochemical reactions. The conventional general staining methods cannot demonstrate the specific granules of the islet cells and can only be used as a guide when attempting to demonstrate these cells. The staining reactions of the general methods are given in Table 6.3. The exocrine granules are also PAS positive.

Autolysis of the pancreas is rapid after death. The longer autolysis continues the less reliable become the staining techniques. In many instances post-mortem material will not be satisfactory. For staining the islet cells, formalin and mercury fixation are probably the best, except in the case of the silver methods of Grimelius also Hellerstrom and Hellman when Bouin is considered superior.

GOMORI'S CHROME ALUM-HAEMATOXYLIN TECHNIQUE (Gomori, 1941)

Notes

This is the traditional method for the islet cells which may, or may not, give good results. In our hands the alpha cells stain well but the beta cells inconsistently. The precise rationale of the technique is obscure.

Table 6.3 Staining reactions of the endocrine pancreas

Cell types	Aldehyde fuchsin light green orange G	Chrome haem. phloxine	Phlox. tart.	Grimelius	Hellerstrom Hellman	Lead haematoxylin	Bodian
A cells (α_2)	Yellow	Red	Yellow	Positive	Negative	Positive	Positive
B cells (β)	Purple	Blue	Red	Negative	Negative	Negative	Negative
D cells (α_1)	Green	Pink	Yellow	Negative	Positive	Positive	Positive

Solutions

Haematoxylin

Mix equal parts of 1% aqueous haematoxylin and 3% aqueous chrome alum. To a 100 ml volume add 5% aqueous potassium dichromate 2 ml and 0.5 M sulphuric acid. Allow to stand for 48 h prior to use. The solution keeps for 4–8 weeks.

0.5% aqueous phloxine.

Technique

1. Take sections to water, and if fixed in for example, formalin, mordant in Bouin's solution overnight.
2. Wash well and treat with equal parts of 0.3% aqueous potassium permanganate and 0.3% sulphuric acid for 1 min.
3. Decolourize in 3% aqueous sodium bisulphite (5% aqueous oxalic acid will do equally well).
4. Wash well, then stain with the haematoxylin solution for 15 min.
5. Wash, differentiate in acid-alcohol. Wash again then blue. The differentiation should be prolonged until only the beta cell granules are stained a clear blue.
6. Stain with the phloxine solution for 5 min.
7. Wash, then treat with 5% aqueous phosphotungstic acid for 1 min.
8. Wash in water for up to 5 min (the phloxine staining will reappear). If the phloxine staining appears too heavy, differentiate in 95% alcohol.
9. Dehydrate, clear and mount as desired.

Results

Alpha cells	red
Beta cells	blue
Exocrine zymogen cells	unstained to red

MODIFIED ALDEHYDE FUCHSIN STAIN
(Halami, 1952)

Notes

This method is an extension of the original Gomori technique. It allows D cells to be demonstrated and, we feel, a better staining of β cells. The sections are oxidized with Lugol's iodine before staining with aldehyde fuchsin. The observations to this stain on page 55 should be noted.

Solutions

Aldehyde fuchsin

See page 55.

Counterstain

Light green	200 mg
Orange G	1g
Phosphotungstic acid	500 mg
Glacial acetic acid	1 ml
Distilled water	100 ml

The solution keeps well.

Technique

1. Sections to water.
2. Oxidize with Lugol's iodine for 10 min.
3. Rinse in tap water and bleach with 2.5% sodium thiosulphate.
4. Wash in tap water followed by 70% alcohol.
5. Stain in aldehyde fuchsin stain for 15–30 min.
6. Wash in 95% alcohol followed by water.
7. Stain nuclei with celestine blue and haemalum.
8. Wash in water, differentiate briefly in acid-alcohol and wash well in tap water.
9. Rinse with distilled water and counterstain with orange G-light green solution for 45 s.
10. Rinse briefly with 0.2% acetic acid followed by 95% alcohol.
11. Dehydrate in absolute alcohol, clear in xylene and mount in DPX.

Results

B cells	purple-violet
A cells	yellow
D cells	green
Nuclei	blue-black

COMBINED PROTARGOL-ALDEHYDE FUCHSIN TECHNIQUE (Cook, unpublished data taken from Bodian, 1936 and Gomori, 1950)

Notes

This method makes use of the argyrophilia of both types of alpha cell to obtain good contrast with subsequent staining of beta granules by aldehyde fuchsin. For the latter a pre-oxidation step is necessary.

The protargol method gives strong argyrophilic demonstration of a number of tissue entities as well, notably nerve fibres and melanin. Sections are treated with protargol (a compound formed of gelatine and silver nitrate) in the presence of metallic copper. Regarding the function of copper it has been suggested that nitric acid is formed, leading to a fall in pH of solution thus producing a slowing down of the reaction, with consequent lessened risk of overimpregnation (G. Cox, personal communication).

Following copper-protargol treatment, the sections are progressively reduced in a hydroquinone-gold chloride-oxalic acid treatment. Background precipitation is not uncommon in this technique, and it is suggested that thorough washing between the various treatments will do much to reduce this.

A number of sources of protargol have been found to be unsatisfactory for this technique and we recommend Messrs. Roques of Paris, obtainable from R. A. Lamb Ltd.

Solutions

Aldehyde fuchsin solution

See page 55.

Acidified potassium permanganate solution

See page 49.

Copper-protargol solution

Prepare fresh 50 ml of 1% aqueous protargol to which are added (in a Coplin jar) 2 g of clean copper foil cut into small (2 mm) pieces.

Primary reducer

Hydroquinone 1 g; sodium sulphite 5 g; in 100 ml distilled water. Prepare fresh (the sodium sulphite acts as a stabilizer allowing the solution to be kept for up to 2 days at 4° C).

Technique

1. Take sections to distilled water.
2. Treat with the copper-protargol solution overnight at 37° C (exact time is not critical but do not leave for more than 18 h).
3. Wash in several changes of distilled water and reduce in the hydroquinone solution for 10 min.
4. Wash well in distilled water. Thorough washing at this stage is most important and it is suggested that one rinses first in distilled water, then in tap water for several minutes and finally in distilled water again.
5. Treat with 1% aqueous yellow gold chloride for 5 min.
6. Wash well in several changes of distilled water.
7. Treat with 2% aqueous oxalic acid for 5 min (only at this stage should silver blackening be evident).
8. Fix in 5% hypo. Wash.
9. Treat with the acidified potassium permanganate solution for 1 min. Wash, then bleach with 5% aqueous oxalic acid. Wash well in water.
10. Rinse in 70% alcohol, and stain with the aldehyde fuchsin solution for 4–6 min.
11. Rinse well in 70% alcohol, then in water.
12. Counterstaining may be carried out in 0.1% light green in 0.2% acetic acid for $\frac{1}{2}$–1 min.
13. Wash, dehydrate, clear and mount in a synthetic resin.

Results

Alpha cells (and nuclei to some degree)	black
Beta cells	purple
Background	green

MITOCHONDRIA

Mitochondria are cytoplasmic organelles which consist of some 40% lipid, so are best preserved by fixatives such as osmium tetroxide and potassium dichromate. A solution we find particularly effective is that of Regaud (3% aqueous potassium dichromate 80 parts; formalin 20 parts). Extended fixation is recommended (4 days or so), and for best results the tissue should be fresh at time of fixing. Tissues such as cardiac muscle, kidney and liver show mitochondria to advantage. Thinner than usual paraffin sections should be used (3–4 mm).

The demonstration of mitochondria at light microscope level is not particularly rewarding, or, indeed of much diagnostic significance.

Providing that the above points regarding fixation are observed, the following techniques can be used to demonstrate mitochondria.

Acid haematein   (see p. 136)
Sudan black   (see p. 132)
Luxol fast blue   (see p. 225)
PTAH (if preceded by treating the section with 5% aqueous ferric chloride for 24 h at room temperature) (see p. 45).

The Heidenhain and Altmann classical methods are described.

IRON HAEMATOXYLIN TECHNIQUE
(Heidenhain, 1896)

Notes

This is the type of technique where a number of structures are simultaneously stained and one differentiates until the desired constituent is shown to greatest advantage. Good results require practice and the novice may well find it of advantage to dilute the differentiator with equal parts of distilled water. This has the effect of slowing down the differentiation making it easier to control. Gentle agitation during differentiation will lead to more even results.

The rationale of the method is following iron alum treatment the section is stained with haematoxylin which allows a tissue-mordant-dye bonding to occur. On subsequent iron alum treatment competition with the bound haematoxylin for the tissue-binding sites occurs and the iron alum being now in excess is successful in progressively replacing the dye.

Solutions

5% aqueous ferric ammonium sulphate (iron alum).

0.5% haematoxylin in 10 ml ethanol and 90 ml distilled water (allow to ripen at least 6 weeks before use).

Technique

1. Take sections to water.
2. Treat with the iron alum solution for 1 h at 56° C.
3. Wash in water, then treat with the haematoxylin solution for 1 h at 56° C.
4. Wash in water and differentiate in the iron alum solution at room temperature. This is best carried out in a Coplin jar and with microscopic control. Differentiate until the mitochondria are well stained against a reasonably colourless background.
5. Wash well in water for several minutes.
6. Counterstaining is optional; suitable counterstains are eosin, tartrazine in Cellosolve, or light green in acetic acid using weak solutions for short periods of time.
7. Dehydrate, clear and mount as desired.

Results

Red blood cells,   blue-black
mitochondria and nuclei
Background   clear or according to the counterstain used

ALTMANN'S TECHNIQUE (Altmann, 1894)

Notes

Whilst Champy's solution (potassium dichromate, osmium tetroxide, acetic acid) is often recommended for this particular method, other fixatives work equally well, e.g. Helly's and Regaud's solutions. Following fixation, postchroming in 3% aqueous potassium dichromate for 3–7 days is usually specified.

Following overstaining in aniline-acid fuchsin there is replacement differentiation with picric acid.

A strong solution of acid fuchsin is necessary for a good result. Also, some variation in differentiation will occur in different parts of the same section.

Solutions

Aniline-acid fuchsin

Add 5 ml aniline to 100 ml of heated distilled water. Mix well and add acid fuchsin to saturation (approximately 14% w/v). Allow to cool. Mix at intervals over 24 h. Filter.

Differentiator I

Saturated alcoholic picric acid	20 ml
30% alcohol	80 ml

Differentiator II

Saturated alcoholic picric acid	10 ml
30% alcohol	80 ml

Technique

1. Take sections to water.
2. Drain, and flood with aniline-acid fuchsin. Heat until the steam rises three times over a period of 5 min (i.e. as for the Ziehl-Neelsen technique).
3. Rinse in water and differentiate in the picric-alcohol I until the excess acid fuchsin staining is removed, then complete differentiation by treating with the weaker differentiator (picric-alcohol II). Control microscopically.
4. Rinse in water, dehydrate rapidly to avoid losing the picric acid background staining. Clear and mount as desired.

Results

Red blood cells, mitochondria and nuclei	red

Background	yellow
(If Champy's fixative is used, fat:	black)

RUSSELL BODIES

Occur in the cytoplasm of plasma cells. They are seen most frequently in cases of myeloma and rheumatoid arthritis. They vary in size and can on occasion fill the cytoplasm of the cell. They stain bright pink with eosin in the same tone as red blood cells, but are distinguished by their smooth round shape. They are PAS positive and mainly protein in content. As they are in plasma cell cytoplasm they contain RNA. The staining reactions of Russell bodies are given in Table 6.4.

Table 6.4 Staining methods for Russell bodies

PAS reaction	Strongly positive
Millon reaction	Positive
Phloxine tartrazine	Bright red
Gram	Positive with xylene-aniline
Methyl green pyronin	Red

LYSOSOMES

Are found in many cells but are particularly numerous in phagocytic cells such as macrophages and neutrophils. They are involved in the enzymic breakdown of phagocytosed material. The lysosomes are membrane bound cytoplasmic organelles which in consequence of their role contain many hydrolytic enzymes and the demonstration of one of these enzymes, acid phosphatase, is used as a lysosomal marker. The large lysosomes within neutrophils can be seen in a Giemsa stain.

REFERENCES

Altmann R 1894 Die Elementarorganismen 2nd edn. Veit, Liepzig
Bodian D 1936 A new method for staining nerve fibres and nerve endings in mounted paraffin sections. Anatomical Record 65: 89

Bower D, Chadwin C G 1968 Demonstration of Paneth cell granules using Naphthalene black. Journal of Clinical Pathology 21: 107

Brookes L D 1968 A stain for differentiating two types of acidophil cells in the rat pituitary. Stain Technology 43: 41

Cook H C 1962 Periodic acid-Schiff-Toluidine blue-aurantia: a stain for the gland cells of the stomach. Stain Technology 37: 317

Dawes R E, Hillier M H 1964 A one stage technique for differentiating the α and β cells of the anterior pituitary. Journal of Medical Laboratory Technology 21: 62

Giemsa G 1902 The azur dyes their purification and physiochemical properties. Zentbl. Bakt., Parasitkde (Abt 1) 31: 429. Cited from Bare: (1970)

Gomori G 1941 Observations with differential stains on human islets of Langerhan's. American Journal Pathology 17: 395

Gomori G 1950 Aldehyde-fuchsin: A new stain for elastic tissue. American Journal of Clinical Pathology 20: 665

Halami N S 1952 Differentiation of the two types of basophils in an adenohypophysis of the rat and the mouse. Stain Technology 27: 61

Ham A W 1969 Histology 6th edn. Lippincott, Philadelphia

Heinenhain M 1896 Noch einmal über die Darstellung der Centralkörper durch Eisenhamatoxylin nebst einigen allgemeinen Bemerkungen über die Hamatoxylinfarben. Z. Wiss Mikrosk. 13: 186

Kerenyi N, Taylor W A 1961 Niagara blue 4B as a fast simple stain for the adenohypophysis. Stain Technology 36: 169

Lendrum A C 1944 The staining of eosinophil polymorphs and enterochromaffin cells in histological sections. Journal of Pathology & Bacteriology 56: 441

Lendrum A C 1947 The phloxine-tartrazine method as a general histological stain and for the demonstration of inclusion bodies. Journal of Pathology & Bacteriology 59: 399

Lendrum A C, Foster D S, Slidders W, Henderson R 1962 Studies on the character and staining if fibrin. Journal of Clinical Pathology 15: 401

Mann G 1894 Ueber die Behandlung der Nerrenzellen fur experimental-histologische Untersuchungen Z.f. Wissensch Mikr. Brnschwg, 1894 xl 671–494

Maxwell A 1963 The Alcian dyes applied to the gastric mucosa. Stain Technology 38: 286

Monroe C W, Frommer J 1966 A basic fuchsin-Alcain blue stain for the human hypophysis. Stain Technology 41: 248

Pearse A G E 1953 Histochemistry, theoretical and applied. Churchill, London

Slidders W 1961a The Fuchsin-Miller method. Journal Medical Laboratory Technology 18: 36

Slidders W 1961b The OFG and Br AB-OFG methods for staining the adenohypophysis. Journal of Pathology and Bacteriology 82: 532

7

Proteins and nucleic acids

Proteins are organic nitrogenous compounds, and form one of the three basic constituents of tissues, along with carbohydrates and lipids. The demonstration of proteins, unlike lipids and carbohydrates does not hold a prominent place in practical histochemistry, with the exception of nucleic acids. Proteins are part of every cell and tissue. On occasions it is necessary to determine whether a given protein is present and the precise nature of that protein. Few of the protein methods are used in routine laboratories and we have decided to give only the most used techniques.

Proteins occur in tissues as either simple proteins (uncombined) or in combination with other constituents (e.g. lipids) as conjugated proteins. As far as histochemistry is concerned the most important proteins are shown in the following table.

Table 7.1 Proteins

Simple	Conjugated
Albumins	Nucleoproteins
Globulins	Mucoproteins
Fibrous, e.g. collagen, fibrin,	Glycoproteins
elastin and keratin	Chromoproteins
	Lipoproteins

Simple proteins are naturally occurring proteins that yield α-amino acids and derivatives on hydrolysis.

Conjugated proteins are compounds of simple proteins in combination with non-protein constituents such as carbohydrates in glycoproteins.

Nucleoproteins are compounds of simple proteins usually basic protein.

DEMONSTRATION

The staining reaction of proteins and protein containing substances depends upon the amino acid composition. The *fibrous proteins* are demonstrated by histological methods based on the physical configuration of their molecules, rather than their chemical composition, i.e. trichrome stains. *Amino acid* methods demonstrate the presence of some of the constituent amino acids and not the whole protein, a positive reaction indicating the presence of the protein, as it is unlikely that free amino acids will remain in the tissue sections. Table 7.1 lists the amino acid methods.

Table 7.2 Amino acid staining methods. This list is not complete — many other methods exist — but it indicates the more common techniques.

Method	Demonstrates	Colour
Millon reaction	Tyrosine (phenyl groups)	Pink
Sakaguchi	Arginine (guanidyl groups)	Orange-red
Mercury orange	Sulphydryl groups	Pale orange
DDD reaction	Sulphydryl groups Disulphide linkages	Reddish-purple
Diazotization with acid	Tyrosine (phenyl groups)	Purple-red
DMAB-nitrite method	Trytophan (indole groups)	Deep blue
Performic acid-alcian blue	Disulphide groups	Dark blue
Ninhydrin-Schiff	Amino groups	Pink

Enzymes are proteins which react upon substrates and are shown by their specific activity (see Ch. 13).

The future for the demonstration of proteins undoubtedly lies in immunohistochemical techniques, at present the immunoglobulins such as IgG, IgA are demonstrated in this way and this technique allows for better localization and is suitable for use at the E.M. level. The basis of the immunohistochemical techniques is described in Chapter 14.

TISSUE PREPARATION

The influence of fixatives on protein methods should always be considered — formaldehyde for instance reacts with α-amino groups. Oxidizing agents used in fixatives will oxidize sulphydryl groups to disulphides. In practical terms formaldehyde fixation should always be used neutral and the time kept to a minimum; osmium tetroxide should be avoided (see Hopwood, 1982). The best localization of proteins is obtained by using freeze dried sections.

STAINING METHODS

The staining methods that follow in some instances give a pale reaction product, also some of the techniques are destructive to tissue sections so care should always be taken. Where possible positive controls should be employed.

NINHYDRIN-SCHIFF METHOD FOR AMINO GROUPS (Yasuma & Itchikwa, 1953)

Notes

Ninhydrin at neutral pH reacts with amino groups to form aldehydes which will recolour Schiff's reagent.

Solutions

0.5 % ninhydrin in absolute alcohol.

Schiff's reagent, see page 102.

Technique

1. Take sections to 70% alcohol.
2. Treat with ninhydrin solution at 37°C overnight.
3. Wash in running tap water.
4. Treat in Schiff's reagent for 45 min.
5. Wash in running tap water.
6. Counterstain with an alum haematoxylin.
7. Wash in tap water; dehydrate through graded alcohols, clear in xylene and mount in DPX.

Results

Amino groups   pinkish purple

BLOCKING METHOD FOR AMINO-GROUPS (Stoward, 1963)

Notes

This is a deamination technique, following which absence of ninhydrin-Schiff reaction is positive confirmation of the presence of amino groups.

Solution

Sodium nitrite	1 g
3% sulphuric acid	30 ml

Technique

1. Sections to distilled water.
2. Immerse in a freshly prepared solution (above) which has been precooled to 4°C for 48 h.
3. Wash in distilled water.
4. Leave sections in distilled water for 4 h at 60°C.
5. Employ the ninhydrin-Schiff method above along with an untreated section.

Result

Amino groups positive after ninhydrin-Schiff method, and negative after blocking method.

MILLON REACTION FOR TYROSINE (Baker, 1956)

Notes

This is a histochemical modification of Millon's (1849) biochemical test. It demonstrates the presence of hydroxyphenyl groups. The phenyl is first converted into nitrosophenol which then combines with mercury to produce a coloured reaction product. Tyrosine is the only amino acid that contains the hydroxyphenyl groups. The colour reaction is usually a very pale pink. Great care and possibly luck is required to keep the sections on the slides, so be sure to take more than one section through the method. Pancreas is a good control tissue.

Solutions

Solution A

10 g of mercuric sulphate is added to a mixture of 90 ml distilled water and 10 ml of conc. sulphuric acid, and dissolved by heating. After cooling to room temperature 100 ml of distilled water is added.

Solution B

250 mg of sodium nitrite is dissolved in 10 ml of distilled water.

Working solution

5 ml of solution (B) is added to 50 ml of solution (A).

Technique

1. Take sections to water.
2. Immerse sections in staining solution in a small beaker and bring to boil gently; simmer for 2 min.

3. Allow to cool to room temperature.
4. Wash in three changes of distilled water, 2 min each.
5. Dehydrate through alcohols, clear in xylene, and mount in DPX.

Result

Tyrosine-containing proteins   red or pink

DIAZOTIZATION-COUPLING METHOD FOR TYROSINE (Glenner & Lillie, 1959)

Notes

This method employs 8 amino-1 naphthol-5-sulphonic acid ('S' acid) as a coupling amine for the diazonium nitrites produced by nitrosation of tyrosine. It is necessary to carry out both incubation stages in the dark and at a low temperature. In our hands this gives better and stronger results than the previous technique.

Solutions

Incubating solution (A)

Sodium nitrite	3.5 g
Acetic acid (conc.)	4.4 ml
Distilled water	47 ml

Incubating solution (B)

8 amino-1-naphthol-5-sulphonic acid	0.5 g
Potassium hydroxide	0.5 g
Ammonium sulphamate	0.5 g
70% alcohol	50 ml

Technique

1. Bring sections to water.
2. Place sections in incubating solution (A) at 4°C for 24 h in the dark.
3. Rinse in four changes of distilled water at 4°C.
4. Transfer sections to incubating solution (B) at 4°C for 1 h in the dark.

5. Wash in three changes of 0.1M HCl, 5 min each.
6. Rinse in running tap water for 10 min.
7. Counterstain if required.
8. Dehydrate through graded alcohols to xylene and mount in DPX.

Results

Tyrosine-containing proteins	purple and red

PERFORMIC ACID-ALCIAN BLUE FOR DISULPHIDE (SS) GROUPS (Adams & Sloper, 1955–56)

Notes

Some proteins contain sulphydryl/disulphide groups. These are produced by the amino acids, cysteine, cystine and methionine. The disulphide linkage is between two sulphur atoms (-S-S-) and the sulphydryl grouping is between a sulphur and a hydrogen atom (-S-H-). Both these sulphur-containing groups can be demonstrated by a number of techniques. This is the best method. It is necessary that the performic acid is freshly prepared and then allowed to stand for 1 h before use. The washing stage following oxidation is critical; the washing needs to be thorough but the sections have a tendency to wash off. Pituitary and keratin make good control tissues. The conventional Schmorl reaction (see p. 148) will also demonstrate sulphur-containing amino acids, but less precisely than this method.

Solutions

Performic acid
98% formic acid	40 ml
100 vol. hydrogen peroxide	4 ml
Conc. sulphuric acid	0.5 ml

Alcian blue solution
Alcian blue	1 g
98% sulphuric acid	2.7 ml
Distilled water	47.2 ml

Technique

1. Take sections to water; blot to remove surplus water.
2. Stand sections in performic acid for 5 min.
3. Wash well in tap water for 10 min.
4. Dry in 60°C oven until just dry.
5. Rinse in tap water.
6. Stain in alcian blue solution at room temperature for 1 h.
7. Wash in running tap water.
8. Counterstain (e.g. neutral red) if required.
9. Wash in tap water.
10. Dehydrate through graded alcohols, clear in xylene and mount in DPX.

Result

Disulphides	blue

The intensity of the blue colour will depend on the amount of disulphide present.

SAKAGUCHI REACTION FOR ARGININE (Baker, 1947)

Notes

Arginine is demonstrated by this method. The guanidyl groups react with α-naphthol and a red colour is developed in the presence of a strong alkali. Sections for this method should be at least 10 μm thick, best results in our hands being obtained with sections 15 μm thick, showing the weak colour better. The method is destructive to sections so they must be handled carefully.

Solutions

Incubating solution
1% sodium hydroxide	2 ml
1% α-naphthol in 70% alcohol	2 drops
1% 'Milton' in distilled water	4 drops

Pyridine-chloroform solution
Pyridine	30 ml
Chloroform	10 ml

Technique

1. Take sections to water.
2. Rinse in 70% alcohol.
3. Flood slide with incubating solution for 15 min.
4. Drain and gently blot dry.
5. Immerse in pyridine-chloroform solution for 2 min.
6. Mount in fresh pyridine-chloroform solution and ring coverslip.

Result

Arginine   orange-red

NUCLEIC ACIDS

Interest in nucleic acids has arisen partly due to their association with chromosomes and partly their involvement in protein synthesis. There are two types of nucleic acid, deoxyribonucleic acid (DNA) and ribonucleic acid (RNA).

The nucleic acids are polynucleotides. A nucleotide is a phosphoric ester of a nucleoside which is the condensation product of a purine or pyrimidine base with a pentose or deoxypentose sugar. The pyrimidine bases include hypoxanthine, xanthine, guanine and adenine (Castleman, 1962).As will be seen it is the sugar that differs in the two types of nucleic acids: in DNA the sugar content is deoxyribose and in RNA ribose. On hydrolysis the nucleic acids yield phosphate groups, sugars and the nitrogenous bases. The demonstration of nucleic acids depends upon:

1. The reaction of dyes with phosphate groups, and
2. The production of aldehydes from the deoxyribose.

Techniques are not available to demonstrate the nitrogenous bases.

DNA DEMONSTRATION

The most reliable histochemical technique for DNA is the Nucleal test, introduced by Feulgen & Rossenbeck.

THE FEULGEN REACTION (Feulgen & Rossenbeck, 1924)

Notes

The method described is the most reliable specific histochemical technique available for DNA. The method utilizes mild hydrolysis using M-HCl at 60°C in which aldehyde groups are liberated by the breaking of the purine-deoxyribose bond. As in the PAS reaction, the aldehydes recolour Schiff's reagent producing the magenta colour in the nuclear chromatin. The RNA is depolymerized by the hydrolysis and takes no part in the reaction. Fixation is important with the method. Bouin's fixative will cause overhydrolysis during fixation and as a result is unsatisfactory as a fixative for this particular reaction. Other fixatives allow the reaction to take place, but the hydrolysis time is adjusted accordingly. Thin rapidly fixed blocks give superior results (Swift, 1953). The hydrolysis stage of the reaction is critical. It is usually carried out at 60° C in M HCl. Although many alternative hydrolysing solutions are available, none produces better results. During hydrolysis a stronger reaction is obtained as the time is increased until the optimum is reached. If the hydrolysis is continued the reaction becomes weaker due to depolymerization of DNA. In cases of doubt a number of

Table 7.3 Hydrolysis times in prewarmed M-HCl at 60° C.

Fixative	Time (min)
Bouin	Unsuitable
Carnoy 6.3.1	8
Chrome-acetic	14
Flemming	16
Formaldehyde vapour	30–60
Formalin	8
Formal-sublimate	8
Helly	8
Newcomer	20
Regaud	14
Regaud-sublimate	8
Susa	18
Zenker	5
Zenker-formal	5

slides should be hydrolysed at different times. Other Schiff positive structures may be present in the tissue section and a control section should be left in distilled water, while the test section is hydrolysed. Remember that active aldehydes occur naturally in the tissues in lipids and connective tissue fibres. The optimum times for hydrolysis are given in Table 7.3.

Solutions

M hydrochloric acid
Hydrochloric acid (conc.)	8.5 ml
Distilled water	91.5 ml

Schiff's reagent, see page 102.

Bisulphite solution
10% potassium metabisulphite	5 ml
M Hydrochloric acid	5 ml
Distilled water	90 ml

Technique

1. Bring all sections to water.
2. Rinse sections in M-HCl at room temperature (1 min).
3. Place sections in M-HCl at 60°C (See Table 7.3).
4. Rinse sections M-HCl at room temperature (1 min).
5. Transfer sections to Schiff's reagent (30 min).
6. Rinse well in distilled water.
7. Counterstain if required in 1% light green (2 min) or tartrazine.
8. Wash in water.
9. Dehydrate through graded alcohols to xylene and mount.

Results

DNA	red-purple
Cytoplasm	green

NAPHTHOIC ACID HYDRAZIDE-FEULGEN FOR DNA (Pearse, 1951)

Notes

This technique utilizes the aldehydes produced by hydrolysis by coupling them to a diazonium salt. The reaction product should be the same as the Feulgen reaction and may be used as a control.

Solutions

M-hydrochloric acid
Hydrochloric acid (conc.)	8.5 ml
Distilled water	91.5 ml

NAH solution
2-hydroxy-3-naphthoic acid hydrazide	50 mg
Absolute alcohol	47 ml
Acetic acid (conc.)	3 ml

Fast blue B solution
Fast blue B	50 mg
Veronal acetate buffer, pH 7.4	50 ml

This solution must be freshly prepared.

Technique

1. Bring all sections to water.
2. Rinse briefly in M-HCl.
3. Place sections in M-HCl at 60°C.
4. Rinse sections in M-HCl at room temperature (1 min).
5. Rinse sections in distilled water (1 min).
6. Rinse sections in 50% alcohol (1 min).
7. Place sections in NAH solution at room temperature (3–6 h).
8. Rinse sections in 50% alcohol (10 min).
9. Rinse sections in 50% alcohol (10 min).
10. Rinse sections in 50% alcohol (10 min).
11. Rinse sections in distilled water (1 min).
12. Place sections in fresh fast blue B solution (3 min).
13. Dehydrate through graded alcohols to xylene and mount in DPX.

Result

DNA	blue to bluish-purple
Protein material	purplish-red

RNA/DNA DEMONSTRATION

Ribonucleic acid methods are not specific: they depend upon the nonspecific property of their affinity for basic dyes. The basophilia is produced by the acidic groups in the nucleic acids. Methyl green appears to be the most selective basic dye for nucleic acids. It is an impure dye and chloroform extraction is necessary to remove the impurities. Methyl green when treated in this way and used at an acid pH appears to be specific for DNA due to spatial aligment of phosphate radicles of the DNA to the NH_2 groups on the methyl green molecules.

METHYL GREEN-PYRONIN METHOD
(Unna, 1902; Pappenheim, 1899)

Notes

This method employs methyl green as discussed above, to demonstrate DNA and pyronin to stain the RNA. The selectivity of pyronin for RNA is not high, but with carefully controlled conditions and careful differentiation the use of pyronin produces acceptable results for RNA. We have found that rinsing in 93% alcohol, followed by absolute alcohol (Warford, 1982) gives better results than the usual acetone-xylene.

Solution

2% methyl green (chloroform washed)	9 ml
2% Pyronin Y	4 ml
Acetate buffer pH 4.8	23 ml
Glycerol	14 ml
Mix well before use.	

Technique

1. Take sections down to water.

2. Rinse in acetate buffer pH 4.8
3. Place in staining solution for 25 min.
4. Rinse in buffer.
5. Blot dry.
6. Rinse in 93% alcohol.
7. Rinse in absolute alcohol.
8. Rinse in xylene and mount in DPX.

Results

DNA	green-blue
RNA	red
Acid mucins	red

The following variation by Ellias (1969) has worked well in our hands.

Solutions

Methyl green

Methyl green	1 g
Acetate buffer pH 4.1	200 ml

Wash in chloroform until completely free of traces of methyl violet.

Staining solution

Methyl green solution	100 ml
Pyronin Y	200 mg

The solution is well stirred and stored at 4° C and filtered before use.

Technique

1. Sections down to distilled water.
2. Place in staining solution at 37° C for 1 h.
3. Rinse in distilled water at 1°C for 2 s.
4. Blot sections dry.
5. Rinse in tert-butanol.
6. Dehydrate in two changes tert-butanol for 5 min
7. Clear xylene and mount in DPX.

Results

DNA	green-blue
RNA	red

HITCHCOCK-EHRICH TECHNIQUE
(Hitchcock & Ehrich, 1930)

Notes

This method is based on the previous technique. It has the advantage of being quick and simple. But is no less capricious than the methyl green-pyronin method. If trouble is being encountered with the M.G-P. it is worth giving this a try. It uses malachite green and acridine red. The authors recommend Zenker-acetic fixation, but the method works after formalin fixation if the staining time is extended.

Solution

Malachite green 300 mg in 15 ml distilled water
Acridine red 900 mg in 45 ml distilled water
Mix before use.

Technique

1. Sections to water.
2. Stain in the solution for 1–5 min.
3. Wash in distilled water.
4. Dehydrate, clear and mount in synthetic resin.

Results

DNA   blue-green
RNA   red

GALLOCYANIN-CHROME ALUM METHOD
(Einarson, 1932, 1951)

Notes

Gallocyanin forms a red cation lake with chromium potassium sulphate. The dye lake combines with the phosphate groups of the nucleic acids to form a tissue-mordant-dye compound. The method demonstrates both types of nucleic acids, so the use of extraction techniques is necessary to isolate a specific nucleic acid. The staining is progressive and should need no differention. It is better not to counterstain. Avoid the use of celloidin. The method is of accepted specificity for the nucleic acids at a low pH (below 1.0).

Solution

Chrome alum   5 g
Distilled water   100 ml
Gallocyanin   150 mg

The chrome alum is dissolved in the distilled water, the gallocyanin added and the solution slowly heated until it boils. It is allowed to boil for 5 min. When the solution has cooled to room temperature, the volume is adjusted to 100 ml. The solution is filtered before use.

Technique

1. Bring sections down to water.
2. Stains in gallocyanin-chrome alum solution (18–48 h).
3. Wash in tap water.
4. Dehydrate through graded alcohols and mount in DPX.

Results

RNA, DNA   blue

EXTRACTION METHODS FOR NUCLEIC ACIDS

Specific control of the staining methods discussed is possible by using extraction techniques (Table

Table 7.4 Extraction of nucleic acids

Solution	Conc.	Temp (° C)	Extracted	Type of method
Ribonuclease	0.1%	37	RNA	Enzyme
Deoxyribonuclease	0.08%	37	DNA	Enzyme
Perchloric acid	5%	60	RNA, DNA	Acidic
Perchloric acid	10%	4	RNA	Acidic
Trichloroacetic acid	4%	90	RNA, DNA	Acidic
Hydrochloric acid	M-HCl	37	RNA, DNA	Acidic

7.4). These techniques remove or denature the nucleic acids, whilst leaving other tissue structures unaffected. The extraction can be carried out in two ways, either enzymatic or chemical. The enzymatic methods using deoxyribonuclease and ribonuclease are specific when used with suitable controls.

Ribonuclease

The enzyme splits RNA into its component nucleotides. It can be produced from fresh beef pancreas (Brachet, 1940). A crude source of the enzyme is found in saliva (Bradbury, 1956). Whilst removing RNA, the Feulgen reaction is unaffected.

Deoxyribonuclease

There is less need for this enzyme as there are specific methods for DNA. It acts only on fixed tissues and is specific for nuclear DNA extraction. The Feulgen reaction will be negative after treatment.

Chemical extraction

Various strong acids can be used to extract nucleic acids from tissue sections. Depending upon the acids and the conditions used, either RNA or both RNA and DNA can be removed.

ENZYME EXTRACTION OF RNA (Brachet, 1940)

Solution

| Ribonuclease | 8 mg |
| Distilled water | 10 ml |

Technique

1. Bring both test and control slides to water.
2. Place test slide in ribonuclease solution, place control slide in distilled water, both at 37° C for 1 h.
3. Wash in distilled water.
4. Apply methyl green-pyronin method (p. 83)

Results

| Test slide | RNA negative, DNA green |
| Control slide | RNA red, DNA green |

ENZYME EXTRACTION OF DNA (Brachet, 1940)

Solution

Deoxyribonuclease	10 mg
0.2 M tris buffer, pH 7.6	10 ml
Distilled water	50 ml

Method

1. Bring both test and control sections to water.
2. Place test section in extraction solution, control in Tris buffer, pH 7.6 both at 37° C for 4 h.
3. Wash in running tap water.
4. Stain both sections by the Feulgen method.

Results

| Test section | DNA negative |
| Control section | DNA red |

EXTRACTION OF NUCLEIC ACIDS WITH PERCHLORIC ACID

Note

Perchloric acid extracts both RNA and DNA. RNA is removed more rapidly. This enables differential extraction of RNA to take place.

1. EXTRACTION OF RNA

Solution

| Perchloric acid conc. | 5 ml |
| Distilled water | 45 ml |

Technique

1. Bring sections to water.
2. Treat sections with 10% perchloric acid at 4°C for 18 h.
3. Rinse in distilled water.

4. Transfer to 1% sodium carbonate for 5 min.
5. Wash in tap water.
6. Employ appropriate staining method.

Results

RNA is extracted.
DNA is not extracted but polymerized, which may affect its staining reaction.

2. EXTRACTION OF RNA AND DNA

Solution

Perchloric acid (conc)	2.5 ml
Distilled water	47.5 ml

Technique

1. Bring sections to water.
2. Treat sections with 5% perchloric acid at 60°C for 20 min.
3. Rinse in distilled water.
4. Transfer to 1% sodium carbonate for 5 min.
5. Wash in tap water.
6. Carry out appropriate technique.

Result

RNA and DNA are extracted.

REFERENCES

Adams C W M 1957 A p-dimethylaminobenza ldehyde-nitrate method for the histochemical demonstration of tryptophane and related compounds. Journal of Clinical Pathology 10: 56

Adams C W M, Sloper J C 1955 Technique for demonstrating neurosecretory material in the human hypothalamus. Lancet 1: 651

Baker J R 1947 The histochemical recognition of certain guanidine derivatives. Quarterly Journal of Microscopical Science 88: 115

Baker J R 1956 The histochemical recognition of phenols especially tyrosine. Quarterly Journal of Microscopical Science 97: 161

Bertalanffy F D, Von, Nagy K P 1962 Fluorescence microscopy and photomicrography with acridine orange. Medical Radiology & Photography 38: 82

Brachet J 1940 La detection histochemique des acides pentose-nucleiques. Comptes Rendus des Seances de la Societe de Biologie et de Sans Filiales 133: 88

Bradbury S 1956 Human saliva as a convenient source of ribonuclease. Quarterly Journal of Microscopical Science 97: 323

Castleman W G B 1962 Histochemical technique. Methuen, London

Einarson L 1932 A method for progressive selective staining of Nissl and nuclear substances in nerve cells. American Journal of Pathology 8: 295

Einarson L 1951 On the theory of gallocyanin-chromalum staining and its application for quantitive estimation basophilia. Acta Pathologica et Microbiologica Scandinavica 81: 256

Elias J M 1969 Effects of temperature, post-staining rinses and ethanolbutanol dehydrating mixtures on methyl green pyronin staining. Stain Technology 44: 201

Feulgen R, Rossenbeck H 1924 Mikroskopisch-chemischer Nachweis einen Nucleinsaurs von Typus der Thymonuclinsaure und die darauf berhende elektive Färbung. Von Zellkernen in Microskopischen Prepäraten Zeitschift Physiology Chemistry 135: 203

Glenner G, Lillie R D 1959 Observations on the Diazotization-coupling reaction for the histochemical demonstration tyrosine: Metal chelation and formazan variants. Journal of Histochemistry & Cytochemistry 7: 416

Hitchcock C H, Ehrich W 1930 A new method for differential staining of plasma cells and of other basophilic cells. Archives of Pathology 9: 625

Hopwood D 1982 In: Bancroft J D, Stevens A (eds) Theory and practice of histological techniques. Churchill Livingstone, Edinburgh

Pappenheim A 1899 Vergleichende Untersuchungen über die elementare Zusammensetzung des rothen Knockenmarkes einiger Säugenthiere. Virchow's Archiv fur Pathologische Anatomie Physiologie 157: 19

Pearse A G E 1951 Review of modern methods in histochemistry. Quarterly Journal of Microscopical Science 92: 393

Unna P G 1902 Eine modifikation der Pappenheimschen Färbung auf Granoplasma. Monatschefte für Praktische Dermatologie 35: 76

Stoward P J 1963 D Phil Thesis. Universtity of Oxford

Yasuma A, Itchikawa T 1953 Ninhydrin-Schiff and alloxon-Schiff staining. Journal of Laboratory and Clinical Medicine 41: 296

8

Amyloid

INTRODUCTION

Amyloid was given its name by Virchow in the eighteen fifties. The name indicates a starch-like appearance. Amyloidosis is a condition where a deposition of amorphous eosinophilic material occurs. It is usually extracellular in tissues. The organs become enlarged, pale and have a 'waxy' appearance. The earliest deposits of amyloid are seen in the walls of blood vessels and if the infiltration continues the structure is replaced and its function lost. It is rare that amyloidosis is not diagnosed at a relatively early stage of the disease. The majority of surgical material contains minimal deposits, often only seen in the walls of blood vessels. In histopathology it is one of the few diseases where the histochemistry can make or break the diagnosis giving the laboratory worker considerable responsibility in that his staining methods will require to be of the highest standard.

In the last 25 years a considerable amount of information regarding the nature and origin has been published; however the aetiology is still largely unknown.

CLASSIFICATION

Many classifications have appeared over the years to keep pace with biochemical, clinical and histopathological developments. The Reimann, Koucky and Eklund (1935) system has stood the test of time and is given below, enlarged by current information.

Primary amyloid is amyloid that occurs spon-taneously without an apparent predisposing illness. It usually affects tissue of a mesodermal origin, viz. muscle, skin, tongue and heart muscle.

Secondary amyloid occurs in association with a wide range of predisposing or co-existent disease. These are usually long-standing chronic infections, such as tuberculosis, osteomyelitis and leprosy. Chronic inflammatory diseases such as rheumatoid arthritis and ulcerative colitis also produce deposits of amyloid. Secondary amyloid is most frequently found in the kidney, spleen, liver and adrenals, but it can also be seen in lymph nodes, intestine and pancreas.

Multiple myeloma associated amyloid is produced with diseases of the immunological system involving plasma cells.

Tumour forming and tumour associated amyloid is found in association with tumours of the amine precursor uptake and decarboxylation (APUD) system. The deposits can be local or systemic.

Familial and hereditary amyloid can be seen in cases of Mediterranean fever, cardiomyopathy and polyneuropathy.

Ageing amyloid can be seen in the heart, brain (in senile plaques and walls of small blood vessels) and seminal vesicles.

Experimental amyloid is produced in animals by repeated casein injections.

CHEMICAL COMPOSITION AND ULTRASTRUCTURE

The composition of amyloid has been a matter of speculation for many years. This has been caused by the reactivity of amyloid to carbohydrate techniques, and the problems encountered in separating a true amyloid deposit from tissue structure. In recent years analyses of pure amyloid have shown that it consists of over 95% protein and between 1 and 5% carbohydrate. The carbohydrate content is mainly mucopolysaccharides, in the form of heparan sulphate, chondroitin sulphate and dermatan sulphate (Bitter & Muir, 1966; Muir & Cohen, 1968). The variable chemical content of amyloid caused presumably by its origin, site and mode of production, affects its histological staining reactions but not its ultrastructure. The protein component has been shown to have high levels of tryptophan and tyrosine.

Amyloid has a unique ultrastructure. Under the electron microscope it appears as unbranched fibrils with no specific orientation. Each fibril consists of two electron dense filaments 2.5–3.5 nm in diameter separated by a 2.5 nm interspace giving the whole fibril a diameter of 8–10 nm and a variable length which may be up to several microns, (Francis, 1982). These fibrils are usually found in extracellular spaces. The amyloid fibril has been subjected to many investigations to locate an amino acid that we could use as a means of demonstration, but to date the histochemist can only identify the proteins mentioned earlier, tryptophan and tyrosine. Eanes & Glenner (1968) showed that the amyloid fibril protein is arranged in an antiparallel β pleated sheet. If the pleated sheet structure is damaged by enzymatic action then the standard characteristics of amyloid, its fibrillar structure and Congo red binding with birefringence and dichroism, is lost. It has become clear that amyloid fibrils can be formed from at least three protein groups, these groups are shown below in Table 8.1 which is modified from Francis (1982).

TECHNIQUE

It is well recognized that amyloid deposits are best shown using cryostat or free-floating frozen sections, but in the routine surgical laboratory this is not usually possible. In our hands fixation does not appear critical, though many of our colleagues prefer mercuric chloride containing solutions. Long fixation over a period of years does seem to reduce the intensity of the staining reaction. Two of the methods we give, the methyl green and DMAB-nitrite method give their best results if applied to unfixed tissue. Cut sections containing amyloid appear to lose some of their reactivity on storage so test and control sections should be freshly cut. As indicated earlier not all deposits will react to staining methods in the same way. Large deposits of amyloid will give a far less intense staining reaction than small deposits in vessel walls. Secondary amyloid gives a brighter and more consistent result to histochemical methods than does primary and other types of amyloid. On occasion primary and experimentally produced amyloid has failed to react with staining methods in our hands despite showing the characteristic ultrastructure. For this reason alone control sections should always be used.

MICROSCOPICAL APPEARANCE

In formalin or mercuric fixed sections amyloid appears as homogeneous material staining pink-red with eosin (eosinophilic). It is weakly PAS positive, staining green or blue with trichromes and khaki with van Gieson. It is weakly autofluorescent and weakly birefringent. None of these methods is specific for amyloid. Using a haematoxylin and eosin stain small amounts of amyloid can easily be confused with other homogeneous pink staining material such as hyaline, old collagen and fibrinoid or missed altogether. These small deposits of amyloid are difficult to see and specialized staining methods must be employed.

Table 8.1 Protein groups in amyloid

Protein group	Origin	Classification
AA amyloid (amyloid of unknown origin)	Dissimilar to any known protein	Secondary Familial Experimental
AL amyloid (immunoglobulin derived)	Immunoglobulin light chains from plasma cells	Primary Multiple myeloma Possible senile
APUD amyloid (polypeptide hormone derived)	Calcitonin, insulin, glucagon, etc.	Insulinomas Medullary carcinoma Pituitary adenomas

DEMONSTRATION OF AMYLOID

At this stage it is probably worthwhile to consider the methods available to demonstrate amyloid (Table 8.2).

Table 8.2 Methods for amyloid

Type of method	Utilizes
Metachromasia and polychromasia	Crystal violet, methyl violet and methyl green
Selective staining	Congo red, sirius red and related dyes
Fluorescence	Thioflavine T. Congo red, Thioflavine S. and other fluorochromes
Polarization	Congo red, sirius red, toluidine blue
Enzyme methods	Pepsin and other enzymes
Protein technique	DMAB-nitrite
Immunochemical	Use of specific antisera
Electron microscopy	Ultrastructure studies using resin embedded material

STAINING METHODS

Amyloid can be demonstrated in fresh tissues with iodine. The tissue is rinsed in 1% acetic acid before being treated with Grams's iodine. Amyloid deposits stain a deep brown colour. Further treatment with 10% sulphuric acid will change the amyloid deposit to blue-violet. This method has traditionally been used in the post-mortem room to demonstrate gross deposits. Fixation affects the reaction but fresh frozen sections can be treated in the same way and as long as they are mounted in an iodine-glycerol mixture will show amyloid as a purple colour.

Metachromatic or polychromatic methods

Methyl violet was first used to demonstrate amyloid as long ago as 1875 by Cornil and, along with crystal violet and dahlia, it has enjoyed considerable popularity. The use of these dyes is often referred to as 'metachromasia' but this is not strictly true as the differential staining of amyloid is almost certainly due to the dye 'mixture' having more than one component (Cohen, 1967).

A more correct term would be 'polychromatic' staining. Conventional metachromatic dyes such as thionin and toluidine blue do not give such good results, although removal of the protein moiety by pepsin digestion will enhance toluidine blue staining (Windrum & Kramer, 1957). Using a 0.1% toluidine blue at pH 5.7 with 0.1 M magnesium chloride and staining for 1 h, Mowry & Scott (1967) obtained a weak red birefringent effect with amyloid. These methods are not very satisfactory as they are nonspecific (mucins also stain purple red), with results that are often less satisfactory when mounted. Frozen sections give brighter and more easily differentiated staining. It is unimportant whether crystal or methyl violet is used. Crystal or methyl violet staining is considered to be unreliable with primary amyloid deposits. The following techniques are the best in our hands.

CRYSTAL VIOLET TECHNIQUE (Hucker & Conn, 1928)

Notes

Ammonium oxalate is added to the crystal violet solution and is said to enhance the polychromatic effect. The slides should be examined wet before mounting as some loss of staining brightness subsequently occurs. Alcohol dehydration destroys the purple-red staining and must be avoided. Aqueous mountant should be used. The recommended one is a modified Apathy's solution, which helps to keep diffusion of dye into the mountant and subsequent fading to a minimum (avoid glycerol-jelly for these reasons).

Solutions

2 g crystal violet is dissolved in 20 ml 95% alcohol. Add 80 ml of 1% aqueous ammonium oxalate. Dissolve with the aid of gentle heat. Cool and filter.

Modified Apathy mountant (Highman, 1946)

Dissolve 20 g gum arabic and 20 g cane sugar in 40 ml of distilled water using gentle heat (56°C).

Then add 20 g potassium acetate and 0.1 g thymol. Mix and allow to stand at room temperature to dissolve. Finally, place in a 56°C oven and filter through a coarse (Green's) filter paper into another container also in the oven. It may be found that the solution will have a tendency to set due to evaporation of the solvent. This can be avoided by adding judicious amounts of prewarmed distilled water.

Technique

1. Take sections to water.
2. Stain with the crystal violet solution for 2–3 min.
3. Wash and differentiate in weak (0.2%) acetic acid. Control differentiation with microscope and by washing in water for 10–30 s. Aim at removing the excess dye only.
4. Wash and mount in the modified Apathy's solution.

Results

Amyloid, certain mucins, colloid, renal hyaline material	red-purple
Background	blue

FORMIC ACID-CRYSTAL VIOLET TECHNIQUE (Fernando, 1961)

Notes

Formic acid is used both as the diluent and differentiator for the dye and serves to accentuate the metachromatic effect. The author recommended that Helly's and Bouin's fixatives be avoided for the best results. He also set out a mountant which is similar in its action to the Highman modification of Apathy's solution, but is nonsetting and requires sealing with varnish. When checking differentiation it is better to rinse in distilled, as opposed to tap water otherwise the amyloid takes on a bluish tinge.

Solutions

1% crystal violet in 3% formic acid.
Mountant:

Dextrin	16.7 g
Sucrose	16.7 g

Sodium chloride	10 g
Thymol	0.01 g
Distilled water	100 ml

Mix constituents and heat in a porcelain dish with constant stirring until dissolved. Cool and filter through a coarse (Green's) filter paper.

Technique

1. Take sections to alcohol.
2. Blot dry. Stain in filtered crystal violet solution for 10 mins.
3. Drain and blot dry.
4. Differentiate in 1% aqueous formic acid for 1–3 min (nearer 1 min). Rinse in distilled water.
5. Mount either in the specified mountant or in modified Apathy's solution.

Results

Amyloid, some mucins, hyaline material	purple-red
Background tissue	blue

METHYL GREEN TECHNIQUE (Bancroft, 1963)

Notes

Following primary staining in methyl violet, partial replacement staining with extracted methyl green is carried out. The methyl green acts as a combined differentiator-counterstain. Only frozen sections give good results; and following methyl violet staining, it is better to carry out partial differentiation in acetic acid prior to the methyl green treatment.

Solutions

1% aqueous methyl violet.

2% aqueous methyl green
Extract with chloroform as for the methyl green-pyronin technique, see page 83.

Technique

1. Take sections to water.

2. Stain with the methyl violet solution for 2 min.
3. Wash in water and briefly (20 s) differentiate in 1% acetic acid. Wash in water.
4. Treat with the methyl green solution for 5–10 min until sufficient differentiation of methyl violet staining of the background has occured.
5. Wash, mount in modified Apathy's solution.

Results

Amyloid, some mucins, hyaline material	purple-red
Nuclei	green
Background	clear

STANDARD TOLUIDINE BLUE (STB) METHOD (Wolman, 1971 from Francis, 1982)

Notes

This method stains many tissue components, including amyloid, an orthochromatic blue colour. Amyloid is distinguished by its dichroism and striking dark red birefringence. Cooper (1974) found the mechanism of binding analogous to that of Congo red. Some tissue components, for example cartilage matrix, mast cell granules, and some connective tissue mucopolysaccharides, stain metachromatically purple with toluidine blue which then gives anomalous yellow-green polarization colours. This is probably electrochemical bonding and can be minimized if staining solution is saturated with sodium chloride (Cooper, 1974). Occasional amyloid deposits, especially those of endocrine origin, are negative with this method and minimal deposits are sometimes difficult to visualize.

Solution

1% toluidine blue in 50% isopropanol.

Technique

1. Well deparaffinized sections are taken to water, removing fixation pigment where necessary.
2. Stain in toluidine blue solution 30 min at 37°C.

3. Blot section carefully then place in absolute isopropanol for 1 min.
4. Clear in xylene and mount.

Results

Amyloid and many other tissue components stain an orthochromatic blue colour but when examined under polarized light amyloid gives a dark red birefringence.

CONGO RED METHODS

That amyloid has an affinity for Congo red has been known for many years. Initially Congo red was used as a clinical test for amyloid. Bennhold (1922) described the first satisfactory Congo red stain. Many modifications have appeared over the years and the most useful and reliable are given below. The dye is highly selective for amyloid but not specific as collagen, elastic fibres, hyaline and corpora amylacea of brain and prostate will also stain. Congo red dye forms nonpolar hydrogen bonds with amyloid. It is also a fluorochrome and will impart a red fluorescence to amyloid.

An important feature of the Congo red staining of amyloid is the red to green (dichroic) birefringence which is given due to the parallel alignment of the dye molecules on the linearly arranged amyloid fibrils (Wolman & Bubis, 1965). This dichroic birefringence effect was first noted by Divry & Florkin (1927), and is widely regarded as being the most effective technique for the demonstration of amyloid (Missmahl & Hartwig 1953; Cohen, 1967). It is not truly specific, however, as cellulose (Puchtler, et al, 1962) and young Haversian bone (Reissenweber, 1969) for example, will also exhibit Congo red dichroic birefringence. Also it has been shown that using fixatives such as Carnoy, alcohol or Bouin, connective tissue fibres can give this effect (Klatskin, 1969). However, in practice, dichroic Congo red birefringence is a reliable index for the presence of amyloid. Heptinstall (1974) reported that the green birefringence may be lacking in thin sections and recommended 6 μm thickness. A weak birefringence with Congo red staining of amyloid may occur and necessitates other confirmatory techniques.

There have been a number of important developments in Congo red technique, and these will be dealt with in chronological order. Other similar dyes have been tried, and of these, Sirius red has been, perhaps the most successful and will be mentioned. Whatever the variant used frozen sections give brighter staining than paraffin sections.

HIGHMAN'S CONGO RED TECHNIQUE
(Highman, 1946)

Notes

An alcoholic solution of Congo red is used. Differentiation is easier to control than in the original Bennhold method and we suggest that Highman's is the method of choice out of the several allied ones in popular use today.

Solutions

0.5% Congo red in 50% alcohol.

0.2% potassium hydroxide in 80% alcohol.

Technique

1. Take sections to water (or alcohol)
2. Stain with the Congo red solution for 5 min. Drain.
3. Differentiate with the potassium hydroxide solution for 15–20 s until the background is clear.
4. Wash in water and stain nuclei with one of the alum haematoxylin solutions. Differentiate and blue.
5. Dehydrate, clear and mount as desired.

Results

Eosinophils, amyloid, elastin	dull red
Nuclei	blue
Background	clear

ALKALINE CONGO RED TECHNIQUE
(Puchtler et al, 1962)

Notes

This is a progressive method, requiring no differentiation step. The added salts act as ionic competitors for the dye, and background (polar)

staining is eliminated; only the non-polar binding of Congo red occurs. The main disadvantages of the method lie in its complexity and the short bench-life of the solutions used.

Solutions

Alcoholic sodium chloride hydroxide stock solution
  Saturated sodium chloride in 80% alcohol (keeps well).

Working solution
Stock solution	50 ml
1% aqueous sodium hydroxide	0.5 ml
Mix and filter, use within 15 min	

Congo red stock solution
  Saturated Congo red in 80% alcohol saturated with sodium chloride (keeps fairly well).

Staining solution
Stock solution (Congo red)	50 ml
1% aqueous sodium hydroxide	0.5 ml

Technique

1. Take sections to water.
2. Stain the nuclei with one of the alum haematoxylin solutions. Differentiate and blue.
3. Treat with the alcoholic sodium chloride-hydroxide solution for 20 min. Drain.
4. Stain with the Congo red solution for 20 min. Rinse in alcohol.
5. Dehydrate, clear and mount as desired.

Results

Eosinophils, amyloid, elastin	orange-red
Nuclei	blue
Background	clear

HIGH pH CONGO RED TECHNIQUE
(Eastwood & Cole, 1971)

Notes

This is an ingenious, but simple technique that uses Congo red at a pH of 10.0, at which level binding of the dye by ionic forces (i.e. background staining) will not occur. In other words, differentiation is minimal. In practice, however, it seems that the post-staining rinsing in alcohol is critical as too long a rinse can give false negative or weak results, whilst too short a rinse can give rise to background staining.

Solution

Dissolve 0.5 g Congo red in 100 ml of 50% buffered ethanol. A suitable buffer is as follows (pH 10.0):

0.1 M glycine (mol.wt. 72.07)	30 ml
0.1 M sodium chloride (mol.wt. 58.5)	30 ml
0.1 M sodium hydroxide (mol.wt. 40)	40 ml

Technique

1. Take sections to water
2. Stain nuclei with one of the alum haematoxylin solution. Differentiate and blue.
3. Stain with the Congo red solution for 10–20 min.
4. Wash in 70% alcohol until background is clear.
5. Dehydrate, clear and mount as desired.

Results

| Eosinophils, amyloid, elastin | orange-red |
| Nuclei | blue |

POTASSIUM PERMANGANATE-CONGO RED METHOD FOR AMYLOID (Romhanyi, 1972: Wright et al, 1977)

Notes

This is a simple technique used in theory for distinguishing different chemical types of amyloid. The method is based on the affinity of amyloid for Congo red after exposure to potassium permanganate and dilute sulphuric acid. Romhanyi (1972) demonstrated that amyloid fibrils were either resistant or sensitive to trypsin digestion. The resistant type was primary or immunoglobulin derived and the sensitive type was that described earlier as secondary amyloid. Wright et al (1977)

modified the technique by using a potassium permanganate oxalic acid sequence instead of trypsin.

Solutions

Acidified potassium permanganate

| 0.5% potassium permangante | 25 ml |
| 0.3% sulphuric acid | 25 ml |

0.5% oxalic acid

Technique

1. Sections to water
2. Treat sections with acidified potassium permanganate (2½ min).
3. Bleach with 0.5% oxalic acid until section is colourless.
4. Rinse thoroughly in tap water.
5. Stain sections by Congo red method (see p. 92)

Results

Primary, senile and familial polyneuropathy-associated amyloids — show positive Congo red staining

Secondary and familial Mediterranean fever-associated amyloids — no Congo red staining

Myeloma associated and casein induced amyloids may react either way

SIRIUS RED TECHNIQUE (Llewellyn, 1970)

Notes

This technique is a variation on the Congo red technique of Puchtler et al (1962) (see above) using the dye Sirius red. The dye is similar to Congo red in that it is a 'direct cotton dye' and was introduced, amongst others, as a suitable alternative to Congo red (Sweat & Puchtler, 1965). The method is similar in principle to the alkaline Congo red technique incorporating various salts to enable progressive staining, but has the added advantage that the solutions are simplified and more stable. Unfortunately, the solutions are not quite as stable as claimed and their preparation requires some expertise. Some workers have also experienced subsequent fading of the stained amyloid.

Solution

Dissolve 0.5 g sirius red F3B in 45 ml distilled water. Add absolute alcohol 50 ml and 1% aqueous sodium hydroxide 1 ml. With vigorous mixing, slowly add sufficient 20% aqueous sodium chloride to just produce a fine precipitate (using a strong backlight) and keeping amount of added salt to the bare minimum (up to 4 ml). Allow to stand overnight and filter.

Technique

1. Take sections to water.
2. Stain the nuclei with one of the alum haematoxylin solutions. Differentiate and blue.
3. Wash in water, then 70% alcohol.
4. Stain with the sirius red solution for 1 h.
5. Wash well in tap water. Dehydrate, clear and mount as desired.

Results

Eosinophils, amyloid, elastin	deep red
Nuclei	blue
Background	colourless

SECONDARY FLUORESCENT STAINING

The first worker to use fluorescent techniques for the demonstration of amyloid was Chiari (1947), who used dyes such as thiazine red, euchrysin 26NV and thioflavine S. This type of method did not become popular, however, until Vassar & Culling (1959) introduced the dye thioflavine T. These two workers claimed specificity of staining for amyloid but it has become increasingly evident that many other substances also exhibit secondary fluorescent staining (Rogers, 1965; Porteous et al, 1966).

Several workers have attempted to increase the selectivity of thioflavine T for amyloid, for example, Mowry & Scott (1967) who used a 0.1% solution of thioflavine T at pH 5.7 containing 0.4 M magnesium chloride. Also Burns et al

(1967) who lowered the pH of the dye solution from 3.6 to 1.2. This latter group of workers found that at this low pH only a few substances other than amyloid, exhibited a yellow fluorescence with short wavelength blue ultraviolet light.

In our experience thioflavine T fluorescence can only be safely used as a confirmatory method in that a substance yielding a negative thioflavine fluorescence is most unlikely to be amyloid. The converse is not necessarily true. However, thioflavine T is frequently used as a screening method.

In a correctly adjusted fluorescence microscope the amyloid deposits fluoresce strongly and can easily be seen at low magnification. Other fluorochromes are used with success notably Congo red and the thioflavine S. Congo red has the advantage over both thioflavine dyes that with careful differentiation little nonspecific staining will be seen. The Congo red method and two versions of the thioflavine T method are given below.

THIOFLAVINE TECHNIQUE (Vassar & Culling, 1959)

Thioflavine T is a fluorochrome with a particular affinity for amyloid and although the rationale has not been definitely established is probably an electrostatic one.

Notes

The thioflavine solution tends to deteriorate over a period of months but will keep better in a dark container. The fluorescence of the stained amyloid will gradually fade on storage of the sections and for best results, examine a recently stained section.

Whilst sections may be mounted in glycerol, perfectly satisfactory results can be obtained by using a DPX-type mountant (avoid Canada balsam as this will exhibit autofluorescence). The fluorescent colour of the thioflavine-stained amyloid will depend very much on the type of barrier filter used — both iodine quartz and mercury vapour systems give equally good results. Paraffin sections are perfectly satisfactory.

Solution

1% aqueous thioflavine T.

Technique

1. Take sections to water.
2. Treat with Mayer's haematoxylin solution for 2 min (this acts merely to mask nuclear fluorescence). Wash.
3. Stain with the thioflavine solution for 3 min. Wash.
4. Differentiate out excess fluorochrome in 1% acetic acid for 20 min.
5. Wash well, blot dry. Dehydrate, clear and mount in a DPX-type mountant.

Results

Using a mercury vapour lamp with a red suppression filter (BG38), exciter filter (UG1) and barrier filter (K430).

Amyloid, elastin, etc.   silver white

Using an iodine quartz or mercury vapour lamp with exciter filter (BG12) and barrier filter (K530).

Amyloid, elastin, etc.   yellow

pH 1.4 THIOFLAVINE T (Burns et al, 1967)

Notes

A low pH increases the selectivity by favouring the fluorochromic fraction binding to amyloid while depressing non-amyloid fluorochrome staining.

Technique

As previous method but using a freshly prepared 0.5% thioflavine T in 0.1 M hydrochloric acid.

Results

Amyloid, Paneth cells   blue or yellow according to filters used

CONGO RED AS A FLUORESCENCE METHOD FOR AMYLOID (Cohen et al, 1959; Puchtler & Sweat, 1965)

Notes

Congo red is a fluorochrome and as such will demonstrate amyloid. Other tissue components will stain, but by using dilute Congo red stain and differentiating, other congophilic material will be barely discernible.

It is possible to overdifferentiate, but this rarely happens.

Preparation of stain

Congo red stain

Congo red	100 mg
Absolute alcohol	50 ml
Distilled water	50 ml

Differentiator solution

Potassium hydroxide	200 mg
Absolute alcohol	80 ml
Distilled water	20 ml

Technique

1. Bring sections to water.
2. Stain in Congo red stain (1 min).
3. Wash in tap water.
4. Differentiate in differentiator solution until all the section appears colourless.
5. Wash in water.
6. Dehydrate through clean alcohol and clear in fresh xylene.
7. Mount in DPX or fluoro-free mountant.

Results

Amyloid deposits fluoresce   orange to red

OTHER STAINING METHODS

Many dyes have been tried in an attempt to find specific methods for amyloid. Most of these attempts have concentrated on staining the mucopolysaccharide content and on a lesser scale the proteins present in deposits.

ALCIAN BLUE TECHNIQUE (Lendrum et al, 1972)

Notes

Pennock et al (1968) used alcian blue at pH 1.0 and 5.7 with magnesium ions. The drawback to the method is the mucin stained by alcian blue. This varies depending upon the pH of the alcian blue and the molarity of the magnesium salt. The method below which uses 0.5% alcian blue and sodium sulphate to suppress background staining has proved reliable in our hands.

Alcian blue at pH 1.0 stains recent amyloids bright green. The colour is rendered fast by alkalisation in borax.

Solutions

Acetic-alcohol (prepare fresh)
95% ethanol	45 ml
Distilled water	45 ml
Acetic acid	10 ml

Alcian blue solution (prepare fresh)
1% alcian blue in 95% ethanol	45 ml
1% aqueous hydrated sodium sulphate	45 ml
Acetic acid	10 ml

Allow to stand for 30 min before use.

Saturated borax in 80% alcohol.

Technique (slightly modified)

1. Take sections to water. Wash.
2. Rinse in the acetic-alcohol solution.
3. Stain with the alcian blue solution for 2 h. Rinse in the acetic-alcohol solution, then in water.
4. Alkalinize in the borax solution for at least $3\frac{1}{4}$ min. Wash.
5. Carry out van Gieson's technique.
6. Rinse in distilled water or alcohol. Dehydrate, clear and mount as desired.

Results

Recent amyloid, some colloids	bright green
Old amyloid	paler green or non-reactive
Collagen	red
Muscle	yellow

POLARIZING MICROSCOPY

An important feature of Congo red and toluidine blue staining of amyloid is the dichroism and birefringence that is produced. Amyloid in unstained sections is weakly birefringent. Under crossed polars, it gives a pale white to yellow colour. In contrast the apple green colour produced in amyloid deposits when stained by Congo red and sirius red is easy to see and was first reported by Divry & Florkin (1927). The birefringence produced is due to the alignment of the dye molecules on the amyloid fibril. The colouration is accepted by many as the most selective test for amyloid fibrils. Green birefringence can also be seen in other situations and conditions. Klatskin (1969) found green birefringence in some connective tissues fixed in Carnoy, Zenker or Bouin's fixatives but rarely formalin. Cellulose (Puchtler & Sweat, 1962), young Haversian bone, prostatic, pulmonary and cerebral corpora amylacea (Reissenweber & Decaro, 1969) and chitin also show the effect. Despite this, dichroic Congo red birefringence is the most reliable method at the light microscope level for demonstrating amyloid.

ENZYME METHODS

Amyloid deposits in paraffin sections seem to be little affected by the use of enzymes. Cooper (1974) tried 11 enzymes and found that the routine staining methods were little changed in their reactivity to amyloid. Work using unfixed cryostat sections shows that some types of amyloid are affected by enzyme activity and others are not. Primary amyloid for instance shows resistance to all types of enzymes whereas secondary amyloid in unfixed sections can be sensitive to digestion. This difference accords with their behaviour in staining methods.

PEPSIN DIGESTION

This is a useful adjunct to the standard techniques. Amyloid is not digested by low pH pepsin treatment, whereas other tissue components are. Absence or presence of digestion can be subsequently confirmed by counterstaining the sections with light green; failure of the background tissues to stain is taken as evidence of digestion.

Notes

Sections should be mounted on slides using an adhesive to prevent loss during treatment. The pepsin should be fairly fresh (several weeks) as we have experienced technique failure due to deteriorated samples.

Solutions

0.2 g pepsin is dissolved in 40 ml of 0.02 M hydrochloric acid to give a solution of pH 1.6.

Highman's Congo red solution and differentiator (see p. 92).

0.2% light green in 0.2% acetic acid.

Technique

1. Take two sections of known control material and two test sections to distilled water.
2. Treat one section of each pair with the preheated pepsin solution and the remaining two sections with 0.2 M hydrochloric acid only for 4 h at 37°C.
3. Wash sections well in water for several minutes.
4. Carry out the Congo red technique on all sections differentiating as appropriate and staining the nuclei with haematoxylin. Wash well.
5. Counterstain all sections with the light green solution for 30 s.
6. Wash, dehydrate, clear and mount as desired.

Results

Amyloid in both treated and untreated sections	pale red
Non-amyloid in the treated section	colourless
Non-amyloid in the untreated section	green
Nuclei	blue

DMAB-NITRITE TECHNIQUE (Adams, 1957)

Notes

If the protein tryptophan is treated with p-dimethylamino-benzaldehyde (DMAB), beta-carboline is formed which, when oxidized by sodium nitrite, forms an insoluble blue pigment. This is of value when a suspected amyloid deposit, although showing Congo red staining, gives a weak birefringence.

Only tryptophan-rich substances such as amyloid and fibrin react, whereas other Congo red-positive material e.g. elastin does not. Deposits giving positive Congo red staining and a positive DMAB-nitrite reaction are most likely to be amyloid (Cooper, 1969). APUD amyloid is low in tryptophan content however, and thus DMAB negative. Lengthy formalin fixation will cause a negative reaction. The technique employs a strong acid and it will be useful to mount sections on slides using an adhesive, and to prepare the reagents in a well-ventilated atmosphere.

Solutions

5% DMAB in conc. hydrochloric acid.
1% sodium nitrite in conc. hydrochloric acid.

Technique

1. Take a known positive control and the test sections to alcohol. Celloidinize.
2. Harden the celloidin film in water, then rinse in distilled water and drain.
3. Treat will the DMAB-HCl solution for 1 min. Drain.
4. Transfer sections to the sodium nitrite-HCl for 1 min with continuous agitation.
5. Wash in water for 30 s, then in 1% acid-alcohol for 15 s. Wash well. Counterstain in 1% aqueous neutral red solution for 5 min.
6. Wash, dehydrate, clear and mount as desired.

Results

Tryptophan, i.e. amyloid, fibrin, fibrinoid, Reinke crystals, Paneth cell granules	dark blue
Nuclei	red

IMMUNOCHEMICAL TECHNIQUES

The future demonstration of amyloid in the surgical laboratory will undoubtedly be by this type of technique. Many workers are producing antibodies to amyloid: some are so specific that they only react with the type of amyloid they were raised from, others react with normal tissue components as well as amyloid. If this book is fortunate to come to a second edition we will be very surprised if there is not an immunochemical method for amyloid included!

ELECTRON MICROSCOPY

As discussed earlier amyloid has an ultrastructure which appears unchanged regardless of the tissue origin, the type of amyloid or the age of the deposit. The amyloid fibril structure is unique, unlike any other fibre seen. Today this allows the electron microscopist to be able to confirm that a deposit is amyloid with conviction.

SUMMARY

In the surgical laboratory today it is rare to receive a case with massive deposits of amyloid as Francis

(1982) states, 'the cases today involve material with minimal deposits often only in the walls of blood vessels'. The needle biopsy and other small biopsy techniques are responsible along with the clinical awareness of the disease. In both our laboratories the rectal biopsy appears to be the clinician's method of choice, with renal biopsies second. The small biopsy has both advantages and drawbacks, as previously mentioned: recently laid down amyloid reacts more intensely with staining solutions than longstanding deposits, so the demonstration is easier. On the other hand the amount of tissue is small and orientation often important. Considerable care is sometimes required. In the staining of rectal biopsies it must be remembered that mucin is also present and will be reactive with polychromatic, metachromatic and possibly other methods.

The laboratory has at its disposal an ever increasing number of staining methods for the demonstration of amyloid, in reality at the present time only the Congo or sirius red with polarization should be used for diagnosis (Table 8.3). The other methods are useful confirmatory techniques, unless of course one is fortunate enough to have access to an electron microscope.

Table 8.3 Amyloid demonstration methods.

Method	Evaluation of method	Comments
Crystal violet	Not sensitive or highly selective	Easy and quick to carry out in experienced hands. Should never be used alone
Toluidine blue	Sensitive with polarization	Positive with polarization. Not to be used alone
Congo red Sirius red	Sensitive and highly selective with polarization	The best the routine lab. has at its disposal. Must always be viewed by polarization
Thioflavine T Congo red as fluorescence dyes	Highly sensitive but not specific	Useful screening method confirmation of positive result required with Congo red polarization
Alcian blue	Moderately sensitive, but not selective or specific	Time consuming. Looks good, not to be used alone
DMAB-nitrite	Moderately sensitive and selective	Confirms a high tryptophan content. Confirmatory use only
Electron microscopy	Highly selective	The final arbiter at present. Not many routine labs. have one. Expensive
Immunochemistry	Specific	Will replace Congo red and electron microscopy in due course

REFERENCES

Adams C W M 1975 A p-dimethylaminobenzaldehyde nitrite method for the histochemical demonstration of tryptophan and related compounds. Journal of Clinical Pathology 10: 56

Bancroft J D 1963 Methyl green as a differentiator and counterstain in the methyl violet technique for the demonstration of amyloid. Stain Technology 38: 336

Bitter T, Muir H 1966 Mucopolysaccharides of whole human spleens in generalised amyloidosis. Journal of Clinical Investigation 45: 963

Burns J, Pennock C A, Stoward P J 1967 The specificity of the staining of amyloid deposits with thioflavine T. Journal of Pathology & Bacteriology 94: 337

Chiari H 1947 Ein Beitrag zur sekundaren Fluoreszenzdesogen localen Amyloids. Mikroscopie 2: 79

Cohen A S 1967 Amyloidosis. New England Journal of Medicine 277: 522

Cohen A S, Calkins E, Levine C I 1959 Analysis of histology and staining reactions of casein induced amyloidosis in the rabbit. American Journal of Pathology 35: 971

Cooper J H 1969 An evaluation of current methods for the diagnostic histochemistry of amyloid. Journal of Clinical Pathology 22: 410

Cooper J H 1974 Selective amyloid staining as a function of amyloid composition and structure. Laboratory Investigation 31: 232

Divry P, Florkin M 1927 Sur les propriétés optiques de l'amyloide. Comptes Rendus de Séances de la Société de Biologie et Ses Filiales 97: 1808

Eanes E D, Glenner G G 1968 X-ray diffraction studies on amyloid dilaments. Journal of Histochemistry & Cytochemistry 16: 673

Eastwood H, Cole K R 1971 Staining of amyloid by buffered Congo red in 50% ethanol. Stain Technology 46: 208

Fernando J C 1961 A durable method of demonstrating amyloid in paraffin sections. Journal of the Institute of Science Technology 7: 40

Francis R J 1982 Amyloid. In: Bancroft J D, Stevens A (eds) Theory and practice of histological techniques. Churchill Livingstone, Edinburgh

Heptinstall R H 1974 Pathology of the kidney, 2nd ed, Vol. 2. Little & Brown, Boston

Highman B 1946 Improved methods for demonstrating amyloid in paraffin sections. Archives of Pathology 41: 559

Hucker G J, Conn H J 1928 A quick stain for staining Gram-positive organisms in the tissues. Archives of Pathology 5: 828

Klatskin G 1969 Non-specific green birefringence in Congo-red stained tissues. American Journal of Pathology 56: 1

Lendrum A C, Slidders W, Fraser D S 1972 Renal hyalin: a study of amyloidosis and diabetic fibrinous vasculosis with new staining methods. Journal of Clinical Pathology 25: 373

Llewellyn B D 1970 An improved Sirius red method for amyloid. Journal of Medical Laboratory Technology 27: 308

Missmahl H P, Hartwig N 1953 Polarisation-optische Untersuchungen an der Amyloidsubstanz. Archive für Pathologische Anatomie 324: 489

Mowry R W, Scott J E 1967 Observations on the basophilia of amyloids. Histochemie 10: 8

Muir H, Cohen A S 1968 In: Mandema E, Ruinen L, Scholten J H, Cohen A S (eds) Symposium on amyloidosis. Excerpta Medica, Amsterdam

Pennock C A, Burns J, Masserella G 1968 Histochemical investigation of acid mucosubstances in secondary amyloidosis. Journal of Clinical Pathology 21: 578

Porteous I B, Beck J S, Curie A R 1966 The pituitary acidophil: A comparison of its staining reactions with anti-human growth hormone and thioflavine T. Journal of Pathology & Bacteriology 91: 539

Puchtler H, Sweat F 1965 Congo red as a stain for fluorescence stain for microscopy of amyloid. Journal of Histochemistry & Cytochemistry 13: 693

Puchtler H, Sweat F, Levine M 1962 On the binding of Congo red by amyloid. Journal of Histochemistry & Cytochemistry 10: 355

Reimann H A, Koucky R F, Eklund C M 1935 Primary amyloidosis limited to tissue of mesodermal origin. American Journal of Pathology 11: 977

Reissenweber N J 1969 Dichroism with Congo red. A specific test for amyloid? Virchow's Archives of Pathology & Anatomy & Physiology 347: 254

Rogers D R 1965 Screening for amyloid with the thioflavin T fluorescent method. American Journal of Clinical Pathology 44: 59

Sweat F, Puchtler H 1965 Demonstration of amyloid with direct dyes. Archives of Pathology 80: 613

Vassar P S, Culling F A 1959 Fluorescent stains with special reference to amyloid and connective tissue. Archives of Pathology 68: 487

Windrum G K, Kramer H 1957 Fluorescent microscopy of amyloid. Archives of Pathology 63: 373

Wolman M 1971 Amyloid its nature and molecular structure: Comparison of a new Toluidine blue polarised light method with traditional procedures. Laboratory Investigation 25: 104

Wolman M, Bubis J J 1965 The cause of the green polarisation colour of amyloid stained with Congo red. Histochemie 4: 351

9

Carbohydrates

The term 'carbohydrate' denotes compounds made up of carbon and water, usually hexose units forming various types of 'saccharide'. In tissue the types of carbohydrate found in demonstrable amounts, i.e. capable of histochemical demonstration, are few in number. They are mostly polysaccharide in nature, of varying importance pathologically and exhibit varying degrees of histochemical complexity.

MUCINS

Mucins, variously described as mucosubstances, proteoglycans, glycoproteins or glycoconjugates, are the chemical components of the secretion delivered by certain types of epithelial cell and connective tissue cells such as fibroblasts and mast cells.

Broadly speaking, these mucins consist of hexosamine sugars covalently bound to varying amounts of protein or lipid. Acid radicals are often present and their type and position on the relevant molecule profoundly influences the histochemical reaction obtained. The following types of mucin may be distinguished and will be described in simple terms.

It is important to appreciate that the following different types of mucin are often present as mixtures of two, sometimes, more entitites.

NEUTRAL MUCINS

Neutral mucins carry no reactive acid radical but there are usually free hexose groups present. They are found in the stomach and prostate and to a variable extent in most goblet cells.

ACID MUCINS: SULPHATED

Strongly acidic (connective tissue)

These mucins with one exception (keratan sulphate), contain sulphated glucuronic acid moieties. They react at low pH levels with cationic dyes, are usually PAS negative and occur in tissues such as skin, cartilage, bone, blood vessel walls and umbilical cord. Included in this group are chondroitin-4-sulphate, chondroitin-6-sulphate (chondroitin sulphates A and C respectively), dermatan sulphate, heparin/heparan sulphate and keratan sulphate.

Strongly acidic (epithelial)

These mucins react similarly to the above group in their reactions with cationic dyes but are usually PAS positive and are epithelial in origin. An example of this type of mucin has been reported in bronchial serous glands (Lamb & Reid, 1970).

Weakly acidic

These mucins are mainly epithelial in origin and react with cationic dyes at a low pH but not as low as the strongly acidic group, i.e. pH 1.0 as oppsed to pH 0.5. They may be found for example, in colonic goblet cells.

ACID MUCINS: CARBOXYLATED

N-acetyl sialomucin (sialidase-labile sialomucin)

These mucins contain a sialic acid molecule which reacts at pH levels of 2.0 and above with cationic dye bonding taking place with carboxyl groups. They are identified by their ready extraction with the enzyme sialidase, occur in salivary and bronchial glands and are PAS positive.

N-acetyl-0-acetyl sialomucin (sialidase-resistant sialomucin)

This is a group which is composed almost entirely of sialomucins which are resistant to sialidase extraction. These mucins are epithelial in origin and react, from a staining point of view, like the enzyme-labile sialomucins. They may be found in colonic goblet cells and are PAS negative.

ACID MUCINS: SULPHATED-SIALOMUCINS

This is a somewhat controversial group, the existence of which has yet to be fully established. Histochemically they give reactions for sulphated mucins and yet are extracted by sialidase. They have been reported in prostatic tumours (Hukill & Vidone, 1967), sheep colon (Kent & Marsden, 1963) and malignant synovioma (Cook, 1973).

MUCINS AND PATHOLOGY

The role of mucins in diagnostic pathology has still to be fully elucidated, although their general demonstration is of accepted usefulness in establishing the presence of mucin-producing malignant tumours. Their precise charaterization is also of some value in a few instances, where secondary tumour identification is necessary in order to establish the identity of the primary, for example, certain gastric carcinomas secrete largely neutral mucin (Cook, 1982) whilst certain breast tumours secrete largely N-acetylated sialomucin (Spicer et al, 1962; Cooper, 1974). In addition, a proportion of adenocarcinomas of the colon and rectum have been shown to contain significant amounts of the 0-acylated form of sialomucin (Culling et al, 1975). Amounts of mucin present in a lesion are sometimes of significances too, e.g. the lessened quan-

tity found in ulcerative colitis as oppsed to Crohn's disease (Filipe, 1969). The presence of a particular entity may be useful diagnostically where such an entity is peculiar to certain conditions, e.g. hyaluronic acid in myxoedema lesions of the skin, or in some mesotheliomas (see p. 108).

In addition to the above, there is a group of related rare congenital disturbances of carbohydrate metabolism known as the mucopolysaccharidoses, where water-soluble mucopolysaccharides are laid down in various tissues such as liver and skin. Special fixation and staining schedules need to be adopted as the component mucins are dissolved out in the conventional aqueous fixatives and stain variably with alcian blue. The most well-known perhaps, of these mucopolysaccharidoses is gargoylism or Hurler-Hunter disease, where the abnormal material laid down is a mixture of dermatan and heparan sulphates. There are, currently, up to 12 recognized mucopolysaccharidoses.

FIXATION AND PROCESSING

With the exception of the component mucins of the mucopolysaccharidoses where either alcohol or acetone fixation should be employed, most routine fixatives are suitable and, in practice, neutral buffered formalin is perfectly satisfactory, Bouin's fluid being rather less so (Cook, 1959; Goldstein, 1962; Allison, 1973). Decalcification procedures can affect the histochemical reactions and must be chosen with care. Charman & Reid (1972), in a survey, considered that the best histochemical results with mucins were obtained following either formic-acid, formic acid-sodium formate or EDTA decalcification.

Whilst freeze-dried material gives undoubtedly the best demonstration of mucins, paraffin processing is satisfactory and is normally used. Floating out on 70% alcohol as opposed to water may, however, be advisable when dealing with the connective tissue mucins, as diffusion from the section may occur.

A selection of the more widely used general techniques for mucins is given below and in Table 9.1.

Table 9.1 Significant techniques for mucins and glycogen. Key: SAB, standard (pH 2.5) alcian blue; LAB, low (0.2) pH alcian blue; PAS, periodic acid — Schiff; BPAS, borohydride-saponification — PAS; HID, high iron diamine; D, diastase digestion; Si, sialidase digestion; Hy, hyaluronidase digestion; dig, digested; V, variable reaction; +, stained; −, unstained; ±, weakly stained.

	SAB	LAB	PAS	BPAS	HID	D	Si	Hy
Polysaccharide: Glycogen	−	−	+	±	−	dig	−	−
Hyaluronic acid	+	−	−	−	−	−	−	dig
Mast cells	±	+	−	−	+	−	−	−
Neutral mucin	−	−	+	−	−	−	−	−
Sialomucin: (a) enzyme labile	+	−	+	−	−	−	dig	−
(b) enzyme resistant	+	−	−	+	−	−	−	−
Strongly sulphated: (a) connective tissue	V	+	−	−	+	−	−	Vdig
(b) epithelial	V	+	+	−	+	−	−	−
Weakly sulphated	+	+	V	−	+	−	−	−

GENERAL TECHNIQUES

PAS TECHNIQUE

The mucins vary in their reactivity to the conventional PAS technique. Neutral mucins are normally postive as are the sialidase-labile sialomucins (Quintarelli, 1960). Weakly sulphated mucins on the other hand vary in reactivity whilst the strongly sulphated mucins and hyaluronic acid are usually negative. It has been shown by Scott & Dorling (1969) that 1 : 4 linked uronic acid-containing mucins such as chondroitin sulphate, may give a positive Schiff reaction by employing a long pre-oxidation step.

For normal demonstration purpose it is of little importance whether the McManus variant (see below) or the Hotchkiss variant is used. It is important to bear in mind that glycogen will react; also (in frozen sections) lipids having a wide distribution in tissue such as sphingomyelin.

PERIODIC-ACID SCHIFF TECHNIQUE
(PAS) (Schiff, 1866; McManus, 1946)

Notes

Substances containing vicinal glycol groups or their amino or alkylamino derivatives are oxidized by periodic acid to form dialdehydes, which combine with Schiff's reagent to form an insoluble magenta compound. Such substances are of the carbohydrate group and this method may be used, therefore, in their identification.

Periodic acid is the oxidant of choice as it does not overoxidize the formed aldehydes to carboxyl groups giving a weak or negative reaction.

Schiff's reagent is one where the chromophoric groups of basic fuchsin are broken by sulphuration to form a colourless solution. In the presence of free aldehyde groups an insoluble coloured compound similar, but not identical, to the original dye is formed.

For basement membranes (basal lamina) rather longer times than for the conventional PAS technique should be used to give brighter results. The use of post-Schiff sulphite rinses to reduce background colouration is not normally necessary, provided that washing in running water is thorough and that the alkalinity of the tap water is not too pronounced.

Solutions

1% aqueous periodic acid.

Schiff's reagent
    Basic fuchsin (for Feulgen and Gomori)1 g
    Distilled water   200 ml

Potassium or sodium metabisulphite	2 g
Analar conc. hydrochloric acid	2 ml
Decolourizing charcoal	2 g

Bring the distilled water to the boil, remove flame (to avoid excessive effervescence), and add the basic fuchsin. Mix, cool to 50°C and add the metabisulphite. Mix and cool to room temperature before adding the hydrochloric acid and charcoal. Leave overnight in the dark at room temperature. Filter and store at 4°C in a dark container.

With use, it will eventually be found that the originally colourless to pale yellow solution will turn pink due to loss of sulphur dioxide causing restoration of the basic fuchsin colour. When this happens the solution should be discarded.

Technique

1. Take sections to distilled water.
2. Treat with the periodic acid solution for 5min (see notes).
3. Rinse well in distilled water.
4. Treat with Schiff's reagent for 15 min (see notes).
5. Wash in running tap water for 5–10 min (this intensifies the colour reaction).
6. Stain nuclei with either an iron haematoxylin solution or Harris's haematoxylin solution. Differentiate and blue.
7. Dehydrate, clear and mount as desired.

Results

PAS-positive material (see below)	magenta
Nuclei	blue or blue-black

PAS-positive substances in tissue

The following is a list compiled from various sources, and in the light of our own experience, of those substances which might be expected to react with the PAS technique:

Basement membranes (basal lamina)
Certain organisms (anthrax, streptococci)
Chitin
Fungi (most)
Cellulose
Collagen (weakly)
Reticulin
Neutrophils
Platelets
Plasma and serum
Pancreatic zymogen granules
Gastric mucous neck cells
Pituitary basophil cells
Cerebrosides and sphingomyelin
Some sialomucins
Glycogen
Amoebae and Balantidium coli
Starch
Corpora amylacea of brain and prostate
Lipofuscins (sometimes)
Paneth cells (sometimes)
Amyloid (weakly)
Alpha-antitrypsin
Thyroid and pituitary colloids
Elastin
Russell bodies
Hyaline degeneration
Fibrin
Fibrinoid
JG cells (sometimes)
Tunicin
Melanin (rarely)
Lymphoblasts
Myelocytes
Megakaryocytes
B and Null lymphocytes

Melanosis coli pigment
Granular cell myoblastoma
Type II striated muscle cells
Neutral mucin

METACHROMASIA

The ability to react metachromatically is a property of both carboxylated and sulphated mucins, the neutral mucins being normally orthochromatic. It is a property exhibited by certain negatively charged entities (polyanions) and certain cationic dyes. These react to form dye polymers which have a different absorption characteristic to the normal dye (monomer) and thus a different colour emission. To give an example, azure A exhibits a purple-red metachromasia and a blue orthochromasia (i.e. non-metachromatic colour). This is known as a *hypsochromic* shift in light absorption, i.e. a shift in absorption towards the shorter wavelengths of light with a consequent shift in colour emission towards the longer wavelengths of light (the opposite reaction is termed bathochromic). Metachromatic dyes such as azure A and toluidine blue may be used at a varying pH in a similar manner to alcian blue. For example, metachromasia below pH 4.0 indicates the presence of sulphated mucins; above 4.0 hyaluronic acid will also react (Spicer, 1960). On the whole, precise mucin identification by metachromatic dyes is difficult and unreliable and is comparatively little used in any critical work. An important use for metachromatic staining, however, is the demonstration of the labile mucins found in the mucopolysaccharidoses, where the usual techniques for mucins give unsatisfactory results.

RELEASING PROTEIN-BOUND CARBOHYDRATE

DEAMINATION TECHNIQUE (from Lillie, 1954)

Notes

Sometimes it occurs that a particular carbohydrate moiety is prevented from reacting histochemically by the protein fraction to which it is chemically bound. This most often is the case when dealing with mucoproteins where removal of the protein amino groups allows the 'unmasked' carbohydrate such as sialic acid to react with suitable dyes.

The technique described is a useful one in this connection and employs van Slyke's reagent to destroy protein groups. The rationale of the technique is that the nitrous acid formed by the action of the acetic acid on sodium nitrite releases nitrogen which converts the primary amino groups to hydroxyl groups. A technique such as the combined alcian blue-PAS, if carried out post-deamination, will show a change from a PAS to an alcian blue reactivity in suitable material. Deamination can be used in general histological practice as a means of blocking acidophilic reactions.

One incidental effect of deamination is that cell nuclei become alcianophilic. This is presumably due to the fact that in the absence of the nuclear proteins the large alcian blue molecules are able to enter the intermicellar spaces of the nucleic acids, and thus link with the negatively charged phosphate radicals.

Celloidinization of slides may be necessary to avoid section loss during treatment.

Solutions

Van Slyke's reagent
  Dissolve 6 g sodium nitrite in 35 ml distilled water. Add 5 ml acetic acid and mix. Prepare fresh.

1% alcian blue in 3% acetic acid.

1% aqueous periodic acid.

Schiff's reagent, see page 102.

Technique

1. Take two test and two positive control sections to distilled water.
2. Treat one section of each with the van Slyke reagent for 15 h at room temperature. The remaining duplicate sections should be treated with 5% acetic acid for the same period.
3. Wash all sections in water for 5–10 min.
4. Carry out the combined alcian blue-PAS technique (see p. 111)
5. Dehydrate, clear and mount as desired.

Results

Deaminated material containing previously masked polyanions will show a loss of PAS positivity and a gain in alcian blue reactivity.

AZURE A TECHNIQUE (Hughesdon, 1949)

Notes

This is one of the more reliable metachromatic techniques in that a reasonably alcohol-fast metachromasia is imparted to a wide range of acidic mucins. The alcohol-fast metachromasia is attributed to the use of a pre-oxidation step using potassium permanganate, and the bright staining effect to the use of uranyl nitrate as a differentiator (the sialomucins giving a particularly bright metachromasia). Poor results can usually be traced to unsatisfactory batches of dye.

Solutions

1% aqueous potassium permanganate.

5% aqueous oxalic acid.

0.2% aqueous azure A.

0.2% aqueous uranyl nitrate.

Technique

1. Take sections to water.
2. Treat with the potassium permanganate solution for 5 min.
3. Wash in water. Bleach with the oxalic acid solution.
4. Wash well in water for several minutes.
5. Stain with the azure A solution for 5 min.
6. Wash briefly in water. Differentiate in the uranyl nitrate solution for 10–30 with agitation until a lighter overall staining effect is achieved.
7. Wash in water and blot dry. Dehydrate, clear and mount in a DPX-type mountant.

Results

Mucins	purple-red
Background	blue

METACHROMATIC TECHNIQUES FOR MUCOPOLYSACCHARIDOSIS-TYPE MUCINS

Notes

Two techniques will be described. They are simple to do but it is important to observe the specified fixation and treatment as these particular mucins are very quickly lost from the tissue.

Paraffin section technique (Gardner, 1968)

1. Fix thin slices of tissue, without delay, in Carnoy's solution for 3 h.
2. Pass straight to the processing alcohols or store until required in 70% alcohol. Continue with a paraffin processing schedule.
3. Paraffin sections are cut and floated-out on alcohol and subsequently dried.
4. Take sections to alcohol and blot dry. Stain with 0.25% aqueous toluidine blue at pH 4.5 for 10 s only (see Buffer Tables).
5. Blot dry, dehydrate, clear and mount in a DPX-type mountant.

Results

The abnormal mucins are stained purple-red and present as finely granular material in fibroblasts or histiocytes. In liver they present as clumped, coarsely granular material which may be either extracellular or intracellular.

Frozen section technique (Haust & Landing, 1961)

1. Cut fresh frozen (cryostat) sections. Fix in equal parts of tetrahydrofuran and acetone for 20 min.
2. Rinse in 2.5% acetone.
3. Stain with 0.5% toluidine blue in 25% acetone for 2 min.
4. Blot dry, rinse in undiluted acetone. Clear in xylene and mount in a DPX-type mountant.

Results

Mucins	purple-red
Background	blue

SOUTHGATE'S MUCICARMINE TECHNIQUE (Mayer, 1896; Southgate, 1927)

Notes

This, one of the earlier empirical techniques, has enjoyed considerable vogue for mucin staining and is useful for staining certain fungi such as *Cryptococcus neoformans*. For practical purposes of mucin demonstration it has little to commend it, for it uses a complex solution, has a relatively lengthy staining time and is imprecise in staining effect. It has been shown (Cook, 1968) that neutral mucins stain weakly or not at all and that the strongly sulphated mucins are variable in their reaction, whilst the other acidic mucins (particularly hyaluronic acid) stain strongly. In its favour is the fact that, like alcian blue, it seems to be specific for mucins.

The solution incorporates aluminium salts and the rationale of staining is presumably one of a positively charged carmine-mordant complex bonding with the negatively charged acid mucins.

The nuclei must be well stained to avoid subsequent masking by the mucicarmine. Ehrlich's haematoxylin should not be used as it also stains some mucins.

Solution

Grind 1 g carmine and place in a large (500 ml) conical flask. Add 100 ml of 50% alcohol and mix. Add 1 g aluminium hydroxide, mix and add 0.5 g anhydrous aluminium chloride. Mix and boil gently for $2\frac{1}{2}$ min. Cool and filter. Store at 4°C where it will keep for 6 months or so.

Technique

1. Take sections to water.
2. Stain the nuclei with one of the alum haematoxylin solutions, (see notes). Differentiate well in acid-alcohol and blue.
3. Stain with the mucicarmine solution for 20 min.
4. Wash in water, dehydrate, clear and mount as desired.

Results

Mucins	red
Nuclei	blue

METHODS FOR CARTILAGE

To demonstrate cartilage it should be borne in mind that this is principally achieved by staining the component mucins of the dense matrix. These mucins are connective tissue in type being mainly of the strongly acidic sulphated group. A minor proportion of hyaluronic acid is also present.

Therefore, techniques such as aldehyde fuchsin (p. 55), high iron diamine (p. 113), low pH alcian blue (p. 110), and high molarity magnesium chloride (p. 110) will all give good results. Rather unexpectedly, cartilage matrix is also PAS-positive, but this is due to the presence of mucoprotein.

Metachromasia is usually strong with dyes such as thionin, toluidine blue and azure A (p. 104). Safranin exhibits a bathochromic metachromasia staining cartilage yellow, as against the non-

cartilaginous elements red. The H and E staining of cartilage is somewhat variable in that the basophilia (haematoxyphilia) is more pronounced when Ehrlich's solution is used.

There are no particularly important aspects of fixation and section to note, but floating out of paraffin sections during microtomy may need to be carried out on warm 70% alcohol, rather than water, to avoid the diffusion of mucoid material which may occur.

METHODS FOR MAST CELLS

Mast cells were first described by von Recklinghausen in the early 1870s and subsequently demonstrated by Ehrlich in 1877. They are regularly found in loose connective tissue such as that of the external muscle layers of the gastro-intestinal tract and in fibroadenosis of the breast. Contrary to belief, they are not found to any great extent in normal human skin, where they can be seen mainly around dermal blood vessels, nerves and skin appendages. Pathologically they are not of great import in diagnostic work except in a skin condition, urticaria pigmentosa. Mast cell tumours may be encountered in animal tissue not infrequently. Other conditions in which there is an increased number of mast cells are neurofibromatosis, mycosis fungoides and basal cell carcinoma (Mikhail & Miller-Milinska, 1964).

The characteristic granules are not easily distinguished in an H and E preparation of human tissue, being more readily distinguished in animal tissue. These granules are rich in heparin, one of the strongly sulphated group of acid mucins; hence their metachromasia and reactions with the low pH alcian blue and aledhyde fuchsin technique. In certain species, e.g. rat, there is also a high content of 5-hydroxytryptamine (5HT) so that the appropriate histochemistry will be obtained (see p. 167). In human tissue this is not a significant factor. Most fixatives are suitable, with mercuric chloride and alcoholic solutions, particularly Carnoy, giving the best results. In addition to the two techniques to be described in detail, the following methods may be used:

PAS (not usually positive in human material).
Alcian blue; either low pH such as 0.2 or 0.5 or
with added electrolyte such as 0.4 M magnesium
chloride (see p. 110)
Giemsa (see p. 63)
Aldehyde fuchsin (see p. 55)
Azure A (see p. 104)
Methyl green-pyronin (see p. 83)
Chloroacetate esterase (see p. 188)

THIONIN TECHNIQUE (Cook, 1961)

Notes

The method makes use of the alcohol-resistant
metachromasia exhibited by mast cell granules to
give highly selective staining. The alkaline pH of
tap water used as a diluent for the stain will
be found to aid the metachromasia. One should
aim at slightly overdifferentiating in the acetic acid
for the best results.

Solution

Prepare a stock 0.6% aqueous thionin solution and
into a Coplin jar filled with tap water filter approximately 0.5 ml of dye solution.

Technique

1. Take sections to water.
2. Stain with the solution for 20–30 min.
3. Wash, then differentiate in 0.2% acetic acid
   until only the cell nuclei and mast cell
   granules are stained purple, controlling
   microscopically.
4. Wash in water then dehydrate, clear and
   mount in a DPX-type mountant. Alternatively
   one may rinse in alcohol and counterstain in
   saturated tartrazine in Cellosolve for 30 s.
   Wash in alcohol, clear and mount.

Results

Mast cell granules	purple
Cell nuclei	blue
Background	clear if not counterstained yellow if counterstained

PINACYANOL TECHNIQUE (Bensley, 1952)

Notes

This method gives clear-cut results allied to a
simple staining technique. Unfortunately, the
staining solution is a complex one and the dye
expensive. Staining is brought about by the inter-
action of pinacyanol with erythrosin; the resultant
precipitate ('erythrosinate') is highly selective
when dissolved in alcohol for mast cell granules.
The reaction is probably a polychromatic one.

Solutions

Stock solution

Allow 0.1 g pinacyanol to dissolve in 100 ml
distilled water overnight in the dark. Dissolve
0.1 g erythrosin in 100 ml distilled water and add
75 ml of this to the pinacyanol solution with
agitation. A precipitate will appear which will
increase as more erythrosin solution is added (a
drop at a time with constant mixing). If too much
erythrosin is added poor results will be obtained.
To determine when the optimal precipitate has
been produced test by adding one drop of solution
to a Whatman number 1 filter paper; when the resultant diffusion ring is just faintly pink then precipitation is complete. If not pink continue adding
a few more drops of erythrosin solution with constant mixing. Do not overshoot. Finally, filter the
solution discarding the filtrate and drying the deposit on the filter paper at 37° C. When dry, dissolve the precipitate in 150 ml of ethanol and store
at 4° C in a dark bottle. The stock solution should
keep for up to 1 year.

Working solution

Stock solution	5 ml
30% ethanol	45 ml
Mix and discard after use.	

Technique

1. Take sections to alcohol.
2. Stain with the solution for 20–30 min.
3. Blot dry, differentiate if necessary in 95%
   alcohol, clear and mount as desired.

Results

| Mast cell granules | purple-red |
| Cell nuclei | blue |

ALCIAN BLUE-SAFRANIN METHOD FOR MAST CELLS (Casba, 1969)

Notes

This method is said to differentiate between the mast cells containing heparin and those with histamine.

Solution

Alcian blue	0.9 g
Safranin	0.045 g
Ferric ammonium sulphate	1.2 g
Acetate buffer pH 1.42 (see Appendix 3)	250 ml

Technique

1. Take sections to tap water.
2. Stain in the alcian blue solution for 15 min.
3. Rinse in tap water.
4. Dehydrate in tertiary butyl alcohol.
5. Clear in xylene.
6. Mount in DPX.

Results

| Mast cells containing biogenic amines | blue |
| Mast cells containing heparin | red |

METHODS FOR MESOTHELIOMA

This most commonly arises in the pleura but may also arise in peritoneum and pericardium, and although not a common tumour, it is of interest histochemically as it may well present diagnostic problems which can sometimes by alleviated by carrying out the appropriate supportive techniques.

It has been shown that hyaluronic acid is present in a small but significant number of cases of mesothelioma (Wagner et al, 1962) also glycogen (Wagner et al, 1962; Cook, 1973), again in a small but significant number of cases.

These tumours show a cellular picture varying from fibroblast-type cells to epithelial-type cells with well marked glandular spaces; often there is a mixture of the two elements. The fibroblastic tumour cells rarely show either hyaluronic acid or glycogen.

Any hyaluronic acid present is likely to be in small amounts and in our experience it is sometimes necessary to conserve the mucin present by floating out paraffin sections on alcohol rather than water, to prevent diffusion of mucin from the tissue. It is also worth carrying out the dialysed iron-Perls' technique in addition to alcian blue, as this is a more sensitive marker for scanty deposits of acid mucin.

The following is a suggested scheme for demonstrating the presence of hyaluronic acid or glycogen in a suspected mesothelioma. It is most important that only mucin contained in — or produced by — the tumour cells be considered and not that present as a nonspecific stromal inflammatory reaction.

Technique

1. Tissue blocks are paraffin processed in the conventional manner. Serial sections (approximately a dozen) are floated out on warm water in the usual way and picked up on serially numbered acid-alcohol washed slides (see p. 24). A duplicate set of sections is floated out on warm 70% alcohol instead. All slides are then heat-dried in the conventional manner.

2. Sections from both sets of slides (alcohol and water floated out) are stained by the standard alcian blue method (p. 109), dialysed iron-Perls' (p. 111) and by alcian blue-PAS and disastase alcian blue-PAS (p. 111). The two sets of alcian blue and dialysed iron-Perls' treated sections are examined microscopically and sections selected for subsequent hyaluronidase digestion based on which method evidenced the greatest amount of mucin. Should the sections floated out on water prove as useful, when stained, as those floated out on alcohol then it is suggested that the former be used, as alcohol flotation may lead to a greater degree of section loss from the slide during staining.

3. Selected test sections, together with positive control sections are subjected to hyaluronidase

digestion (p. 119) followed by either the alcian blue or dialysed iron-Perls technique (whichever had proved better).Any material digested by the enzyme may then be suitably stained to differentiate sulphated from carboxylated acid mucin using further slides, i.e. to confirm that it is hyaluronic acid (carboxylated) present rather than sulphated; this is, however, rarely necessary.

INTERPRETATION OF HISTOCHEMICAL RESULTS

Alcian blue and dialysed iron Perls' techniques

Positive staining by tumour cells which is abolished by prior hyaluronidase digestion is most likely to be due to the presence of hyaluronic acid. This finding would support a diagnosis of mesothelioma. Acid mucin present in the tumour cells which was not digested by the enzyme, would indicate an epithelial neoplasm, possibly secondary adenocarcinoma.

Alcian blue-PAS technique

It is the PAS result which is significant in this instance. A positive reaction which was abolished by prior diastase digestion indicates glycogen in the tumour cells. This finding would support a diagnosis of mesothelioma.

Alternatively, should the PAS positive material be undigested by diastase treatment, then it would denote the presence of neutral mucin. This finding would not support a diagnosis of mesothelioma and, in fact, would indicate an epithelial neoplasm, possibly a secondary adenocarcinoma. Such a conclusion would be further supported if, in addition to neutral mucin, the tumour cells contained acid mucin which was unaffected by hyaluronidase digestion.

METHODS FOR ACID MUCINS

ALCIAN BLUE TECHNIQUE

Notes

The dye, first used in the dyeing of cotton, was introduced by Haddock (1948) being subsequently presented as a histochemical technique by Steedman (1950). Alcian blue, together with the related dye alcian yellow and the mixtures of the two forming alcian green 2 GX and alcian green 3 BX, is a copper phthalocyanin dye and contains positively charged groups capable of salt linkage with certain polyanions.

These polyanions consist of the sulphate and carboxyl radicals of the acid mucins — the phosphate radicals of the nucleic acid do not react. Consequently, only the acid mucins are stained and moreover intensely and permanently. Although certain insoluble calcium deposits in tissue also stain (through their non protein-bound phosphate radicals), the staining of mucins by the alcian dyes can be safely regarded, in practice, as being specific. The standard solution for staining acid mucins in general is 1% alcian blue in 3% acetic acid.

By varying the pH of the solution more information can be gained concerning the types of acid mucin present. At a pH of 0.2 only the strongly sulphated mucins will be ionized and thus react; at pH 1.0 both weakly and strongly sulphated mucins react, whilst at pH 2.5 most acid mucins with stain. A word of caution: using pH staining variation it is not always possible to obtain clear-cut demarcation of the different mucins. Better results may sometimes by obtained using varying electrolyte molarities of alcian blue solutions — the so-called critical electrolyte concentration (CEC) effect. The CEC-type techniques rely, according to the originators of this approach, on the fact that electrolytes such as magnesium chloride, if incorporated into the staining solution will compete with the alcian blue molecules for the points of attachment with the acid mucins. The point at which staining ceases, due to this electrolyte competition, is the CEC point and varies according to the substrate used. For example, below a molarity of 0.06 magnesium chloride both carboxyl and sulphate groups will stain with alcian blue. Above a molarity of 0.2–0.3 only sulphate radicals should stain (Scott & Dorling, 1965; Dorling, 1969; Scott et al 1968).

Alcian blue solutions slowly deteriorate with age and should be discarded after 6 months; as an additional precaution one should always filter before use. Celloidin is strongly stained by the alcian dyes and should be avoided, i.e. remove any celloidin films prior to staining.

Staining times are not, on the whole, critical and the ones specified will be found ample. Counterstaining should be minimal to avoid masking any weak alcian blue reactions.

VARYING pH TECHNIQUE

Solutions

pH 3.1: dissolve 1 g alcian blue in 0.5% acetic acid. pH 2.5: dissolve 1 g alcian blue in 3% acetic acid. pH 1.0: dissolve 1 g alcian blue in 0.1M hydrochloric acid. pH 0.2: dissolve 1 g alcian blue in 10% sulphuric acid.

0.5 per cent aqueous neutral red.

Technique

1. Take sections to distilled water.
2. Filter on the appropriate dye solution and leave for 5 min.
3. If the lower pH solutions are being used, drain and blot dry to prevent any alteration in staining due to water washing. Otherwise wash in water briefly.
4. Counterstain in 0.5% aqueous neutral red for 2–3 min.
5. Wash in water. Dehydrate, clear and mount as desired.

Results

At pH 3.1 and 2.5 most acid mucins (excepting some of the strongly sulphated group)	blue
At pH 1.0 only weakly and strongly sulphated acid mucins	blue
At pH 0.2 only the strongly sulphated group	blue
Nuclei	red
Background	very pale red or colourless

CRITICAL ELECTROLYTE CONCENTRATION (CEC) TECHNIQUE (SCOTT & DORLING, 1965)

Solutions

These should be prepared fresh for use.

0.05% alcian blue in 0.2M acetate buffer pH 5.8 (see Appendix 3).

Prepare a range of different molarity of electrolyte solutions with the above, using magnesium chloride ($MgCl_2$, $6 H_2O$ M.W. = 203·30) Having calculated the amount of salt required, add to the 0.05% alcian blue solution, mix well then filter. Note that the magnesium chloride is a deliquescent salt and will need to be stored under airtight conditions.

The following range of varying molarity magnesium chloride-alcian blue solutions is suggested as a useful workable scheme:

0.06 M
0.02–0.3 M
0.5–0.6 M
0.7–0.8 M
0.9–1.0 M

Technique

1. Take five identical sections to water.
2. Stain a section in each of the different alcian blue solutions overnight (i.e. 16–18 h).
3. Wash in water and counterstain in 0.5% aqueous neutral red, 2–3 mins.
4. Wash in water, dehydrate, clear and mount as desired.

Results

0.06 M magnesium chloride-alcian blue	all acid mucins stain blue (there will also be a weak background reaction)
0.2/0.3 M magnesium chloride-alcian blue	weakly and strongly sulphated mucins stain blue only
0.5/0.6 M magnesium chloride-alcian blue	strongly sulphated acid mucins stain blue only
0.7/0.8 M magnesium chloride-alcian blue	heparin/heparan sulphate and keratan sulphate stain blue only
0.9/1.0 M magnesium chloride-alcian blue	keratan sulphate stains blue only

DIALYSED IRON-PERLS TECHNIQUE

Notes

The use of a dialysed iron-Prussian blue reaction to visualize the acid mucins is a more sensitive technique than alcian blue, but tends to give nonspecific staining (Casselman, 1962; Korhonen & Makela, 1968). Whilst strong colouration of acid mucins is certainly afforded, we prefer the much simpler alcian blue technique for routine use, although the dialysed iron-Perls technique is useful for scanty deposits of acid mucins (see section dealing with mesothelioma identification p. 108). As with the alcian blue technique, it is possible to combine with PAS to afford a similar tinctorial distinction between acid and neutral mucins.

The rationale of the method is that at a low pH (1.9) colloidal iron is selectively adsorbed on to the acidic groups of mucin. The adsorbed iron is subsequently visualized by forming Prussian blue with potassium ferrocyanide. As any haemosiderin present in the tissue will also react, it is important to also take through a duplicate control section which is treated with the ferrocyanide-hydrochloric acid mixture only. Any consequent colouration should be borne in mind when assessing the results of the test section.

It will be found that a shorter-than-usual application of ferrocyanide-hydrochloric acid is necessary to avoid an undesirable heavy reaction with the colloidal iron and consequently heavier background. The dialysed iron solution will deteriorate with time and should not be used when more than 3 months old.

Solutions

Dialysed iron solution

Mix equal parts of dialysed iron (obtainable from British Drug Houses as a BPC 1949 preparation) and 2 M (12%) acetic acid.

2% aqueous potassium ferrocyanide.

2% hydrochloric acid.

1% aqueous neutral red.

Technique

1. Take the test and a duplicate control section to distilled water.
2. Treat the test section only with the dialysed iron-acetic solution for 10 min.
3. Wash well in several changes of distilled water.
4. Treat both test and control sections with the filtered solution consisting of equal parts of potassium ferrocyanide and hydrochloric acid for 10 min.
5. Wash well in distilled water.
6. Counterstain with neutral red for 5 min.
7. Dehydrate, clear and mount in a synthetic resin.

Results

Acid mucins, haemosiderin	dark blue
Collagen	pale blue
Nuclei	red

In the duplicate control section (not treated with dialysed iron) only haemosiderin will be blue.

SEPARATING ACID FROM NEUTRAL MUCINS

COMBINED ALCIAN BLUE-PAS TECHNIQUE (Mowry, 1956)

Notes

This is a most useful technique in that apart from distinguishing between acid mucins and neutral mucins, it also serves to demonstrate most mucins in the one preparation. This means in practice that a negative result, i.e. alcian blue negative and PAS negative, can be taken to mean that a given substance is unlikely to be a mucin.

The rationale of the method is that by first treating with alcian blue the acid mucins will stain and thus be unable to react with the subsequent PAS. By following on with the PAS only neutral mucins and carbohydrates such as glycogen will stain red.

Should a haematoxylin nuclear stain be used it is important to stain lightly to prevent cytoplasmic staining action as a potential source of confusion with the alcian blue. Mayer's haematoxylin solution is particularly suitable in this connection. The alcian greens or alcian yellow are unsuitable for this combined technique as they are more easily masked by the PAS.

Solutions

1% alcian blue in 3% acetic acid.

1% aqueous periodic acid.

Schiff's reagent, see page 102.

Technique

1. Take sections to distilled water.
2. Treat with the alcian blue solution for 5 min.
3. Wash well in distilled water.
4. Treat with the periodic acid solution for 5 min.
5. Wash well in distilled water. Then wash in Schiff's reagent for 15 min.
6. Wash in running water for 10 min.
7. Stain the nuclei with Mayer's haematoxylin solution. Differentiate and blue (see Notes)
8. Dehydrate, clear and mount as desired.

Results

Acid mucins	blue
Neutral mucins	red
Mixtures	purple
Nuclei	pale blue

METHODS FOR NEUTRAL MUCINS

These are widely occurring carbohydrates of epithelial origin which do not possess histochemically demonstrable anionic radicals so that for example, they do not stain with alcian blue. The reactive side chain hexose groups, however, permit their demonstration with PAS based techniques. One such has already been described (the combined alcian blue-PAS technique p. 111) and a blockade-PAS reaction will now be given, together with a technique employing carmine staining. Although neutral mucins and mucopro-

tein react in a similar manner histochemically, it should be appreciated that there are fundamental differences. The latter substance, in contrast to neutral mucin, may be derived from epithelium *or* connective tissue and also has a dominant protein moiety which may mask a reactive polyanion such as sialic acid (see p. 116).

PHENYLHYDRAZINE-PAS TECHNIQUE FOR NEUTRAL MUCIN (Spicer, 1961)

Notes

Aldehydes produced from neutral mucins can be blocked by phenylhydrazine so that they are subsequently Schiff negative. Acid mucins are not blocked. The rationale of this differential blockade is considered to devolve on the negatively charged phenylhydrazine molecules being repelled by negatively charged polyanions such as those of n-acetylated sialomucin and thus not blocked. Neutral mucins, on the other hand, being electrostatically neutral do not repel the phenylhydrazine with which they condense, and so become Schiff negative. Other normally PAS-positive substances such as glycogen and mucoproteins, will also be blocked.

The phenylhydrazine solution should be prepared fresh for use, although the dry reagent has a reasonably long room temperature shelf life. As is usual with this type of method one set of slides is treated with phenylhydrazine and another set with solvent only so that final comparisons can made.

Solutions

1% aqueous periodic acid

5% phenylhydrazine hydrochloride

Schiff's reagent, see page 102.

Technique

1. Take positive control and test sections to distilled water.

2. Treat all sections with periodic acid for 5 min.
3. Wash well in distilled water and treat the positive control and test sections with phenylhydrazine for 1 h. Duplicate sections are allowed to remain in distilled water for that period.
4. Wash the treated sections in running water for 5 min or so, then rinse well in distilled water.
5. Treat *all* sections with Schiff's reagent for 15 min.
6. Wash in running tap water for 5–10 min.
7. Stain the nuclei with a suitable haematoxylin such as Harris's solution. Differentiate and blue as per usual.
8. Dehydrate, clear and mount as desired.

Results

Neutral mucins	negative
Periodate-reactive acid mucins	magenta
Nuclei	blue

CARMINE TECHNIQUE FOR NEUTRAL MUCINS (Berger & Pizzolato, 1976)

Notes

A simplified Best's carmine solution is employed in this technique for neutral mucin which is stained a bright red colour — along with glycogen and, to a lesser extent cell nuclei, elastin and keratin. The authors suggested rationale is that of hydrogen bonding of the carmine by hydroxyl groups on the neutral mucin complexes. As with Best's carmine technique (p. 122) the high (12.0) pH of the solution prevents dye to tissue binding based on ionic interactions alone.

Staining may be by the carmine solution alone, or (as we prefer) preceded by alcian blue staining to give a combined demonstration of acid and neutral mucins in a similar manner to the combined alcian blue-PAS technique (p. 111). The technique is easy to perform and seems, in our limited experience, to give reproducible results.

Solutions

1% alcian blue in 3% acetic acid.

Carmine solution

Dissolve 1 g potassium carbonate in 70% alcohol, then add 1 g carmine and mix thoroughly. Filter. The solution remains stable for upto 3 days at 4° C.

Technique

1. Take sections to water.
2. Stain with alcian blue for 5 min.
3. Wash in water, then in 70% alcohol.
4. Stain with the carmine solution for 30–45 min.
5. Wash in 95% alcohol (washing in water will extract the stain), then in absolute alcohol. Clear and mount as desired.

Results

Neutral mucin and glycogen	red
Cell nuclei, keratin and elastin	pale red
Acid mucins	blue

METHODS FOR SULPHATED MUCINS

HIGH IRON DIAMINE TECHNIQUE FOR SULPHOMUCINS (Spicer, 1965)

Notes

Sulphated mucins are clearly and specifically demonstrated by this method which has become the standard technique for the demonstration of this large and somewhat complex group of substances. The rationale is treating sections with a mixture of certain diamine salts and ferric chloride, a black/brown cationic complex is formed which bonds to sulphate-containing moieties. The accepted specificity of the technique is largely due to the low (1.4) pH of the reactant solution, at which pH level carboxylated moieties are non-ionized. It is important that the stated times of treatment are not exceeded, as otherwise non-sulphated mucins also progressively react.

Following the demonstration of sulphomucins with high iron diamine, counterstaining with a pH 2.5 alcian blue solution will then stain carboxylated mucins a contrasting blue colour. It is convenient to purchase the ferric chloride as a 60% solution, but discard when more than a few weeks old.

Solutions

High iron diamine

N, N-dimethyl-meta-phenylene-diamine dihydrochloride*	120 mg
N, N-dimethyl-para-phenylenediamine dihydrochloride*	20 mg
Distilled water	50 ml
Ferric chloride (60 % BDH solution)	1.4 ml

Dissolve the two diamine salts simultaneously in the distilled water, then add to the ferric chloride solution and mix. (The mixing is conveniently done in a Coplin jar.)

1% alcian blue in 3% acetic acid.

0.5% aqueous neutral red.

Technique

1. Take a positive control and the test sections down to distilled water.
2. Treat all sections with the high iron diamine solution for 18–24 h.
3. Wash well in running water.
4. Stain with the alcian blue solution for 5 min.
5. Wash in water, stain nuclei with the neutral red solution for 2–3 min.
6. Wash in water, dehydrate, clear and mount as desired.

Results

Sulphated mucins	black/brown
Carboxylated mucins	blue
Nuclei	red

*Obtainable from: Kodak Ltd., Industrial and Research Chemical Sales, Kirkby, Liverpool.

COMBINED ALDEHYDE FUCHSIN-ALCIAN BLUE TECHNIQUE (Spicer & Meyer, 1960)

Notes

This method depends on the greater affinity of sulphated mucins for aldehyde fuchsin as opposed to that of the carboxylated mucins (neutral mucins do not stain unless pre-oxidants such as periodic acid are used). If alcian blue staining follows then the sulphated mucins will not stain as they will have taken up the aldehyde fuchsin comparatively strongly, only the carboxylated mucins stain blue. Pre-oxidants, such as iodine or potassium permanganate, are unnecessary for the reaction. (For a discussion of the rationale of aldehyde fuchsin staining see p. 55).

Bearing in mind the fact that the aldehyde fuchsin staining is not specific for sulphated mucins (elastin will also stain), it is nonetheless a successful technique and one that we have found reliable.

The general points appertaining to the preparation of aldehyde fuchsin apply here (p. 56).

Solutions

Aldehyde fuchsin solution, see page 55.

1% alcian blue in 3% acetic acid.

Technique

1. Take sections to 70% alcohol.
2. Treat with the aldehyde fuchsin solution for 20 min.
3. Rinse well in 70% alcohol, then in water.
4. Stain with the alcian blue solution for 5 min.
5. Wash in water. Dehydrate, clear and mount in a synthetic mountant.

Results

Strongly sulphated mucins	deep purple
Elastin, weakly sulphated mucins	purple
Carboxylated mucins	blue

ALUMINIUM SULPHATE-ALCIAN BLUE TECHNIQUE (Heath, 1961)

Notes

Certain dyes, such as thionin, toluidine blue, methylene blue, nuclear fast red and alcian blue when dissolved in an aluminium sulphate solution, will stain only sulphated mucins. Heath attributed this to the formation of mordant-type chelate bonds. However it seems more likely that this is a CEC type reaction (see p. 110), in which competition of the aluminium ions with alcian blue for binding with carboxyl groups takes place.

We have found it to be a reasonably reliable technique although not infallible, and of undoubted use as a screening method. Of the various dyes specified alcian blue is probably the best due to its comparative insolubility in the post-staining dehydrating alcohols. The staining solutions do not keep well and it is advisable to prepare fresh ones when more than 3–4 weeks old.

There are two points to note: a known positive control should always be taken through with the test section; and amounts of positively-staining material may be scanty so that it is important not to over-counterstain with neutral red.

Solution

Dissolve 0.1 g alcian blue in 100 ml of boiling 5% aqueous aluminium sulphate. Cool and filter.

Technique

1. Take sections to distilled water.
2. Drain the slide and stain with the alcian blue solution for 30 min.
3. Wash in distilled water.
4. Counterstain with 0.5% aqueous neutral red for 2–3 min.
5. Wash in water, dehydrate, clear and mount as desired.

Results

Sulphated mucins	blue
Nuclei	red

Carboxylated mucins will also often stain red.

37° C ('MILD') METHYLATION TECHNIQUE (Spicer, 1960)

Notes

Strictly speaking, carboxylated mucins are also identified but by exclusion of staining rather than positive staining, so this particular technique will be placed in the 'sulphated only' group. The technique involves the use of methanol (plus hydrochloric acid as a catalyst for the reaction) and brings about the blockade of carboxyl groups by forming methyl esters, so that if subsequent alcian blue staining is carried out only sulphated mucins will stain. In practice, the reactivity of the strongly sulphated mucins may also be blocked.

This method, the so-called 'mild methylation' technique is a reasonably reliable one but it is important to methylate for no longer than 4 h. Controls are also important as will be detailed.

For critical work it is always better, with this type of technique, to cut serial sections numbering them so that only adjacent sections are used.

Solutions

0.1 M (0.8%) hydrochloric acid in methanol (prepare fresh).

1% alcian blue in 3% acetic acid.

Technique

1. Take two positive control and two test sections to distilled water.
2. Drain and treat one positive control and one test section with preheated reagent for 4 h at 37° C. The remaining two sections may be left in distilled water for the same time and temperature.
3. Wash all sections well in water for 5 min or so.
4. Stain with the alcian blue solution for 5 min.
5. Wash in water. Counterstain in 0.5% aqueous neutral red for 2–3 min.
6. Wash in water. Dehydrate, clear and mount as desired.

Results

Sulphated mucins only	blue (the untreated sections should show no loss of staining)
Nuclei	red

METHODS FOR CARBOXYLATED MUCINS

METHYLATION-SAPONIFICATION TECHNIQUE (Spicer & Lillie, 1959)

Notes

The rationale of this technique is that both carboxylated (i.e. sialomucin and hyaluronic acid) and sulphated mucins are blocked by methylation at 60° C, the former being esterfied and the latter hydrolysed. Subsequent 'saponification' in a strong alkali will break the methyl-carboxyl ester bonds allowing subsequent restoration of the alcian blue staining. The sulphated mucins having been hydrolysed will not show this restoration of staining.

The technique is popular amongst workers in this field; why this is so we find hard to comprehend as the results are known to be of dubious reliability. In our experience, and those of other workers, both false positive and false negative post-saponification staining can occur.

There are two practical points to bear in mind when carrying out the technique. Firstly, the sections tend to come off the slide, particularly during saponification. It is wise, therefore, to use a section adhesive and to cover the section with celloidin (remove before staining!): although according to Sorvari & Stoward (1970) section loss may be minimized by saponifying for 2 h at 4° C. Secondly, during the methylation stage phosphate groups of the nucleic acids will also be hydrolysed so that the normal nuclear basophilia will be lost. Because of this, final counterstaining in neutral red will prove difficult and we have found eosin to give a background of acceptable contrast.

Control sections are again essential and will be described.

Solutions

0.1 M hydrochloric acid in methanol.
1% potassium hydroxide in 70% alcohol.
1% alcian blue in 3% acetic acid.
1% aqueous eosin (ws).

Technique

1. Take three sections each of positive control and test material down to distilled water. Label one test section and one of control material 'A', another similar pair of sections 'B' and the third pair of section 'C'. Celloidinize all slides.
2. Place sections 'A' and 'B' in preheated methanol-hydrochloric acid for 5 h at 60° C. Place the 'C' sections in distilled water for the same time and temperature.
3. Wash all sections well in water for 5 min or so. Rinse in distilled water.
4. Treat sections 'A' with the alcoholic potassium hydroxide solution for 30 min at room temperature, leaving the B and C sections in 70% alcohol only for this period.
5. Wash all sections well in water for 5 min or so.
6. Remove the celloidin film from the slides and stain with the alcian blue solution for 5 min.
7. Wash in water. Stain with 1% aqueous eosin for 15–20 s.
8. Wash in water. Dehydrate, clear and mount as desired.

Results

Sections A	only carboxylated mucins should stain blue
Sections B	both sulphated and carboxylated mucins are blocked and there should be no alcian blue staining at all
Section C	all acid mucins should be stained blue
Background	pink

SIALIDASE (NEURAMINIDASE) DIGESTION FOR N-ACETYLATED SIALOMUCINS (Spicer et al, 1962)

Notes

Sialidase digestion, when followed by alcian blue staining, will give reliable presumptive evidence of

N-acetylated sialic acid moieties by loss of alcian-ophilia. As mentioned, it is indeed a reliable technique if carefully carried out but it should be remembered that a proportion of sialomucins are sialidase-resistant (see following techniques).

Should the combined alcian blue-PAS technique follow digestion it will be seen that the sialidase-labile sialomucins, whilst losing their normal alcianophilia, will be stained red. This is due to the fact that sialomucins are PAS-positive, a feature not normally shown by the undigested material in the combined stain because they first take up alcian blue.

Calcium ions, in the form of calcium chloride, are incorporated into the enzyme solution as a necessary activator for the reaction.

Celloidinization of paraffin sections may block the action of the enzyme and is better avoided.

Solutions

Sialidase

1 unit per 1 ml sialidase (neuraminidase) ex *Vibrio cholerae** diluted to 1 in 5 with pH 5.5 acetate buffer, with 1% calcium chloride w/v added.

1% alcian blue in 3% acetic acid.

0.5% aqueous neutral red.

Technique

1. Take two duplicate test and two duplicate positive control sections to distilled water.
2. Treat one test and one positive control section with the preheated buffered enzyme in a damp chamber for 16 h at 37° C. The remaining duplicate sections are treated with the buffer only for the stated time and temperature.
3. Wash all sections well in water.
4. Stain with the alcian blue solution for 5 min. Wash in water.
5. Counterstain in the 0.5% aqueous neutral red for 2–3 min.
6. Wash in water. Dehydrate, clear and mount as desired.

*Obtainable from Koch Light Ltd., Haverhill, Suffolk.

Results

N-acetylated (sialidase-labile) sialomucins	loss of alcianophilia
All other acid mucins	blue
Nuclei	red

BOROHYDRIDE-SAPONIFICATION-PAS TECHNIQUE FOR O-ACETYLATED SIALOMUCINS (modified from Culling et al, 1975)

Notes

We are concerned, here, with the N-acetyl O-acetyl form of sialomucin which, in contrast to the N-acetylated form, is not only resistant to the action of the enzyme sialidase but is also PAS negative.

This PAS negativity of O-acetylated sialomucin was utilized by the above workers to demonstrate, in specific PAS terms, this particular entity. This was done primarily for the purpose of identifying secondary colo-rectal adenocarcinomas, in which this particular type of mucin was considered to be a significant feature.

The rationale of the method is that initial sodium borohydride treatment following periodic acid oxidation blocks the formed aldehydes from a wide range of normally PAS positive substances. Alkaline hydrolysis (saponification) follows which breaks the PAS inhibitory O-acyl bond of the resistant form of sialomucin. Thus a subsequent periodic acid-Schiff reaction will only now stain magenta the previously negative sialomucin.

There are two practical points of importance. Firstly sections may become detached from the slide during the borohydride or saponification stages. Therefore section adhesives (see p. 24) should be used and/or celloidinization of the slides. The second point to note is that glycogen staining may well still be evident at the conclusion of the technique. To minimize this, it is important to use an increased initial oxidation time, so that as many aldehydes as possible will be blocked by the subsequent borohydride blockade. Even so, weak glycogen staining is often present in the final result.

A suitable positive control is that of paraffin sections from colon or rectum.

Solutions

Sodium borohydride

Sodium borohydride	0.1 g
Disodium hydrogen phosphate (anhyd.)	1 g
Distilled water	100 ml

Dissolve the phosphate salt in the water, followed by the sodium borohydride; the working pH should be 9.4.

Saponification

Potassium hydroxide	0.5 g
70% ethanol	100 ml

1% aqueous periodic acid.

Schiff reagent (see, p. 102)

Technique

1. Take test sections plus positive control sections to distilled water. Label one positive control and one of each test section 'A'; and equivalent set 'B' and a third set 'C'.
2. Treat all sections (A, B and C) with periodic acid for 30 min.
3. Wash well in distilled water, then treat the A and B sections only with the borohydride solution for 30 min.
4. Wash well in running water, then A sections only in 70 % alcohol followed by the potassium hydroxide solution for 30 min. Finally, the A sections are washed in 70 % alcohol, then in several changes of distilled water followed by periodic acid treatment for 5 min.
5. Treat all sections A, B and C with Schiff reagent for 15 min.
6. Wash well in running water and counterstain with haematoxylin as per the standard PAS technique (p. 102).

Results

Sections A — only O-acetylated sialomucin stains magenta (but see notes)
Sections B — these should be negative

Sections C — all normally PAS positive substances will stain magenta.

SULPHURIC ACID HYDROLYSIS TECHNIQUE FOR SIALOMUCINS (Lamb & Reid, 1969; Allen, 1970)

Notes

Both sialidase-resistant and sialidase-labile forms of sialomucin are demonstrated by this technique, which employs sulphuric acid hydrolysis to destroy their normal affinity for alcian blue. By carrying out this technique in conjunction with the sialidase digestion technique, it will readily be determined whether or not a given sialomucin is in the enzyme-labile or enzyme-resistant form. It is a reasonably reliable technique but the hydrolysis does tend to slightly weaken the subsequent basophilia of the acid mucins generally. Minor losses of alcian blue staining should be discounted. On occasion, a sialomucin may be present which is relatively resistant to sulphuric acid hydrolysis and will need extended times of treatment before the alcianophilia is destroyed.

The original technique of Lamb and Reid called for a 1 h treatment at 80° C. This somewhat drastic treatment has been modified by Allen and employs a temperature of 60° C. Even so, section loss may occur and it is prudent to not only use a section adhesive but also to celloidinize the sections.

Due to the concomitant acid hydrolysis of the nucleic acids nuclear-type counterstains such as neutral red are not successful; it is better to use one of the cytoplasmic dyes such as eosin. The sulphuric acid solution should be preheated to the desired temperature using a Coplin jar placed in a water bath at the appropriate temperature.

Solutions

0.5 M sulphuric acid.
1% alcian blue in 3% acetic acid.
1% aqueous eosin (ws).

Technique

1. Take two positive control and two test sections to distilled water.

2. Treat one of the test and one of the positive control sections (celloidinized) with the preheated sulphuric acid for 2 h at 60° C. The remaining test and control sections should be placed in distilled water for the stated time and temperature.
3. Wash in water for 5–10 min. Remove any celloidin films in alcohol-ether.
4. Stain with the alcian blue solution for 5 min. Wash in water.
5. Counterstain briefly (20 s or so) in 1% aqueous eosin.
6. Wash in water, dehydrate, clear and mount as desired.

Results

Sialidase-labile and siali-
dase-resistant sialomucins — loss of alcian blue staining

All other acid mucins — blue
Background — pink

HYALURONIDASE DIGESTION FOR HYALURONIC ACID (modified from Pearse, 1953)

Notes

The most easily obtainable form of the enzyme is that derived from bovine testis. Using this, chondroitin sulphates A and C are digested as well as hyaluronic acid, so that the appropriate techniques for those entities may need to be carried out to determine exactly what has been digested (see (see Fig. 2.1). The principle of the method, which is normally a reliable one, is that following treatment with hyaluronidase the sections are stained with alcian blue. Loss of staining, when compared to a non-treated duplicate section, establishes the

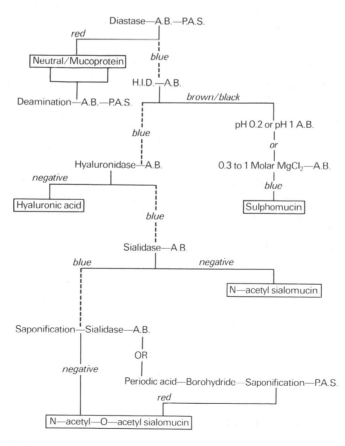

Fig. 2.1 Mucins and their identification.

presence of one or more of the three hyaluroni-dase-labile mucins. If only scanty deposits of mucin are present, it may be advantageous to use the more sensitive dialysed iron-Perls' technique (p. 111). If the presence of the highly sulphated mucins is suspected, a low pH alcian blue should be done. An alternative form of the enzyme is that produced from various bacteria such as staphylococci and pneumococci. This bacterial hyaluronidase is much more selective in its action as only hyaluronic acid and hyaluronosulphate (an uncommon mucin found in cornea) are digested. Unfortunately the bacterial enzyme is obtained commercially only with difficulty.

The pH prescribed (6.7) whilst optimal is not ciritcal and minor deviations from this may safely be made.

Solutions

Hyaluronidase
   Dissolve 1 mg Type IV testicular hyaluronidase★ in 1 ml of pH 6.7 phosphate buffer.

1% alcian blue in 3% acetic (1% alcian blue in 0.2 M hydrochloric acid at pH 0.5 may also be used; see Notes). Alternatively, the dialysed iron-Perls' technique may be used (see Notes).

Technique

1. Take two duplicate test and two duplicate positive control sections to distilled water.
2. Treat one section only of test and control material with the preheated buffered enzyme for 3 h at 37° C. The remaining sections are placed in buffer only for the stated time and temperature.
3. Wash all sections well in water.
4. Stain with the alcian blue solution for 5 min. Wash in water.
5. Counterstain with 0.5% aqueous neutral red for 2–3 min.
6. Wash in water. Dehydrate, clear and mount as desired.

Obtainable from Sigma Chemical Company Ltd., Poole, Dorset.

Results

Hyaluronic acid (also hyaluronosulphate, chondroitin sulphates A and C)	loss of alcianophilia
Other acid mucins	blue
Nuclei	red

GLYCOGEN

The term 'glycogen' is derived from 'glycogenic' substance coined by Bernard in 1849. A more contemporary synonym is 'homoglycans' which is much less often used than the older, more established term. Chemically it is a simple polysaccharide consisting of branched glucose chains of two types: (1) lyoglycogen, a water-soluble form; (2) desmoglycogen a water insoluble and protein bound form. The association of glycogen to protein is almost certainly on a physical basis, rather than a chemical one (Meyer & Jeanloz, 1943).

Under normal conditions glycogen is usually (but not exclusively) intracytoplasmic and found in cardiac and voluntary muscle, liver, hair follicles, retina, early secretory endometrium, cervical and vaginal epithelium; also in cells such as megakaryocytes and leucocytes.

From a pathological aspect the demonstration of glycogen is, on the whole, a contributory factor to diagnosis, rather than as an essential part of diagnosis. Its greatest use, in our experience, is in the identification of secondary deposits of renal carcinoma, where the often considerable quantities of intracellular glycogen serve as a very useful marker. Glycogen may be found intranuclearly in liver cells and in the cytoplasms of renal tubule cells in diabetes. Certain other types of tumour cell show demonstrable quantities also; such as those of squamous carcinoma, transitional cell carcinoma, lymphosarcoma and primary hepatic carcinoma (hepatoma).

A group of allied congenital disorders of glycogen metabolism must also be mentioned. These are the glycogenoses of which there are currently types I to IX inclusive. The glycogenoses are associated with various enzyme deficiencies and exhibit varying degrees of excessive glycogen deposition in liver and other organs such as the heart.

FIXATION AND PRESERVATION

Fixation and preservation of glycogen is an important aspect of glycogen histochemistry.

There seems general agreement that fixatives such as Rossman's solution, Gendre's solution (see Appendix for formulae), 10% formal-alcohol or 80% alcohol give the most satisfactory preservation. Zenker-acetic or the Heidenhain 'Susa' fixatives seem to be contraindicated (Manns, 1958; Murgatroyd, 1971). Due to the solubility of free glycogen it was traditional to avoid aqueous fixatives such as formalin but glycogen loss in these fixatives is, in practice, minimal due probably to its close association, in tissue, with protein (Manns, 1958). It should be noted, however, that the component glycogen of the glycogenoses is water soluble, and thus formalin should be avoided.

Fixation should be prompt and preferably carried out at 4° C. At this temperature glycogen loss is reduced and the characteristic 'streaming' or polarization effect, seen with room temperature fixation, avoided. The polarization of glycogen is absent with freeze drying or freeze substitution techniques. The absence of glycogen polarization at low temperatures is presumably due to the slower penetration rate of the fixing fluids presenting minimal stress forces to the glycogen. Therefore, displacement is lessened. The type of fixative employed will affect the presentation of the glycogen in stained preparations. Alcohol and picric acid fixation tend to produce a coarser granule than say, formalin, whilst acidification of alcoholic fixatives seems to accentuate clumping of the glycogen granules.

Decalcification of calcium-containing tissue can cause loss of glycogen and in a series to determine the optimal combination of fixative and decalcifying agent Ferraz et al (1966) recommended Gendre fixation followed by 5% trichloracetic acid.

Regarding the preparation of sections for glycogen demonstration Murgatroyd (1969) recom-

mended freeze drying for maximum preservation and preferred paraffin to frozen sections. However, Lake (1970) stated that unfixed cryostat sections are to be preferred when demonstrating the abnormal glycogens of the glycogenoses. In our experience paraffin sections are usually suitable for most purposes of glycogen demonstration, although there is undoubtedly a variable loss of glycogen with paraffin processing following formalin fixation. To counter this, it will be found efficaceous to secondary fix the tissue blocks in Rossman's solution (see Appendix) for 24 h, prior to paraffin processing.

Celloidinization of sections

Celloidinization has enjoyed considerable vogue in the past, but there now seems to be considerable doubt as to the necessity for its use when dealing with the usual glycogen deposits in tissue (Manns, 1958; Murgatroyd, 1969). Originally it was considered that coating slides with celloidin prevented any loss of glycogen from the sections, particularly when they were in contact with water. As was mentioned previously, glycogen is held in a protein matrix and is thus not easily dissolved out, as was once thought to be the case. Lillie (1965), for example, considered that celloidinization of sections for glycogen demonstration served no useful purpose other than, perhaps, to retard section loss during staining with highly alkaline solutions such as Best's carmine. However, when dealing with fresh cryostat sections celloidinization is undoubtedly necessary as translocation of glycogen will otherwise occur.

DEMONSTRATION

In addition to the technique to be described one may use the Grocott-Gomori hexamine-silver (see p. 212) or the Langhans (1890) iodine technique. The latter technique stains glycogen a dark brown colour. It is, however, impermanent and nonspecific and nowadays very little used for glycogen demonstration.

The main techniques for glycogen are still the PAS and Best's carmine techniques. Which of these is to be used we suggest is a matter of practical convenience, for whilst Best's carmine undoubtedly gives the more intense and selective colouration of glycogen, the staining solution does not keep well and is rather time-consuming to prepare. So that unless glycogen demonstration is to be regularly carried out, it is probably simpler to perform the PAS technique as it is a rare laboratory that does not maintain a constant supply of Schiff's reagent.

BEST'S CARMINE TECHNIQUE (Best, 1906)

Notes

This is a popular, highly selective technique for glycogen staining as it dyes the carbohydrate a distinctive red colour. Unfortunately it is prone to dye precipitation artefact and is rather time-consuming in terms of reagent preparation.

The rationale of the technique has been assiduously studied by several workers, who attribute the staining of glycogen by carmine to the formation of hydrogen bonds between OH groups on the glycogen and H_2 bonds on the carmine molecule (Goldstein, 1962; Murgatroyd, 1969).

The dye used in the rather complex solution is carmine. This is obtained from extracted cochineal and contains some 56% carminic acid which is the active staining ingredient. Carmine, as such, was first used in biological work as long ago as 1778, but was not employed in microtechnique until 1849. Not until 1884 was pure carminic acid used widely. The function of the potassium salts is attributed to that of inhibiting nonspecific (background) staining due to ionic attraction between the negatively charged carminic acid, and any available tissue cations such as the basic proteins. The ammonia used in the solution appears to have the twin functions of acting partly as a solvent for the carminic acid, and partly to maintain a high (10.0) pH; below this pH level staining is less selective (Murgatroyd, 1969).

There are several practical points worthy of note. The dye precipitation on to the section which not uncommonly occurs, is due to evaporation of the ammonia in which the carminic acid is highly soluble. It is sound practice to filter the working solution and to use it only in a closed container. For similar reasons it is unwise to allow the slide to dry following staining and before washing in alcohol. Whilst Best's differentiatior is often prescribed, both methanol and industrial methylated spirit can be used equally well. The stain solution fairly quickly deteriorates, even if stored at 4 °C and the staining time will need to be lengthened when it is more than 2–3 weeks old.

Of interest is the use of dyes such as alizarin and haematein, having potential hydrogen bonding properties, to stain glycogen when used in a Best carmine-type solution. Successful results have been claimed (Murgatroyd & Horobin, 1969). We have tried out the haematein variant for glycogen, but considered the results inferior to those given by Best's solution.

Best's carmine is not specific for glycogen as fibrin and neutral mucin also stain, albeit more weakly (Casselman, 1962; Lauren & Sovari, 1967). The latter group of workers, incidentally, were able to stain Paneth cell granules using Best's carmine, preceded by a methylation treatment for 6 h at 56° C. We have been unable to reproduce their results.

Although diastase-digested controls are not perhaps as essential with Best's technique as for the PAS technique, on account of the former's high selectivity for glycogen, it is probably good practice to have controls bearing in mind that Best's technique is not truly specific. What is more important is that sections of positive control material should also be taken through in order to establish the efficacy of the staining solution.

Solutions

Carmine stock solution

To 60 ml distilled water, add 2 g carmine; 1 g potassium carbonate and 5 g potassium chloride. Boil gently in a large flask (to avoid spillage due to the resultant effervescence) for 6 min. Cool and add 20 ml concentrated ammonia. Filter and store in a dark container at 4° C where it will keep for 1–2 months.

Working solution

Stock solution	15 ml
Conc. ammonia	12.5 ml
Methanol	12.5 ml

The staining time to be given is for the freshly prepared solution. It is worth increasing this time as the stock solution ages.

Best's differentiator

Methanol	40 ml
Ethanol	80 ml
Distilled water	100 ml

Technique

1. Take test and positive control sections to water.
2. Treat duplicate sections only of test and control material with diastase (see p. 124) subsequently washing well in water.
3. Stain the nuclei of all sections well using one of the iron haematoxylin solutions. Differentiate and blue so that the background is clear.
4. Treat with the carmine solution for 10 min.
5. Without delay transfer the slides to a Coplin jar of differentiating solution (see notes).
6. Wash in fresh alcohol, clear in xylene and mount as desired.

Results

Glycogen	bright red
Neutral mucin, mast cells, fibrin	pale red
Nuclei	blue

CHROMIC ACID-SCHIFF TECHNIQUE (CAS) (Bauer, 1933)

Notes

This is the oldest of the more popular oxidant-Schiff reactions, and uses chromium trioxide as the oxidant. The colour reaction obtained is weaker and more selective than that given by the conventional PAS technique. Because PAS-positive substances such as collagen, reticulin and basement membranes (basal lamina) are not shown in the Bauer-Schiff method (due to the lessened dialdehyde formation of chromic acid, as opposed to periodic acid, oxidation) some workers favour the technique as giving more easily interpreted results. However, Lillie (1947) considered the technique to be unreliable in that small glycogen deposits are not demonstrated. Our own feeling is that nothing is to be gained by using the CAS as opposed to the PAS.

Diastase controls should again be used, as substances of the mucin group will also react.

Solutions

5% aqueous chromium trioxide.

Schiff's reagent, see page 102.

Technique

1. Take test and control sections to distilled water. Diastase digest (p. 124)
2. Wash well in water for 5–10 min. Rinse in distilled water.
3. Oxidize with the chromium trioxide solution for 1 h.
4. Wash well in several changes of distilled water.
5. Treat with Schiff's reagent for 10 min.
6. Wash in running water for 5–10 min.
7. Stain with haematoxylin (Harris's or an iron haematoxylin). Differentiate and blue.
8. Dehydrate. clear and mount as desired.

Results

Glycogen, neutral mucins, certain acidic mucins	magenta
Glycogen only will be diastase-labile	
nuclei	blue

POTASSIUM PERMANGANATE-ALCIAN BLUE TECHNIQUE (Cook, 1974)

Notes

It is a fairly well-established fact that certain oxidants will, unlike periodic acid, overoxidize aldehydes formed from vic glycol-containing substances to carboxylic acids. Use is made of this in the following technique to form carboxyl groups in glycogen capable of binding electrostatically with alcian blue. Prolonged potassium permanganate oxidation is used and the results, whilst inferior to those of the conventional PAS technique, are sufficiently strong to serve as practical proof of a theoretical premise.

Any mucin present will also stain, but again, diastase digestion can be carried out on duplicate sections.

Solutions

1% aqueous potassium permanganate.

5% aqueous oxalic acid.

1% alcian blue in 3% acetic acid.

1% aqueous neutral red.

Technique

1. Take sections to distilled water.
2. Treat with the potassium permanganate solution for 1 h.
3. Wash in water and bleach with the oxalic acid solution for 10–30 s.
4. Wash well in water for 5–10 min.
5. Stain with the alcian blue solution for 5 min. Wash in water.
6. Counterstain in the neutral red solution for 5 min.
7. Wash in water. Dehydrate, clear and mount as desired.

Results

Glycogen, mucins	blue
Nuclei	red
Background	pale blue

DIGESTION TECHNIQUES

DIASTASE/AMYLASE-PAS

Notes

Diastase digestion is often employed to render moderately selective methods for glycogen, such as PAS, highly-selective or specific in practice. According to Bernfeld (1951) the rationale hinges on the hydrolysis of the glycogen to water-soluble maltose, which dissolves out in the aqueous solvent used. Malt diastase or alpha-amylase can be used, although it must be said that human saliva is equally effective if one disregards the aesthetic aspects. We prefer to use a fairly strong (1%) diastase solution and have experienced little or no increase in section loss during treatment or subsequent staining. Any starch granules which may be present as an incidental feature will show a PAS positivity which is also diastase-labile, albeit much less readily.

There are several points to note with regard to glycogen digestion.

1. Celloidinization of sections inhibits digestion.
2. Using the PAS technique poststaining digestion is not effective unlike the Best's carmine technique where digestion of glycogen can be carried out either preceding or following staining.
3. The fixation employed will affect the rate, or indeed, the ability of the enzyme to digest glycogen. For example, it has been shown that following Gendre and glutaraldehyde fixation the digestion times may need to be increased (Byron, 1970) whilst osmium tetroxide has been shown to inhibit digestion (Sasse, 1965).
4. Control sections are essential.

There seems little point in using the Hotchkiss PAS as opposed to the McManus variant—again this devolves around contemporary rethinking of glycogen fixation/solubility processes. An interesting point is that according to Ovadia & Stoward (1971) only 23–24% of glycogen is oxidized by conventional periodate solutions even after prolonged treatment. They suggested that an increase in Schiff reaction may be obtained by incorporating an electrolyte with the iodate solution. (This would presumably result in a decreased repulsion of the negatively charged periodate ions and glycogen molecules).

Solutions

1% aqueous malt diastase.*

1% aqueous periodic acid.

* Obtainable from R. A. Lamb, London, N.W. 10.

Schiff's reagent, see p. 102.

Technique

1. Take two test section and two positive control sections to distilled water.
2. Treat one of the test sections and one control section with the aqueous diastase solution for 1 h at 37° C.
3. Wash well in water for 5–10 min.
4. Treat all sections with periodic acid and Schiff's reagent and counterstain with haematoxylin in the usual way (see p. 102).
5. Dehydrate, clear and mount as desired.

Results

Glycogen (or starch)	red staining material present in the undigested sections but absent in the digested sections
Nuclei	blue

PECTINASE

Notes

Whilst normal glycogen deposits in tissue are fairly readily digested by diastase, there occurs in the rare type IV glycogenosis (amylopectinosis) a polysaccharide which is only readily extracted by the enzyme pectinase (Ishak et al, 1978).

Solutions

0.4% pectinase* in pH 4.0 acetate buffer (see Appendix).

1% aqueous periodic acid.

Schiff's reagent, see page 102.

---

* Obtainable from Sigma Chemical Company Ltd., Poole, Dorset.

Technique

(taken from Lillie, 1965)

1. Test and control sections are taken to water. Rinse in pH 4.0 buffer.
2. Treat a positive control section and test sections with the enzyme solution for 48 h at 37° C. Duplicate sections are treated with buffer solution only under similar conditions.
3. Carry out the standard PAS technique (p. 102).
4. Dehydrate, clear and mount as desired.

Results

Glycogen (both normal and abnormal) also some mucins are rendered PAS negative by the enzyme treatment.

STARCH

Starch is a polysaccharide consisting of two major components: amylose and amylopectin.

Starch granules are often present as contaminants from starch-containing surgical glove powders in sites of surgical operations. Very occasionally these granules may set up an inflammatory reaction resulting in a starch granuloma. Starch is not easily discerned in H and E preparations: therefore, its demonstration in such a lesion is of importance.

DEMONSTRATION

Starch granules vary from round to polyhedral in shape and are roughly 15–20 μm in size and a typical feature is the presence of a central refractile 'droplet' in each granule. Staining varies from pale pink (usually) to blue with H and E preparations and they are PAS positive and hexamine silver positive (p. 102 and 212 respectively). The granules stain blue with iodine solutions. Starch is slowly digested with diastase, and with the polarizing microscope exhibits a Maltese cross-type of birefringence.

Table 9.2 Techniques for starch, cellulose and chitin

Polysaccharide	Technique						
	E	I	PAS	C	B	G	AB
Starch	±	+	+	V	+	+	−
Cellulose	V	+	+	+	+	+	−
Chitin	+	−	+	V	±	+	−

Key: E, eosin (as in H and E). I, iodine. PAS, periodic acid-Schiff. C, Congo red. B, birefringence. G. Grocott. AB, alcian blue. V, variable reaction. +, positive reaction. ± weak reaction. −, negative.

LANGHANS IODINE TECHNIQUE
(Langhans, 1890)

Notes

The following slightly modified technique, whilst impermanent, gives results which are stable for a few days at least. After this period the blue colour of the starch reverts to the normal brown of the iodine. The production of the blue colour with iodine is, of course, the classical test for starch and presumably involves an oxidation process by the iodine. On eventual mounting this oxidation is reversed by reduction processes.

The dehydrating alcohols contain iodine to minimize loss of this from the section, as the iodine is highly soluble in alcohol.

Solution

Lugol's iodine, see page 204.

Technique

1. Take sections to water.
2. Stain with Lugol's iodine for 10 min.
3. Drain and blot dry.
4. Dehydrate rapidly in absolute alcohols which are saturated with iodine. Clear in xylene and mount in a DPX-type resin.

Results

Starch	blue
Glycogen, amyloid, cellulose	brown
Background	yellow-brown

CELLULOSE

The demonstration of cellulose in human tissue is of very little consequence in diagnostic pathology. Usually the only occasions where this is to be seen is where the cellulose presents as undigested food particles in the lumen of an appendix. As such material is on rare occasions implicated in inflammatory lesions, e.g. foreign bodies in skin and intestinal fistulae, the necessity for cellulose demonstration occasionally arises.

DEMONSTRATION

The cellulose particles will adopt a variety of appearances, depending on origin (plant material, wood splinters etc.) A fairly typical presentation is that of fenestrated bodies or fibres.

In an H and E preparation, the cellulose may be stained blue, pink or may fail to stain with either dye. It is PAS positive and hexamine silver positive (p. 102 and 212 respectively), stains brown with iodine, and under polarizing microscopy is birefringent. An interesting staining characteristic is the ability of cellulose to stain with Congo red and related dyes and to, sometimes, exhibit a dichroic birefringence. The use of the enzyme cellulase conjugated with FITC for the specific demonstration of cellulose, has been reported by Seibert et al (1978).

CHITIN

Chitin is of the mucoprotein family and is also known by the somewhat indigestible term of homopolyaminosaccharide. As mentioned, chitin is a carbohydrate and found in association with protein and calcium, but such is its physical and histochemical characteristics that it is usually dealt with under a separate heading.

In human tissue it is of relevance only in cases of hydatid cyst formation. These cysts have a wall formed of chitin which has been laid down by the contained larvae of the dog tapeworm — *Echinococcus granulosus*. Hydatid cyts may be found in either the lungs or liver.

DEMONSTRATION

Chitin is a dense hyaline material which stains a bright pink in H and E preparations. It is PAS positive, hexamine-silver positive (see p. 102 and 212 respectively), and variably Congo red positive (see p. 92). Rather like the use of a specific enzyme for the demonstration of cellulose so too with chitin, where the enzyme chitinase has been employed conjugated with FITC (Benjaminson, 1969).

REFERENCES

Allen M G 1970 The effect of acid hydrolysis on sialomucins at selected epithelial sites. Thesis for Fellowship of the Institute of Medical Laboratory Technology

Allison R T 1973 The effects of fixation on the subsequent demonstration of mucopolysaccharides. Medical Laboratory Technology 30: 27–31

Bauer H 1933 Microskopisch-chemischer Natwer's von Glykogen und einigen anderen Polysaccharden. Zeitschift für mikroskopische-anatomische Forschung 33: 143

Benjaminson M A 1969 Conjugates of chitinase with Fluorescein isothiocyanate or lissamine rhodamine as specific stains for chitin in situ. Stain Technology 44: 27–31

Bensley S H 1952 Pinacyanol erthyrosinate as a stain for mast cells. Stain Technology 27: 269

Berger C, and Pizzolato P 1975 The staining of Brunner's gland and other neutral mucins by carmine, haematoxylin and orcein in alkaline solutions. Stain Technology 50: 383–6

Bernfeld P 1951 Enzymes of starch degradation and synthesis. Advances in Enzymology 12: 379

Best F 1906 Uber Karminfarbung des Glykogens und der Kerne. Zeitschrift für wissenschaftkiche Mikroskopie und für Mikroskopische Technik 23: 319–22

Byron F M 1970 Demonstration of glycogen in glycogenosis Types 1, 2 and 4. Journal of Medical Laboratory Technology 27: 43–8

Casselman W G B 1962 Histochemical technique 2nd edn. Methuen, London

Charman J, Reid L 1972 The effect of decalcifying fluids on the staining of epithelial mucins by alcian blue. Stain Technology 47: 173–8

Cook H C 1959 A comparative evaluation of the histological demonstration of mucin. Journal of Medical Laboratory Technology 16: 1–6

Cook H C 1961 A modified thionin technique for mast cells in tissue sections. Journal of Medical Technology 18: 188–9

Cook H C 1968 Some observations of the demonstration of mucin in human tissue. Journal of Medical Laboratory Technology 25: 13–24

Cook H C 1973 A histochemical characterization of malignant tumour mucins as a possible aid in the identification of

metastatic deposits. Medical Laboratory Technology 30: 217–24

Cook H C 1974 Manual of histological demonstration technique. Butterworths, London

Cook H C 1982 Neutral mucin content of gastric carcinomas as a diagnostic aid in the identification of secondary deposits. Histopathology 6: 591–9

Cooper D J 1974 Mucin histochemistry of mucous carcinomas of breast and colon and non-neoplastic breast epithelium. Journal of Clinical Pathology 27: 311–4

Csaba G 1969 Mechanism of the formation of mast cell granules. Acta Biologicae Academicae Scientianum Hungariae 20: 205

Culling C F A, Reid P E, Burton J D, Dunn W L 1975 A histochemical method of differentiating lower gastro-intestinal tract mucin from other mucins in primary or metastatic tumours. Journal of Clinical Pathology 28: 656–8

Dorling J 1969 Critical electrolyte concentration method in histochemistry. Journal of Medical Laboratory Technology 26: 124–30

Ferraz Correa A C, Merzel J 1966 Histochemical behaviour of polysaccharide methods on tissue submitted to decalcification. Acta Histochemica 25 Band, 233–8

Filipe M I 1969 Value of histochemical reactions for mucosubstances in the diagnosis of certain pathological conditions of the colon and rectum. Gut 10: 577–86

Gardner D G 1968 Metachromatic cells in the gingiva in Hurler's syndrome. Journal of Oral Surgery 26: 782

Goldstein D J 1962 Correlation of size of dye particle and density of substrate with special reference to mucin staining. Stain Technology 37: 79–93

Haddock N H 1948 Alcian blue, a new phthalocyanine dyestuff. Research 15: 685–9

Hale C W 1946 Histochemical demonstration of acid mucopolysaccharides in animal tissues. Nature, London 157: 802

Haust M D, Landing B H 1961 Histochemical studies in Hurler's disease: a new method for localization of acid mucopolysaccharide and an analysis of lead acetate fixation. Journal of Histochemistry and Cytochemistry 9: 79

Heath I D 1961 Staining of sulphated mucopolysaccharides. Nature, London 191: 1370

Hughesdon P E 1949 Two uses of uranyl nitrate. I. Permanent metachromatic staining of mucin. Journal of the Royal Microscopical Society 69: 1–7

Hukill P B, Vidone R A 1967 Histochemistry of mucus and other polysaccharides in tumours. Laboratory Investigation 16: 395–406

Kent P W, Marsden J O 1963 A sulphated sialoprotein from sheep colonic mucin. Biochemistry Journal 87: 38–9

Korhonen L, Makela V 1968 Carbodydrate-rich tissue components in lung cancer and normal bronchial tissue: a histochemical study. Histochemical Journal 1: 124–40

Lake B D 1970 The histochemical evaluation of the glycogen storage diseases. A review of techniques and their limitations. Histochemical Journal 2: 441–50

Lamb D, Reid L 1969 Histochemical types of acidic glyocprotein produced by mucous cells of the tracheo-bronchial glands in man. Journal of Pathology 98: 213–29

Lamb D, Reid L 1970 Histochemical and autoradiographic investigation of the serous cells of the human bronchial glands. Journal of Pathology 100: 127–38

Langhans C 1890 Ueber Glykogen in pathologischen Neubildungen und den menschlichen Eithauten. Virchow's Archives of Pathology, Anatomy and Physiology 120: 28

Lauren A P, Sorvari T E 1967 Staining of Paneth cells with Best's carmine after methylation. Stain Technology 42: 311–5

Lillie R D, Laskey A, Greco J, Jacquier H 1947 Studies on the preservation and histologic demonstration of glycogen. Bulletin of the International Association of Medical Museums 27: 23

Lillie R D 1954 Histologic technic, 2nd edn. McGraw-Hill, New York

Lillie R D 1965 Histopathologic technic and practical histochemistry, 3rd edn. McGraw-Hill, New York

McManus J F A 1946 Histological demonstration of mucin after periodic acid. Nature 158: 202

Manns E 1958 The preservation and demonstration of glycogen in tissue sections. Journal of Medical Laboratory Technology 15: 1–12

Mayer P 1896 Uber Schleimfarbung. Mitteilungen aus der Zoologischen Station zu Neapel 12: 303

Meyer K H, Jeanloz R W 1943 Recherches sur Loamidon XXV. Le glycogene due muscle natif. Helvetica Chimica Acta 26: 1784

Mikhail E R, Miller-Milinska A 1964 Mast cell population in human skin. Journal of Investigative Dermatology 43: 249

Mowry R W 1956 Observations on the use of sulphuric ether for the sulphation of hydroxly groups in tissue sections. Journal of Histochemistry and Cytochemistry 4: 407

Murgatroyd L B 1969 Studies on the histochemical demonstration of glycogen. Thesis for Fellowship of the Institute of Medical Laboratory Technology

Murgatroyd L B 1971 Chemical and spectrometric evaluation of glycogen after routine histological fixatives. Stain Technology 46: 111–9

Murgatroyd L B, Horobin R Q 1969 Specific staining of

glycogen with haematoylin and certain anthraquinone dyes. Stain Technology 44: 59–62

Pearse A G E 1953 Histochemistry, theoretical and applied. Churchill, London

Quintarelli G, Tsuiki S, Hashimoto Y, Pigman W 1960 Histochemical studies of bovine salivary glands. Biochemistry, Biophysics Research Communications 2: 423

Sassa D 1965 Untersuchungen zum Cytochemischen Glykogenachweis. VII Mitteilung. Histochemie 5: 378–83

Schiff U 1866 Eine neue Reihe organischer Diamine. Justus Liebigs Annin Chem 140: 92

Scott J E, Dorling J 1965 Differential staining of acid glyosaminoglycans (mucopolysaccharides) by alcian blue in salt solutions. Histochemie 5: 22–33

Scott J E, Dorling J 1969 Periodate oxidation of acid plysaccharides. (III) A PAS method for chondroitin sulphates and other glycosamino-glucuronans. Histochemie 19: 295–301

Scott J E, Dorling J, Stockwell R A 1968 Reversal of protein blocking of basophilia in salt solutions: implication in the localization of polyanions using alcian blue. Journal of Histochemistry 16: 38–6

Siebert G R, Benjaminson M A, Hoffman H 1978 A conjugate of cellulase with fluoroscein isothiocyanate: a specific stain for cellulose. Stain Technology 53: 103–6

Sovari T E, Stoward P J 1970 Saponification of methylated mucosubstances at low temperature. Stain Technology 46: 49–52

Southgate H W 1927 Note on preparing mucicarmine. Journal of Pathology and Bacteriology 30: 729

Spicer S S 1960 A correlative study of the histochemical properties of rodent acid mucopolysaccharides. Journal of Histochemistry and Cytochemistry 8: 18–35

Spicer S S 1965 Diamine methods for differentiating mucopolysaccharides histochemically, Journal of Histochemistry and Cytochemistry 13: 211

Spicer S S 1961 The use of cationic reagents in the histochemical differentiation of mucopolysaccharides. Americal Journal of Clinical Pathology 36: 393–407

Spicer S S, Lillie R D 1959 Saponification as a means of selectively reversing the methylation blockade of tissue basophilia. Journal of Histochemistry and Cytochemistry 7: 123–5

Spicer S S, Meyer D B 1960 Histochemical differentiation of acid mucopolysaccharides by means of combined aldehyde fuchsin-alcian blue staining. Americal Journal of Clinical Pathology 33: 453–60

Spicer S S, Neubecker R D, Warren L, Henson J G 1962 Epithelial mucins in lesions of the human breast. Journal of the National Cancer Institute 29: 963–70

Steedman H F 1950 Alcian blue 8 GS; a new stain for mucin. Quarterly Journal of Microscopic Science 91: 477–9

Wagner J C, Munday B E, Harington J S 1962 Histochemical demonstration of hyaluronic acid in pleural mesotheliomas. Journal of Pathology and Bacteriology 84: 73–8

10

Lipids

Lipids can be defined as substances that may be extracted from the tissues by the use of several or all of the usual fat solvents and are insoluble or only colloidally soluble in water (Baker, 1946). Lipids are normal constituents of tissues found in the adipose tissue as stored lipid for energy production, or as specialist lipid structures such as myelin. As well as other tissue constituents (e.g. carbohydrates and proteins) lipids are rarely found in a pure state in tissue sections; they are usually in combination with carbohydrates in glycolipids or proteins in glycoproteins. This results in the histochemical methods yielding less specific information than we would like. The advantage of histochemistry over biochemistry is that it shows the localization of the lipid at a cytological level or in some cases an ultrastructural level. It is only recently that we have been able to identify individual lipids with any precision, specific histochemical methods having become available.

CLASSIFICATION OF LIPIDS

The classification of lipids has been somewhat confused in the past, a detailed table is given by Bayliss-High (1982). The following is a simplified working version.

UNCONJUGATED LIPIDS

Free fatty acids; cholesterol.

CONJUGATED LIPIDS

1. Ester lipids
    cholesterol esters; triglycerides.

2. Phospholipids
    glycerol based lecithins, cephalins (phosphoglycerides) and plasmalogens.
3. Sphingosine based
    Sphingomyelins, cerebrosides, sulphatides, gangliosides.

LIPID HISTOCHEMISTRY AND DIAGNOSIS

In a routine laboratory a request for a fat stain is usually required for identifying the presence of lipid material. Lipids are found in a number of pathological conditions including liposarcoma, thecoma, atheroma, xanthoma and lipid pneumonia.

In exceptional cases, precise localization and identification is required, notably in the lipid storage diseases (Table 10.2). In these cases due to an enzyme defect, lipids become stored abnormally. The diagnosis of the disease is often dependent upon the identification of the stored lipid. The more common storage disorders are listed in Table 10.2 along with their known staining reactions.

DEMONSTRATION OF LIPIDS

PHYSICAL PROPERTIES

The surface property of lipids is an important factor in their demonstration. For staining purposes they can be described as either 'hydrophilic lipids' — lipids that have an affinity for absorbing water, i.e. they are water miscible.

Table 10.1 Lipids and methods for their demonstration

Method	Lipid
Bromine sudan black	All lipids
Sudan black, oil red O	All lipids in a liquid state
Nile blue sulphate	Acidic and neutral lipids
Copper-rubeanic acid	Free fatty acids
Perchloric acid-naphthoquinone*	Cholesterol and esters*
Digitonin-PAN*	Free cholesterol*
Ultraviolet Schiff	Unsaturated lipids
Osmium tetroxide	Unsaturated lipids
Calcium lipase	Triglycerides
Acid haematin	Choline-containing phospholipids
Sodium hydroxide-acid haematin	Sphingomyelin
Plasmal reaction	Plasmalogen phospholipids
Modified PAS	Cerebrosides
Copper-orcinol	Gangliosides
Acriflavine-DMAB	Sulphatides

*In our hands the demonstration of cholesterol histologically is difficult and often more than one attempt is required. It is essential to include a known positive control, sections of the adrenal cortex are recommended.

Alternatively, they can be 'hydrophobic lipids' — lipids that repel water. These assume the typical globular shape in an aqueous environment. The hydrophobic lipids react strongly with the Sudan related dyes whereas the hydrophilic do not, and are best demonstrated by other methods, see Table 10.3.

Table 10.3 Surface properties of lipids

Hydrophilic	phospholipids gangliosides cerebrosides sulphatides
Hydrophobic	unconjugated simple esters

FIXATION

Unfixed cryostat sections undoubtedly give the best results for the majority of techniques. Fixation is required however in some histochemical methods to protect the lipid and the section from the reagents used. Baker's formal calcium (see Appendix 1) appears to be the best routine fixative. In many instance simple lipids are not fixed or removed by treatment with formalin.

EXTRACTION

The definition given by Baker and quoted at the beginning of this chapter indicates that lipids can be removed by solvents. Lipids do show a differential solubility in organic solvents: unfortunately lipids are rarely found in a pure form and this severely affects the results. Fixation will affect the way a lipid reacts to a solvent. Therefore any extraction techniques should be applied to unfixed sections. Use has been made of extraction, notably in Baker's acid haematim method, where pyridine is used to specifically remove phospholipids. It is also used as a control, when treatment in

Table 10.2 Lipid storage diseases and their staining reactions. This table is based on Bayliss-High (1982) and other workers.

Storage disease	Lipid stored	PAS	Sudan black	Oil red O	Luxol fast blue	Tol. blue	Feyrter thionin
Batten's	Retinoic acid	++	++	+	++	−	−
Fabry's	Ceramide trihexoside	++	++	++	++	−	−
Gaucher's	Gluco-cerebroside	+	±	±	−	−	−
Metachromatic leucodystrophy	Sulphatide	+	+	+	−	++	++
Niemann-Pick's	Sphingomyelin and cholesterol	±	++	++	−	−	−
Krabbe's	Galacto-cerebroside	++	±	±	−	−	−
Tay Sach's	Ganglioside	++	+	+	++	(+)	++
Wolman's	Cholesterol and triglycerides	±	++	++	−	−	−

choloroform-methanol (1:1) at 56° C for 1 hour will remove all lipids.

MELTING POINT

Not all lipids are liquid at room temperature. Some hydrophobic lipids, particularly fatty acids, are crystalline at this temperature and elevated temperatures are necessary for their demonstration.

BIREFRINGENCE

If a section is viewed in polarized light after staining with a Sudan dye, the unstained crystalline lipid will be birefringent. Stained lipids and liquid lipids do not exhibit this effect.

It is unwise to attempt to derive too much information from the birefringent effects of lipids as their optical properties vary according to their physical state. Examining cryostat sections at room temperature usually shows:

Monorefringent lipids: triglycerides
free fatty acids
Birefringent lipids: phospholipids
cerebrosides
sphingomyelin
free cholesterol (notched corner plates)
esterified cholesterol (Maltese cross)

OIL SOLUBLE DYES

The lipids seen in tissues as fats are normally demonstrated by the Sudan dyes. Not all lipids are stained by these dyes, free fatty acids and phosphoglycerides are often unstained.

The oil soluble dyes are virtually insoluble in water and only slightly so in alcohol. As indicated they are soluble in most lipids and require a vehicle for their use. A number of solutions have been tried: 70% alcohol (Daddi 1896), 70% alcohol and acetone mixture of Herxheimer (1903) were used originally, but they are likely to remove small amounts of lipid. The solvents of choice are isopropyl alcohol (Lillie & Ashburn, 1943),

propylene glycol (Chiffelle & Putt, 1951) and triethyl phosphate (Gomori, 1952). We have found that 60% isopropyl alcohol or 60% triethyl phosphate give the best results.

The oil-soluble dyes stain lipids by being more soluble in the lipids than in their solvent. Most of them are not dyes in the accepted sense, i.e. they contain no auxochromic groups but are chromogens. An exception to this is Sudan black which contains the amino group auxochrome. This probably accounts for the more sensitive fat staining occurring with this dye, which is particularly apparent during staining of phospholipid-rich tissues, where some degree of salt binding undoubtedly occurs. The original method employed Sudan III (Daddi, 1896) but was supplanted in popularity by the deeper red Sudan IV (Michaelis, 1901). Other oil-soluble dyes are Sudan black, brown, blue or green, and also oil red O, oil blue NA and oil brown D.

Counterstaining presents problems as most dyes diffuse or are bleached by the aqueous mountants used. For the red lipid dyes haematoxylin is the usual counterstain but tends to fade in time. The Sudans blue and black present greater problems as the normally recommended dye, carmalum, requires long staining periods and, at best, stains the nuclei only weakly. A possible alternative once suggested to us was to first carry out the Feulgen-Schiff reaction to colour the DNA before staining with Sudan black!

There are several mountants available, e.g. glycerol-jelly, Farrant's solution or Apathy's solution. There is not much to choose between them, and we usually prefer the modified Apathy mountant (see p. 89) which can be hardened by placing the mounted sections for a short period in the 37° C incubator.

SUDAN BLACK METHOD FOR LIPIDS
(Lison & Dagnelie, 1935; Lillie, 1954; Bayliss & Adams, 1972; Bayliss-High, 1981)

Notes

Lillie (1954) introduced a bromination stage to depress the solubility of unsaturated lipids in organic solvents. Bayliss & Adams (1972) noted that the fatty acids and phosphoglycerides were rendered insoluble in the dye bath and that crystalline cholesterol was converted to derivatives that were liquid at room temperature and hence demonstrated. Bayliss-High (1981) showed that following bromination only phospholipids will survive extraction and appear to be selectively stained. These modifications provide an easy and sensitive method for staining all lipid classes. Bayliss-High (1982) recommends it as a screening method; for morphology she advises the oil red O method which is also useful in combination with other dyes such as Baker's acid haematin.

STANDARD SUDAN BLACK TECHNIQUE

Technique

1. Mount sections on to slides and allow to dry.
2. Rinse in 70% ethanol.
3. Stain in a saturated solution of Sudan black in 70% ethanol for 15 min. Filter before use.
4. Remove excess stain in 70% ethanol.
5. Stain nuclei with 2% Carmalum for 5 min.
6. Wash well in water and mount in glycerin jelly.

Results

Unsaturated cholesterol esters, triglycerides, phospholipids	blue-black

BROMINATION — SUDAN BLACK

Technique

1. Mount sections on to slides and allow to dry.
2. Immerse sections in 2.5% aqueous bromine for 30 min at room temperature in a fume cupboard.
3. Wash in water (10 min).
4. Treat with 0.5% sodium metabisulphite for 1 min.
5. Wash in distilled water, three changes.
6. Proceed with standard Sudan black method above.

Results

As previous method plus lecithin, free fatty acids and free cholesterol	blue-black.

BROMINATION — ACETONE — SUDAN BLACK

Technique

1. Follow steps 1–5 in previous method and allow sections to dry.
2. Treat sections with anhydrous acetone for 20 min at 4° C.
3. Follow steps 3–6 in the standard Sudan black method above.

Results

Only phospholipids stain blue-black.

OIL RED O TECHNIQUE (French, 1926; Lillie & Ashburn, 1943)

Notes

The deep red staining of lipids given by this method makes it one of the most popular techniques for lipids in present in use. Always use a covered container and ample amounts of solution when staining and use care in washing.

Of the two alternative staining solutions presented below we prefer the isopropanol variant as although the triethyl phosphate solution of oil red O gives brighter staining, it can also lead to a dye precipitate forming during long storage of the stained sections.

Solutions

Variant 1

Dissolve 0.5 g of oil red O in 200 ml of isopropyl alcohol. Warm the solution in a long-necked container (2 litre volumetric flask) in a 56° C water bath for 1 h. Cool. The working solution is prepared prior to use by adding four parts of distilled water to six parts of the stock solution. Mix and allow to stand for 10 min. Filter through a fine filter paper (No. 42 Whatman).

Variant 2 (Gomori, 1952)

Dissolve 1 g of oil red O in 100 ml of triethyl phosphate by heating in a 56° C water bath for several hours. Filter (No. 1 Whatman). The working solution is prepared by adding four parts of distilled water to six parts of the stock solution. Mix well and filter through a fine filter paper as before.

Technique

1. Rinse frozen sections in water.
2. Rinse in either 60% isopropyl alcohol or 60% triethyl phosphate (both dilutions prepared with distilled water) as appropriate.
3. Stain in either dye variant for 10 min.
4. Wash briefly in either 60% isopropyl alcohol or 60% triethyl phosphate. Wash well in water.
5. Stain the nuclei in Mayer's haematoxylin solution for $1-1\frac{1}{2}$ min. Wash and blue.
6. Wash in water and mount in one of the aqueous mountants.

Results

Unsaturated hydrophobic lipids i.e. triglycerides, cholesterol esters.   red
Phospholipids   pink
Nuclei   blue

NILE BLUE SULPHATE TECHNIQUE
(Smith, 1907)

Notes

The following technique, which is slightly modified from the original, gives good separation of acidic from certain of the non-acidic lipids. The phospholipids in particular are stained blue, deeper than the fatty acids (Dunnigan, 1968).

The Nile blue sulphate solution contains two oxazines (the salt and its free base) which stain acidic structures such as phosphate groups blue by salt linkage, and an oxazone moiety which is oil-soluble and red in colour. It must be appreciated that the staining of acidic lipids is nonspecific as other acidic tissue moieties, e.g. nucleic acids, also stain. The temperature at which the reaction is carried out is important, as the various fatty acids have different melting points so that the temperature of reaction should be near or above this point. For example, the melting point of stearic acid is 70° C, palmitic 63° C and oleic acid 14° C. The tempera-

ture suggested for this technique is 60° C (Cain, 1947).

Solution

1% aqueous Nile blue sulphate (syn. Nile blue)

The dye should be rich in oxazone content in order to achieve good results and should be tested as follows:

Add a little of the powdered dye, or a few drops of the aqueous solution to 5–10 ml of xylene in a test tube and mix well. The oxazone fraction will go into solution and appear red. Should a negative or weak red colour result the dye oxazone content may be increased by sulphuric acid oxidation as follows. Make up a 1% solution of Nile blue sulphate in 5% aqueous sulphuric acid. Boil in a reflux condenser for 1–2 h. Cool and retest in xylene. If positive, use the oxidized solution as it is.

Technique

1. Take frozen sections to distilled water.
2. Stain with the Nile blue sulphate solution for 10 min at 60° C. (preheat the solution).
3. Wash in distilled water at 60° C for a few seconds.
4. Differentiate in 1% acetic acid at 60° C until the excess blue staining is removed (approximately 30 s).
5. Wash in tap water at room temperature and mount in an aqueous mountant.

Results

Neutral fats, cholesterol esters   red
Fatty acids, phospholipids, nuclei,   blue
some lipofuscins, acidic mucins

COPPER-RUBEANIC ACID METHOD FOR FREE FATTY ACIDS (Holczinger, 1959)

Notes

The free fatty acids will bind heavy metal ions to form soaps. Benda (1900) & Holczinger's (1959) technique uses copper acetate to bind the fatty acids and rubeanic acid to demonstrate the copper soaps. EDTA is used to remove nonspecific absorbed copper. M HCl is employed initially to desaponify calcium salts.

Technique

1. Treat duplicate sections with M HCl at 20° C for 1 h.
2. Wash well in distilled water and then air dry.
3. Treat one section with acetone at 4° C for 20 min.
4. Immerse both sections in 0.005% cupric acetate for 3 h.
5. Wash in 0.1% EDTA pH 7.0 (adjust pH with NaOH) for 10 s.
6. Repeat wash.
7. Wash in distilled water.
8. Treat sections with 0.1% rubeanic acid in 70% ethanol for 10 min.
9. Rinse in 70% ethanol.
10. Counterstain nuclei in Mayer's Carmalum.
11. Wash in water and mount in glycerine jelly.

Results

Free fatty acids	dark green
Acetone extracted section	negative

PERCHLORIC ACID-NAPHTHOQUINONE (PAN) FOR CHOLESTEROL (Adams, 1961)

Notes

This method is more precise and sensitive than the classical Schultz method and is included to the exclusion of the former. In the Adams method perchloric acid is used to condense cholesterol to cholesta-3:5 diene, which is converted by 1:2 naphthoquinone to a red or blue pigment. The colour variation being due to the different physical state of the cholesterol (Bayliss-High, 1982). The oxidation of the cholesterol is an important stage of the method and should not be omitted or the time reduced.

Solution

1:2 Naphthoquinone-4-sulphonic acid	40 mg
Ethanol	20 ml
60% Perchloric acid	10 ml
Formaldehyde	1 ml
Distilled water	9 ml

Mix and use the same day.

Technique

1. Air dry sections on to slides.
2. Oxidize sections in 1% ferric chloride for 4 h.
3. Wash well in distilled water.
4. Coat the sections with above solution with a brush, place slides on a hotplate at 70° C, keep coating the sections with the solution until the colour develops for 1–5 min.
5. Rinse in 60% perchloric acid.
6. Mount in 60% perchloric acid.

Results

Cholesterol and esters	red or blue

DIGITONIN REACTION FOR CHOLESTEROL (Windaus, 1910, Modified)

Notes

Cholesterol and cholesterol esters will form a compound with digitonin. The resultant digitonide forms birefringent needles or rosettes. Free cholesterol can be differentiated from its esters by the fact that the esters will be coloured by an oil soluble dye or by using the PAN method after completing the technique. Alternatively the esters can be extracted in acetone.

Technique

1. Dry sections on to slides.
2. Immerse in 0.5% digitonin in 4% ethanol for 2 h.
3. Extract esters in acetone for 1 h (optional).
4. Proceed with method of choice.

Results

Using an oil soluble dye; no extraction

Free cholesterol	unstained
Cholesterol esters	stained

After acetone extraction and PAN technique

Free cholesterol   red or blue
Cholesterol esters   negative

After polarization and precipitation with digitonin

Free cholesterol and esters   birefringent

ULTRA-VIOLET — SCHIFF METHOD FOR UNSATURATED LIPIDS (Belt & Hayes, 1956)

Notes

A highly selective technique. Ultraviolet light oxidizes double bonds to aldehydes, allowing subsequent Schiff staining.

Technique

1. Mount sections on to slides and expose to a source of ultraviolet light for 2 hs.
2. Treat with Schiff's reagent for 15 min, together with a non-irradiated control section to exclude non-lipid aldehydes.
3. Wash well in tap water and rinse in distilled water.
4. Mount sections in glycerine jelly.

Result

Unsaturated lipids appear magenta.

SECONDARY FLUORESCENCE METHOD (Popper, 1944)

Note

This is a useful screening method. The fluorochromes being in aqueous solution will not dissolve any lipid material.

Technique

1. Wash sections in distilled water.
2. Stain for 3 min in 0.1% aqueous phosphine 3R.
3. Rinse quickly in distilled water and mount in 90% glycerol.

Results

Simple lipids, including triglycerides, cholesterol esters and all compound lipids — silvery-white fluorescence.
Fatty acids and cholesterol are negative.

OSMIUM TETROXIDE

Notes

The use of osmium tetroxide to demonstrate lipids is probably the oldest technique of all. It depends on the reduction of the osmium tetroxide to lower (black) oxides by an ethylene linkage mechanism. It should be appreciated, however, that certain reducing substances such as melanin will also blacken (Lillie, 1965). Osmium tetroxide will blacken only unsaturated fatty acids and their esters such as those of oleic acid. In order to demonstrate the saturated fats, the tissue should be treated with alcohol following osmium tetroxide treatment, a process known as 'secondary staining.'

It is as well to bear in mind the toxicity of osmium tetroxide vapour.

Frozen section technique

1. Fix tissue in formalin and cut frozen sections.
2. Wash in distilled water then treat with 1% aqueous osmium tetroxide for 1 h in a dark container.
3. Wash in running water.
4. Mount in an aqueous mountant.

Results

Unsaturated lipids   brown-black
Background   yellow-brown

OSMIUM TETROXIDE METHOD FOR THE DEMONSTRATION OF LIPID IN PARAFFIN SECTIONS

Notes

See previous method.

Technique

1. Fix thin slices of tissue in Flemming's fluid (see Appendix 1) for 24–48 h.
2. Wash in running water for 12–16 h.
3. Dehydrate in 70%, 90% and absolute alcohol, clear in chloroform or toluene and embed in paraffin wax.
4. Cut sections at 5–10 μm, mount on slides and dry.
5. Remove wax with xylene and mount with a synthetic resin medium. Counterstaining with neutral red or safranin is optional.

Results

Lipids are blackened as are other reducing substances.

CALCIUM LIPASE METHOD FOR TRIGLYCERIDES (Adams et al, 1966)

Notes

Calcium will also stain with this method. Suitable controls must be used. Pancreatic lipase hydrolyses the triglycerides into fatty acids. In the presence of calcium ions the insoluble soaps are converted to lead soaps and visualized by treatment with ammonium sulphide.

Solution

Tris buffer at pH 8.0	15 ml
2% calcium chloride	10 ml
Distilled water	25 ml
Porcine pancreatic lipase	50 mg

Warm solution to 37° C and filter before use.

Technique

1. Incubate free-floating frozen, or slide mounted cryostat sections, in the lipase medium at 37° C for 3 h.
2. Wash sections well and mount on to slides.
3. Together with a duplicate section, not subjected to enzyme, treat with 1% lead nitrate for 15 min.
4. Wash very thoroughly in several changes of distilled water.

5. Immerse for 10 s in dilute ammonium sulphide (three drops to a Coplin jar of water).
6. Wash well, counterstain with Mayer's haemalum for 3 min.
7. Wash in tap water, followed by a rinse in distilled water.
8. Mount sections in glycerine jelly.

Results

Triglycerides	brown

ACID HAEMATEIN TECHNIQUE (after Baker, 1946)

Notes

The rationale of this technique is following treatment with a dichromate solution, phospholipids and certain other acidic tissue components form a mordant-type linkage with haematoxylin which is relatively resistant to borax-ferricyanide differentiation. If a duplicate piece of tissue is first subjected to pyridine extraction, only phospholipids will be extracted and show subsequent loss of staining (Casselman, 1962). Provided that an extracted control block is taken through, this is probably the most reliable technique for phospholipids.

Solutions

Picro-formal-acetic

Saturated aqueous picric acid	50 ml
Formalin	10 ml
Acetic acid	5 ml
Distilled water	35 ml

Calcium-dichromate

Dissolve 5 g potassium dichromate and 2 g of hydrated (1 g anhydrous) calcium chloride in 100 ml of distilled water.

Haematoxylin

Add 0.05 g haematoxylin and 1 ml of 1% aqueous sodium iodate to 48 ml of distilled water. Bring to the boil, cool to 37° C and add 1 ml of acetic acid. This solution does not keep and should be prepared prior to use.

Differentiator

Dissolve 0.25 g potassium ferricyanide and 0.25 g borax (sodium borate or tetraborate) in 100 ml distilled water.

Technique

1. Fix one block of the tissue in formal-calcium (1 g calcium chloride in 10% formalin) overnight, then transfer to the calcium-dichromate solution for 18 h. Following this, transfer the tissue to fresh calcium-dichromate solution but at 60° C for 24 h. Wash in running water overnight then cut frozen sections.
   Alternatively, cut fresh-frozen sections and fix in formal-calcium for 1–2 h. Wash in water briefly, then treat with the 60° C calcium-dichromate solution for 12–16 h. Wash in several changes of distilled water for 30 min.
2. A duplicate control block or fresh-frozen section is fixed in the picro-formal-acetic solution for 20 h. Wash in 70% alcohol for 1 h then in 50% alcohol for 30 min and running water for 30 min. Place in pyridine at room temperature for two changes of 1 h each, then into pyridine for 24 h at 60° C. Wash well in running water (2 h or so) then treat in a similar manner to the test block as from the room temperature calcium-dichromate stage in step 1.
3. Take all sections into water and place into the calcium-dichromate solution for 1 h at 60° C (this step may be omitted if the calcium-dichromate-treated section method has been used). Wash sections in several changes of distilled water.
4. Stain in the haematoxylin solution for 2 h at 37° C.
5. Rinse in distilled water and differentiate in the borax-ferricyanide solution for 2 h at 37° C. Wash well in water.
6. Mount in an aqueous mountant.

Results

In the unextracted tissue sections phospholipids, some cerebrosides, nuclei, acidic mucins, red blood cells — dark blue.
In the extracted tissue sections the phospholipids will have been extracted and thus not stained.

SODIUM HYDROXIDE-ACID HAEMATEIN METHOD FOR SPHINGOMYELIN (Adams & Bayliss, 1963)

Notes

This is a specific method; it is a development of the acid haematein method. Cryostat sections tend to lift. Hydrolysis removes phosphoglycerides but leaves sphingomyelin unaffected allowing for its demonstration by the acid haematein method.

Technique

1. Subject free-floating frozen sections (or slide mounted crystat sections) to 2M NaOH for 1 h at 37° C.
2. Wash well in water and rinse in 1% acetic acid.
3. Mount sections on to slides and proceed as for the acid haematein method (p. 136).

Results

Sphingomyelin   blue

THE PLASMAL TECHNIQUE (Feulgen & Voit, 1924; Terner & Hayes, 1961)

Notes

Both acetal phosphatides and plasmalogens are demonstrated by this technique. Mercuric chloride hydrolysis is employed to liberate fatty aldehydes which recolours Schiff's reagent to form magenta compounds.

The technique is simple to do but of questionable specificity. As a control, take through a duplicate section and omit the mercuric chloride step. Any fixation of tissue should be for short (6 h) and only in formalin.

Solutions

1% aqueous mercuric chloride.

Schiff's reagent, see page 102.

Technique

1. Take either fixed frozen sections to distilled water; or better still unfixed frozen sections.
2. Treat the test section only with mercuric chloride for 7 min.
3. Transfer all sections to Schiff's reagent for 10 min.
4. Wash in distilled water.
5. Wash in tap water for 10 min. Counterstain in 2% aqueous methyl green (extracted).
6. Wash and mount in an aqueous mountant.

Results

Plasmals	magenta
Nuclei	green

The negative control section should show no Schiff reaction.

MODIFIED PAS REACTION FOR CEREBROSIDE (Adams & Bayliss, 1963)

Notes

This can be a difficult method to use. The chloramine T converts amino groups to carbonyls and must be handled with care as it can become explosive. Periodic acid is used to convert the hexose groups within cerebrosides to aldehydes. Blocking techniques are used to suppress other aldehyde reactivity.

Solution

Performic acid

98% formic acid	45 ml
100 vols hydrogen peroxide	4.5 ml
Conc. sulphuric acid	0.5 ml

Prepare an hour before use and stir occasionally with a glass rod, inside a fume cupboard, to release bubbles of gas from the solution.

Technique

1. Mount duplicate sections on to separate slides and extract one of these with chloroform-methanol (2:1 v/v) for 1 h at room temperature.
2. Deaminate both sections in 10% aqueous chloramine T for 1 h at 37° C.
3. Wash slides vigorously and as rapidly as possible, one at a time, in a large volume of water before transferring them immediately to performic acid for 10 min. The washing must be swift yet thorough to prevent detachment of sections from slides.
4. Wash well in distilled water.
5. Treat with a filtered saturated solution of 2:4 dinitrophenylhydrazine in M HCl at 4° C for 2 h.
6. Wash well in water.
7. Treat with 0.5% periodic acid for 10 min.
8. Wash in distilled water.
9. Stain in Schiff's reagent for 15 min
10. Wash in tap water for 15 min to develop colour.
11. Counterstain nuclei with Mayer's haemalum if wished.
12. Wash in tap water, distilled water and finally mount sections in glycerine jelly.

Results

Cerebrosides — magenta, indicated by the difference in staining intensity between the extracted and unextracted sections.

COPPER-ORCINOL-HCL METHOD FOR GANGLIOSIDES (SIALIC ACIDS) (Ravetto, 1964)

Notes

The hydrochloric acid used for this method must be fresh; preferably from a newly-opened bottle (Lake, 1968). The method uses a modified Bial reagent. The resultant colour is pale, but is sufficient to see moderate deposits in brain.

Solution

Orcinol	200 mg
0.1M copper sulphate	0.25 ml

Distilled water 20 ml
Conc. hydrochloric acid 80 ml
Allow the solution to mature for 4 h before use.

Technique

1. Mount sections on to slides and dry thoroughly.
2. Spray the sections with the solution, using a very fine spray.
3. Transfer slides to a screwcap polythene container containing HCl vapour, for 10 min at 70° C. A thin layer of concentrated HCl is poured into the jar, which is heated to 70° C before inserting the sections.
4. Remove slides and rapidly dry them in a current of air from a compressor or cylinder.
5. Rinse in xylene and mount in Canada balsam.

Results

Gangliosides pink

ACRIFLAVINE-DMAB METHOD FOR SULPHATIDES (Hollander, 1963)

Notes

Mast cells will also stain red. Sulphatide is stained by an acidic acriflavine solution, the reaction product is converted to an insoluble red dye by using DMAB.

Solutions

Acriflavine stock solution

Acriflavine 100 mg
Distilled water at 80° C. 20 ml
Store in the dark at 4° C.

Acriflavine working solution

0.1M citrate-HCl buffer pH 2.5 99 ml
Stock acriflavine solution 1 ml

DMAB Solution

p-dimethylamino-benzaldehyde 0.6 g
20% hydrochloric acid 30 ml
Isopropanol 70 ml

Technique

1. Mount sections on to slides.
2. Stain for 6 min in acriflavine solution.
3. Differentiate for 1 min in two changes of 70% isopropanol.
4. Treat with DMAB reagent for 30–45 s.
5. Rinse in distilled water for 2–3 min.
6. Counterstain nuclei in Mayer's haemalum for 3 min.
7. Blue the haemalum in tap water, rinse in distilled water and mount sections in glycerine jelly.

Results

Sulphatide red

REFERENCES

Adams C W M 1961 A perchloric acid-naphthoquinine method for the histochemical localisation of cholesterol. Nature (London) 193: 331
Adams C W M, Bayliss O B 1963 Histochemical observations on the localisation and origin of sphingomyelin, cerebroside and cholesterol in normal and atherosclerotic human artery. Journal of Pathology and Bacteriology 85: 113
Adams C W M, Abdulla Y H, Bayliss O B, Weller R O 1966 Histochemical detection of triglyceride esters with specific lipases and a lead sulphide technique. Journal of Histochemistry and Cytochemistry 14: 385
Baker J R 1946 The histochemical recognition of lipine. Quarterly Journal of Microscopical Science 87: 441
Bayliss O B, Adams C W M 1972 Bromine Sudan black

(BSB) A general stain for lipids including free cholesterol. Histochemical Journal 4: 505
Bayliss-High O 1982 In: Bancroft J D, Stevens A (eds) 'Lipids' in theory and practice of histological techniques 2nd edn. Churchill Livingstone. Edinburgh
Belt W D, Hayes E R 1956 An ultra-violet Schiff reaction for unsaturated lipids. Stain Technology 31: 117
Benda C 1900 Eine makro- und mikrochemisch Reaction der fett Gewebsnekrose. Virchow's Archiv fur pathologische Anatomie und Physiologie und fur klinische Medizin 161: 194
Cain A J 1947 Use of Nile blue in the examination of lipoids. Quarterly Journal of Microscopical Science 88: 383
Casselman W G B 1959 Histochemical techniques. Methuen, London

Chiffelle T L, Putt F A 1951 Propylene and ethylene glycol as solvents for Sudan IV and Sudan black B. Stain Technology 26: 51

Daddi L 1896 Nouvelle methode pour colorer la graisse dans les tissues. Archives Italiennes de Biologie 26: 143

Dunnigan M G 1968 The use of NBSO$_4$ in the histochemical identification of phospholipids. Stain Technology 43: 249

Feulgen R, Voit K 1924 Ueber einen Weitverbreiteten festen Aldehyd seine Entstehung aus einer Varstufe, sein mikrochemischer Nachweis und die Wege zu seiner proparativen Darstellung. Pflügers Archiv für die Gesamte Physiologie des Menschen und der Tiere 206: 389

Feyrter F 1936 Über ein sehr einfaches Verfahren der markscheiden Fürbüng, zugleich neue Art der Färberei. Virchow's Archiv fur Pathologische Antomie und Physiologie und fur Klinische Medizin 296: 645

French R W 1926 Azure C as tissue stain. Stain Technology 1: 79

Herxheimer G W 1903 Zur Fettfürbung. Zeitbl. All. Pathologie Anatomie 14: 841

Holczinger L 1959 Histochemischer Nachweis freier Fattsäuren. Acta Histochemica 8: 167

Hollander H 1963 A staining method for cerebroside-sulphuric esters in brain tissue. Journal of Histochemistry and Cytochemistry 11: 118

Lillie R D 1954 Histopathologic technique and practical histochemistry, 2nd edn. Blakiston, New York

Lillie R D 1965 Histopathologic technique and practical histochemistry, 3rd edn. Blakiston, New York

Lillie R D, Ashburn L L 1943 Supersaturated solutions of fat stains in dilute isopropanol for demonstration of acute fatty degeneration not shown by Herxheimer's technique. Archives of Pathology 36: 432

Lison L, Dagnelie J 1935 Methodes nouvelles de colouration de la myéline. Bulletin d'Histologie Apliquée à la Physiologie et à la Pathologie et de Technique Microscopique 12: 85

Michaelis L 1901 Ueber Fett-Farbstoffe. Virchow's Archiv fur Pathologische Anatomie und fur Klinische Medizin 164: 263

Popper H 1941 Histologic distribution of vitamin A in human organs under normal and pathological conditions. Archives of Pathology 318: 766

Ravetto C 1964 Histochemical demonstration of sialic (neuraminic) acids. Journal of Histochemistry & Cytochemistry 12: 306

Smith J L 1908 On the simultaneous staining of neutral fat and fatty acids by oxazine dyes. Journal of Pathology & Bacteriology 12: 1

Terner G Y, Hayes E R 1961 Histochemistry of plasmalogens. Stain Technology 36: 265

Windaus T 1909 Ueber die quantitative Bestimmung des Cholesterins und der Cholesterinester in einigen normalen und pathologischen Nieren. Z. Phys. Chemistrie 65: 110

11

Pigments

INTRODUCTION

The pigments that we deal with in this chapter are those which are classed as artefact or fixation, and the large group of pigments known as endogenous. A third group, the exogenous pigments are briefly discussed. The demonstration of this third group is far from satisfactory; the histochemical methods for some of the metallic salts are far from specific and no methods exist for others.

Pigments are produced by the body under normal conditions. They are also found in pathological conditions when their site and quantity may be changed. There is no simple sound classification of pigments, partly due to minerals being classed as pigments. However, the classification given below will be found useful if not scientifically precise. Many of the pigments to be described are shades of yellow-brown in colour in unstained or H and E sections, and it is important to appreciate that the same pigment can adopt a variety of presentations and the laboratory worker should be beware of rash bets on an H and E section!

Pigments can be conveniently split into two groups. Firstly, those that can be coloured, i.e. haemosiderin, lipofuscin, etc., and secondly those that are not coloured, i.e. they are unreactive to dyes and include formalin, carbon, etc. but are identified by their solubility in acid or alkaline solutions, or their sensitivity to bleaching solutions. Overall they are classified as:

Artefact: fixation pigments
Endogenous: produced within the tissues
Exogenous: gain access to the tissues

FIXATION PIGMENTS (Table 11.1)

FORMALIN

The full name for this birefringent pigment is acid formaldehyde haematin and its formation is favoured by long-term fixation of highly vascular tissue in acid pH formalin, although we have also experienced the formation of a formalin pigment at alkaline pH levels. The pigment may exhibit a variety of forms varying from a fine diffuse dark brown granule to a yellow needle-like crystal occurring in clusters. Whilst formalin pigment is usually extracellular it may occasionally be found in macrophages. Formalin pigment is said to be positive to the Perls' technique following micro-incineration.

Unquestionably the most effective means of removing the pigment is by the use of alcoholic picric acid, although the rationale is obscure. Other methods tend to be long and capricious.

Solution

Saturated alcoholic picric acid.

Technique

1. Take sections to alcohol or water.
2. Treat with the alcoholic picric acid solution for 10–30 min.
3. Wash well in water for 5 min.
4. Carry out desired staining procedure.

If preferred treat with 0.1% sodium or potassium hydroxide in 70% alcohol, or 10 volumes hydrogen peroxide but for much longer periods (1–24 h).

Formalin pigments can be largely prevented by using a buffered solution with a pH over 6.5.

MERCURIC CHLORIDE

Mercuric chloride is found to a variable extent after fixation in mercuric chloride-containing fixatives, being most pronounced with long fixation. As with the formalin pigment, mercuric chloride pigment can vary in appearance although it is usually a large irregular brown crystal. It is extracellular. The pigment is monorefringent but may be found in a birefringent form, particularly if the tissues were primarily fixed in formalin, then in mercuric chloride ('secondary fixation').

Another interesting feature is that following long storage of sections containing mercuric-chloride pigment, the crystal form changes to a globular one and exhibits a Maltese cross-type birefringence.

The almost universal removal technique is that forming soluble iodides and chlorides with iodine treatment, followed by hypo bleaching. The iodine treatment is attributed to both Mayer and Vigelius in 1886; whilst hypo bleaching was introduced in 1909 by Heidenhain. Lugol's iodine is used at a reasonably standard treatment time; alternatively, one may use an 0.5% iodine in 70% alcohol solution.

Solutions

Lugol's iodine solution, see page 204.

Technique

1. Take sections to water.
2. Treat with Lugol's iodine solution for 5 min.
3. Wash, bleach with 5% hypo for 10–30 s.
4. Wash well in water. Carry out proposed staining technique.

MALARIA PIGMENT

An alternative name for malaria pigment is haemozoin. It is a blood-derived pigment which is found in reticulo-endothelial cells of organs such as liver, spleen and brain in cases of malaria. It is a fine, dark brown pigment and reacts histochemically like formalin precipitate in that it is birefringent and soluble in alcoholic picric acid. Unlike formalin pigment, however, it is invariably intracellular.

Like haemoglobin, some of the protein-masked iron fraction of malaria pigment can be made available for the Perls' reaction, by treating with hydrogen peroxide. Schistosome infestation may produce a pigment histologically identical to haemozoin.

CHROMIC OXIDE

Chromic oxide is a fine yellow-brown precipitate which results in tissues due to the omission of washing in water following fixation in chromic acid or potassium dichromate-containing fixative. The subsequent processing alcohols reduce the chrome salts to lower oxides resulting in the precipitation of insoluble chromic oxides. It is rarely met with in practice and is difficult to produce even intentionally!

Chromic oxide pigment is monorefringent, extracellular and is removed from sections by treatment with 1% acid-alcohol for 30 min or more.

Table 11.1 Artefact pigments

Pigment	Removed by	Identified by
Formalin	Alcoholic picric acid	Dark brown to yellow granules Birefringence Site
Mercury	Alcoholic iodine	Coarse brown crystals Distribution
Malaria	Alcoholic picric acid	Dark brown granules Birefringence Site
Chromate	Acid-alcohol	Fine yellow-brown deposits

ENDOGENOUS PIGMENTS

This is the largest group of pigments and by definition it should include all those produced by the body. But it is here that a simple classification fails, because the body also produces or utilizes iron, calcium and copper which in pathological conditions may be increased and located in abnormal situations. They are often identified separately as minerals but we will consider them here under the heading 'endogenous.' The majority of endogenous pigments are derived from the blood and can be referred to therefore as haematogenous pigments.

HAEMOGLOBIN

Haemoglobin is involved in the transport of oxygen and carbon dioxide within the blood stream. The red pigmented component is called haem and contains ferrous iron. This cannot be readily demonstrated, unless freed from the protein by treatment with hydrogen peroxide. Other iron containing pigments are less intensely bound to protein. Under normal conditions haemoglobin is confined to red blood cells and as such does not require histological demonstration. In pathological states it can be found in casts in renal tubules in haemoglobinuria or in active glomerulonephritis.

Demonstration

There are two types of demonstration method. Either the component enzyme, haemoglobin peroxidase, can be stained or the haemoglobin itself can be demonstrated. The enzyme is moderately stable and is able to withstand short fixation and paraffin processing. Other peroxidase enzymes will also stain. The method using Patent blue is given below. Due to the basic structure of haemoglobin it is well stained by acid dyes, eosin for example stains it a vivid orange colour in a well differentiated section; other acid dye techniques are listed in Table 11.2. Haemoglobin is monorefringent and

Table 11.2 Methods for haemoglobin

Technique	Colour	Element stained
Dunn-Thompson	Green	Haemoglobin
Amido black	Dark blue	Haemoglobin
Kiton red-almond green	Red	Haemoglobin
Leuco patent blue	Blue	Enzyme
Solochrome cyanine	Blue	Lipoprotein envelope
PTAH	Blue	Lipoprotein envelope

nonfluorescent. Fixation is best in formalin or mercuric chloride. Drury & Wallington (1980) state that Susa preserves it poorly. The following techniques demonstrate haemoglobin well.

DUNN-THOMPSON TECHNIQUE (Dunn-Thompson, 1945)

Notes

This is a modified van Gieson method. Fixation in neutral formalin gives the best result. The double haematoxylin staining gives a stronger colouration to haemoglobin.

Solutions

0.25% haematoxylin in 5% aqueous ammonium alum.

Van Gieson solution, see page 41.

4% aqueous iron alum.

Technique

1. Take sections to water.
2. Stain in haematoxylin solution for 15 min.
3. Wash in tap water.
4. Mordant in 4% iron alum for 1 min.
5. Stain in haematoxylin solution for 10 min.
6. Rinse in tap water.
7. Stain in van Gieson's solution for 15 min.
8. Rinse in 95% alcohol for 2 min.
9. Dehydrate, clear and mount in DPX.

Results

| Haemoglobin casts | green |
| Red blood cells | greenish black |

KITON RED-ALMOND GREEN TECHNIQUE (Lendrum, 1949)

Notes

This is a highly selective technique which gives colourful results after a little practice. The nuclei should be strongly stained with haematoxylin to avoid subsequent masking by the green counter-stain. Lendrum specified 'almond green' stain, but most contrasting anionic dyes will serve.

Solutions

Saturated brilliant kiton red B in Cellosolve.

Almond green stain

Saturated tartrazine in Cellosolve   equal parts
Saturated lissamine green BN 200
in Cellosolve
Dilute 1 : 2 with Cellosolve prior to use.

Technique

1. Take sections to water.
2. Stain the nuclei with one of the iron haematoxylin solutions. Differentiate and blue.
3. Rinse in Cellosolve. Stain with the kiton red solution for 20–30 min.
4. Differentiate in tap water. The haemoglobin will become a progressively brighter red and the background clearer; this stage may take several minutes.
5. Drain and counterstain with the almond green solution for a few seconds only.
6. Rinse with Cellosolve. Clear in xylene and mount as desired.

Results

Nuclei	blue-black
Haemoglobin (red blood cells)	red
Background	green

AMIDO BLACK TECHNIQUE (Puchtler & Sweat, 1962)

Notes

Using a tannic acid-phosphomolybdic acid mordanting sequence the amido black is strongly bound by haemoglobin. It is not a capricious technique and does not require great expertise. The authors recommend Zenker-formal fixation, but this is not by any means essential in practice.

Solutions

5% aqueous tannic acid.
1% aqueous phosphomolybdic acid.
Saturated amido black 10B (synonym: naphthalene black) in nine parts methanol to one part acetic acid conc.

Technique

1. Take sections to water. The authors recommend mordanting sections overnight in Zenker-formal should the tissue not have been fixed in this solution (see above).
2. Treat with the tannic acid solution for 5 min.
3. Wash well in distilled water. Treat with the phosphomolybdic acid solution for 10 min.
4. Wash well in distilled water, drain and blot dry.
5. Filter on the amido black solution and leave for 5 min.
6. Rinse in methanol-acetic (9 : 1) then in water.
7. Counterstain in the neutral red solution for 5 min. Wash, dehydrate, clear and mount as desired.

Results

Oxyhaemoglobin and methaemoglobin	dark blue
Nuclei	red

LEUCO PATENT BLUE TECHNIQUE (Lison, 1938; Dunn, 1946)

Notes

Patent blue is reduced to the leuco form by nascent hydrogen, and in the presence of the enzyme (haemoglobin peroxidase) is recolourized by hydrogen peroxide oxidation. (Aniline blue may be used in place of the patent blue.)

The method is specific and usually reliable. However, it is important to appreciate that poorly fixed tissue and tissue fixed longer than 48 h in formalin, may give a negative result due to loss of the enzyme. It is recommended that a positive control section be taken through with the test sections.

Solutions

Stock leuco patent blue

To 100 ml of a 1% aqueous patent blue V solution add 10 g powdered zinc and 2 ml acetic acid. Boil until the solution turns a pale straw colour (approximately 10 min). Cool and filter.

This solution will keep for 8 months.

Working solution

To 10 ml stock solution add 2 ml acetic acid and 1 ml of 10 volumes hydrogen peroxide.

Technique

1. Take sections to distilled water.
2. Stain with the leuco patent blue solution for 3–5 min.
3. Wash well in distilled water.
4. Counterstain with 1% aqueous neutral red for 5 min. Wash.
5. Dehydrate, clear and mount as desired.

Results

Haemoglobin peroxidase (red blood cells and neutrophils)   blue
Nuclei   red

PORPHYRIN PIGMENTS

Porphyrin pigments are normally involved in haemoglobin synthesis and very rarely may be found deposited in tissue. This deposition usually occurs in familial porphyria, an uncommon disease in which the patient passes a port wine-coloured urine due to the presence of large amount of porphyrins. The liver is usually affected and the porphyrins appear as dark brown intracellular granules.

The most effective way to demonstrate the pigment is to examine fresh frozen sections with a fluorescence microscope, when a brilliant orange primary fluorescence will be seen.

For further details see Cripps & Scheuer (1965) and Cripps & MacEachern (1971).

BILE PIGMENTS

The breakdown process of red blood cells occurs in the reticulo-endothelial system. During the process haemoglobin is released from the red cells and iron is removed from the haem leaving biliverdin. This is produced in phagocytic cells in the spleen and bone marrow and then is transported to the liver: in this form it is insoluble in water. When in the liver it is reduced from biliverdin to bilirubin which is also insoluble in water until it is conjugated with glucuronic acid. The conjugated bilirubin is passed through the liver to its reservoir, the gall-bladder. It is obvious that in histological sections various stages of bile production can be present. It is important to remember this, for while we all refer to the substances as 'bile pigments' they are chemically different and may not react histologically and histochemically in the same manner. The term 'bile pigments' is used because in the normal course of events sections of liver containing bile will invariably contain a mixture. In addition to the above, a related pigment haematoidin occurring in tissue is classed as a bile pigment. This is usually found in old haemorrhagic areas, most often in the spleen and brain. It is thought that haem has undergone a chemical change at its site and has not been transported to the liver. The bile pigments in summary consist of:

Biliverdin
Bilirubin — unconjugated
Bilirubin — conjugated
Haematoidin

IDENTIFICATION

The first step is to consider the normal localization of the substances. Biliverdin will be found in phagocytic cells in the spleen, bone marrow and lymph nodes. The unconjugated bilirubin in liver cells and the conjugated form in bile canaliculi and the gall-bladder. Colour can also be used in identification, i.e. biliverdin appears as a green pigment, bilirubin as a dark brown pigment while haematoidin is a yellow amorphous deposit.

Demonstration

Although the brown and yellow colour of bilirubin and haematoidin respectively are well seen in an H and E section, the green colour of biliverdin is often masked by eosin. In these instances an unstained paraffin or frozen section or a haematoxylin nuclear stain only is called for. Bile pigments are not autofluorescent and are monorefringent. Their solubilities when in fixed tissue sections are unhelpful, although it has been reported that haematoidin is partly soluble in fat solvents (Ria & Scheuer, 1968). The majority of the techniques for demonstrating bile pigments are oxidation methods, the classical ones of Gmelin, Stein and Fouchet follow. The Schmorl reaction, the van Gieson method and on occasion the PAS technique will also demonstrate the pigments, blue, green, magenta, respectively.

GMELIN TECHNIQUE (Tiedemann & Gmelin, 1826)

Notes

When tissue containing a bile pigment is treated with nitric acid a spectrum of colours is produced. This colour spectrum is brought about by the oxidation of bilirubin to biliverdin, then to an admixture of biliverdin and purpurins, finally to a mixture of these plus yellow choletins.

The method tends to be capricious, is impermanent and gives best results with the larger bile pigment deposits.

Solution

Conc. nitric acid.

Technique

1. Take sections to distilled water and mount.
2. Place one or two drops of the concentrated nitric acid to one side of the coverslip and draw under the coverslip by means of a piece of blotting paper placed at the opposite side.
3. Wipe off excess solution and examine immediately.

Results

In the presence of bile pigment the following colour spectrum will gradually appear: green — red — blue — purple.

STEIN TECHNIQUE (Stein, 1935)

Notes

Bilirubin is oxidized by iodine to form green biliverdin, although in practice this is not readily observed. What happens is that the bile pigments tend to take up the iodine and stain a dark brown. Although the method is slow and nonspecific it clearly demonstrates even small bile pigment granules. A method similar in principle to Stein's is the use of pH 2.2 potassium dichromate to achieve oxidation of bilirubin to green biliverdin (Glenner, 1957).

The final dehydration is carried out in acetone as ethanol will extract the iodine colouration.

Solutions

Lugol's iodine, see page 204.

Tincture of iodine

Iodine	2 g
Potassium iodide	2 g
Distilled water	25 ml
Absolute alcohol	75 ml

Mix 3 parts of Lugol's iodine with 1 part of the tincture of iodine.

Technique

1. Take sections to water.
2. Stain with the iodine solution for 6–12 h.
3. Wash in water and differentiate in 5% hypo for 15–30 s.
4. Wash in water and counterstain lightly with 1% aqueous neutral red solution for 1–2 min. Wash.
5. Dehydrate in acetone, clear and mount as desired.

Results

Bile pigments   green (or brown)
Nuclei   red

Any amyloid or glycogen present will be stained brown.

FOUCHET TECHNIQUE (Fouchet, 1917)

Notes

In the presence of trichloracetic acid the bile pigments are oxidized by ferric chloride to form a mixture of green bilirubin and blue cholecyanin. The technique is quick and simple to do, and will demonstrate both coarse and fine pigment deposits. We consider it to be the method of choice. While counterstains such as neutral red are suitable, van Gieson's solution seems to accentuate the green-blue reaction product.

Solutions

Fouchet's reagent
    25% aqueous trichloracetic acid   100 ml
    10% aqueous ferric chloride   100 ml

Van Gieson's solution, see page 41.

Technique

1. Take sections to distilled water.
2. Stain with Fouchet's reagent for 5 min.
3. Rinse in distilled water.
4. Counterstain with van Gieson's solution for 2–3 min.
5. Rinse in distilled water, or drain and wash in alcohol. Dehydrate, clear and mount as desired.

Results

Bile pigments   blue-green
Collagen   red
Muscle   yellow

LIPOFUSCINS

These pigments are produced from the process of oxidation of lipids and lipoproteins. They have a variable structure that differs with the distribution throughout the body. The oxidation of the lipid material is said to be progressive and this accounts for the variable staining reactions and the different colours, shape and size of the pigments. Lipofuscin is normally laid down during the ageing process. It also occurs abnormally in vitamin E deficiency.

There are many sites for these pigments. The more common are those of liver, cardiac muscle cells, the inner layer of the adrenal cortex, the interstitial cells of the testis and the cytoplasm of neurones. During the progressive oxidation, the first produced lipofuscins are only partly oxidized; these include ceroid. Ceroid and the other 'early lipofuscins' retain some of the staining characteristics of lipids but can fail to stain by other methods. The histochemical reactions vary by the amount of oxidation that has occurred. The further the oxidation the stronger the staining with the reduction type methods. It is necessary therefore to use more than one method to demonstrate lipofuscin. At this point it will be worth remembering that other pigments are also capable of reducing solutions, melanin being the most important. Lipofuscins are mainly formed from lysosomes but also from mitochondria.

DEMONSTRATION

The staining techniques for lipofuscins are many. The two most precise depend upon the lipid content, staining with Sudan dyes (sudanophilia) and acid-fastness with the Ziehl-Neelsen technique. The more oxidized lipofuscins give a strong result with the Schmorl reaction due to their increased reducing ability. Some of the early lipofuscins are PAS positive although we are not certain of the reason for this. Other methods are shown in Table 11.3.

Table 11.3 Methods for lipofuscins

Method	Colour/reaction
Long ZN	Magenta
Sudan black	Black
Schmorl	Dark blue
Masson-Fontana	Black
PAS	Magenta
Giemsa	Greenish
Aldehyde Fuchsin	Purple
Basic dyes	According to dye
Thionin pH 3.0	Dark green
Primary fluorescence	Yellow
Bleaching	Removal

SUDAN BLACK TECHNIQUE

Technique

1. Take paraffin sections to 70% alcohol.
2. Stain overnight at room temperature in saturated Sudan black B in 70% alcohol (filter the desired quantity into a Coplin jar).
3. Wash and differentiate out the excess background dye in 70% alcohol.
4. Wash in water and mount in an aqueous mountant such as Apathy's mountant.

Results

Lipofuscin pigment, red blood cells	black
Background	weak grey

LONG ZIEHL-NEELSEN TECHNIQUE
(Pearse, 1953)

Notes

Victoria blue may be used to advantage in place of basic fuchsin in the staining solution.

Solutions

Carbol fuchsin, see page 206.

0.2% aqueous methylene blue.

Technique

1. Take sections to water.
2. Stain in filtered carbol fuchsin for 3 h at 56° C.

3. Wash well in water.
4. Differentiate in 1% acid-alcohol until the excess background staining is lost (1–3 min).
5. Wash well in water and counterstain in the aqueous methylene blue solution for ½–1 min. Wash.
6. Dehydrate and differentiate the counterstain in alcohol. Clear and mount.

Results

Lipofuscin	bright magenta
Nuclei	blue
Background	pale magenta to pale blue

SCHMORL TECHNIQUE (taken from Golodetz & Unna, 1909)

Notes

There are two often-quoted rationales for the Schmorl technique. The potassium ferricyanide is reduced to the ferrous salt, which in the presence of the ferric ions forms Prussian blue or the ferric chloride is reduced to the ferrous salt which reacts with the potassium ferricyanide to form Turnbull blue.

At all events, an insoluble blue pigment is formed by the reducing agents in situ. The time of reaction depends on the substance to be demonstrated. In this instance, for lipofuscin 5 or 6 min is usually enough. Melanin requires a shorter incubation time.

Ferric sulphate may be used in place of the ferric chloride and seems to result in a lighter background to the section.

A control section should be taken through with the test sections.

Solution

1% aqueous potassium ferricyanide (prepare fresh) 1% aqueous ferric chloride or 1% aqueous ferric sulphate	equal parts

Use within 30 min of mixing.

Technique

1. Take sections to distilled water.
2. Treat with the reagent mixture for 30 s to 10 min.

3. Wash well in water for several minutes.
4. Counterstain in 1% aqueous neutral red solution for 5 min.
5. Wash, dehydrate, clear and mount in a synthetic resin.

Results

Argentaffin cells, chromaffin
cells, melanin, some
lipofuscins, thyroid colloid,
sulphydryl groups   dark blue
Nuclei   red

CONTROLLED pH THIONIN TECHNIQUE (Lillie, 1954)

Notes

At a pH of 3.0 thionin will selectively stain lipofuscin; the blue dye combining with the brown pigment to give a dark green colouration.

Technique

1. Take sections to distilled water.
2. Stain with 0.25% thionin in pH 3.0 buffer (see Buffer Tables) for 3 min.
3. Wash in distilled water, blot dry, clear in xylene and mount in a DPX-type mountant.

Results

Lipofuscin   dark green
Nuclei   blue

MELANIN

Melanin is an intracellular pigment that varies in colour from light brown to black. The colouration depends upon the amount of melanin at any one site. It is normally located in the skin, retina, substantia nigra of the brain and hair shafts. Pathologically it is found in benign naevus cell tumours and malignant melanomas. Melanin is produced from tyrosine (see p. 192). The active sites of melanin production are well demonstrated by the DOPA oxidase reaction (see p. 192). The melanins are bound to proteins and these complexes are located within cells.

DEMONSTRATION

The identification of melanin can be by:

1. Staining methods utilizing the reducing capabilities of melanin with silver (Masson-Fontana) and ferricyanide (Schmorl).
2. The active sites demonstrated as described above by enzyme methods.
3. The solubility of melanin in strong alkali.
4. The bleaching effect with potassium permanganate.
5. Fluorescence produced by the treatment of melanin precursor cells with formaldehyde.

See also Table 11.4.

MASSON-FONTANA TECHNIQUE (Masson, 1914; Fontana, 1912)

Notes

This technique by Masson which utilizes Fontana's silver solution does not employ a reducing bath and will only demonstrate substances capable of silver-salt reduction. It is simple to do and the success or otherwise, of the technique devolves on the

Table 11.4 Methods for melanin

Method	Type of method	Colour	Comments
Masson-Fontana	Silver reduction	Black	Other substances will stain
Schmorl	Ferricyanide reduction	Blue	Other substances will stain
DOPA reaction	Enzyme	Brown	Specific
Potassium permanganate	Bleaching	Colourless	Selective
Sodium hydroxide	Solubility	Removed	Selective
Formaldehyde-induced fluorescence	Fluorescence	Yellow	Selective

preparation of the ammoniacal silver solution. A positive control section should always be taken through with the test. We prefer the longer room-temperature treatment for more precise results.

Solution

Add concentrated ammonia drop by drop to 20 ml of 10% aqueous silver nitrate, mixing well between each drop, until the formed precipitate almost redissolves. A faint opalescence will be evident when the end point is reached. Should the ammonia addition be overshot, add 10% aqueous silver nitrate drop by drop with constant mixing, until a faint opalescence is obtained. Finally, add 20 ml of distilled water, mix and filter. Store in a dark container. The solution may be used repeatedly for up to 1 month, although a fresher solution gives better results for lipofuscin and argentaffin granules.

Technique

1. Take sections to distilled water.
2. Treat with the ammoniacal silver solution in a dark container (e.g. a Coplin jar painted black) for either 20–40 min at 56° C or overnight at room temperature.
3. Wash well in several changes of distilled water.
4. Treat with 0.5% hypo for 2 min (a stronger solution tends to bleach the reduced silver).
5. Wash, counterstain in 1% aqueous neutral red for 3–5 min.
6. Wash, dehydrate, clear and mount as desired.

Results

Melanin, argentaffin, chromaffin, some lipofuscin pigment	black
Nuclei	red

FORMALDEHYDE-INDUCED FLUORESCENCE TECHNIQUE (Eranko, 1955)

Certain aromatic amines, e.g. dopamine, catecholamines, 5HT, when exposed to formaldehyde form non-fluorescent isocarboline derivatives which after spontaneous dehydrogenation become fluorescent. This means in practice that mast cells, enterochromaffin cells, adrenal chromaffin cells, C cells of thyroid and melanin-producing cells, if fixed in formalin or formaldehyde vapour, will exhibit a yellow primary fluorescence. This is particularly useful when demonstrating a secondary amelanotic melanoma, as this type of lesion can be difficult to diagnose and yields a negative melanin reaction, but as melanoma cells contain dopamine they are capable of showing the formalin-induced fluorescence as a means of identification.

The best results are achieved using freeze-dried slightly humid paraformaldehyde vapour-fixed material but the following technique gives acceptable results using formalin-fixed frozen sections. Paraffin processed material may also be used.

Technique

1. Deparaffinize formalin-fixed paraffin sections in xylene. Frozen sections are rinsed in distilled water.
2. Rinse in clean xylene and mount in a DPX-type mountant (avoid Canada balsam as this is autofluorescent), or mount frozen sections in 50% glycerol.
3. Examine the sections using a mercury vapour ultraviolet emission lamp incorporating a red suppression filter (e.g. BG 38), ultraviolet exciter filter (e.g. UG1) and colourless barrier filter (e.g. K430).

Results

Melanin-precursor cells	weak yellow fluorescence
Other naturally fluorescing material e.g. elastin	silver-white

Alternatively (Hoyt et al, 1979)

Prepare a solution of 6% paraformaldehyde in pH 7.2 phosphate buffer at 90° C Cool and filter. Fix blocks 1–3 days and section, etc.

Also note (Corrodi et al, 1964)

The FIF of biogenic amines but *not* that of other autofluorescent substances can be destroyed by treating the aldehyde-fixed sections (prior to microscopy) with 0.5% sodium borohydride for 30 min.

IRON AND HAEMOSIDERIN

Iron is absorbed from the gastro-intestinal tract and is combined with a protein molecule for its transportation to the bone marrow where it is incorporated into the haemoglobin molecule. Iron is also stored in the bone marrow and spleen in its ferric state as haemosiderin when it is loosely combined with protein. When haemoglobin is broken down in tissues haemosiderin is produced. If excess iron is given to the body haemosiderin becomes deposited in the organs involved with iron storage, i.e. bone marrow, spleen and liver. This condition is called haemosiderosis. If iron is absorbed indiscriminately into the body a condition called haemochromotosis exists in which large amounts of haemosiderin are deposited in many tissues. The fine golden brown pigment in tissue sections is usually derived from damaged red cells and occurs in macrophages.

DEMONSTRATION

Not all the iron in tissues can be demonstrated. On occasions metallic iron introduced into the tissues by exposure will fail to react with staining methods. Iron that is firmly bound with protein as in haemoglobin will also fail to react unless released from the protein by treatment with hydrogen peroxide. It is rarely necessary to demonstrate this type of iron in the routine laboratory.

Perls' reaction is used to demonstrate ferric iron (ferritin is also demonstrated by Perls' reaction). It is one of the classical histochemical methods introduced by Perls' in 1867. The Schmeltzer technique (1933) will demonstrate both ferric and ferrous iron, although the latter is rarely found in tissues.

PERLS' TECHNIQUE (Perls, 1867)

Notes

Hydrochloric acid splits off the bound protein, allowing the potassium ferrocyanide to combine specifically with ferric iron to form ferric ferrocyanide (Prussian blue). Weak solutions used for a lengthy period give more precise results; Bunting (1949) found that 2% solutions were best. Whilst stronger results are given by carrying out the reaction at raised temperature (e.g. 56° C), false positive results can be obtained and it is therefore recommended that room temperature be employed. A control section of positive material should always be taken through with the test material.

Following reaction with ferrocyanide-hydrochloric acid the sections should be well washed in water otherwise, particularly with a neutral red counterstain, a heavy dye precipitate will be formed on the section. Mounting should be in a DPX-type mountant to obviate the eventual fading of the Prussian blue which occurs in mountants such as Canada balsam.

In this technique a common artefact is the presence of blue granules, either on or around the section, following treatment with the hydrochloric-ferrocyanide mixture. In our experience this may be due to one of two things: (1) an old deteriorated potassium ferrocyanide solution — the remedy is obvious; (2) iron contaminants in the floating-out water (rust, etc.) during sectioning. The simplest remedy here is to have a suitably-sized beaker containing distilled water to one side of the bath. The distilled water will be maintained at the correct temperature and it is a simple matter to float out sections to be subsequently stained by the Perls' reaction.

Solutions

2% aqueous potassium ferrocyanide.
2% hydrochloric acid.
1% aqueous neutral red.

Technique

1. Take the test sections and a control section to distilled water.

2. Mix equal parts of the hydrochloric acid and potassium ferrocyanide solutions and filter on to the sections. Leave for 30 min at room temperature, changing to fresh solution after 15 min.
3. Wash for several minutes in water.
4. Stain with the neutral red solution for 5 min. Wash in water.
5. Dehydrate and differentiate in alcohol. Clear and mount in a DPX-type mountant.

Results

Haemosiderin (ferric iron salts)	blue
Nuclei	red
Background	pale red

QUINKE TECHNIQUE (Quinke, 1880)

Both ferric and ferrous iron salts are converted to a black ferrous sulphide by treating with yellow ammonium sulphide. This method is not specific for iron salts as both silver and lead deposits are also blackened.

TIRMANN TECHNIQUE (Tirmann, 1898)

This is similar in principle to the Perls' reaction, but the ferrous iron haemosiderin is converted to ferrous ferricyanide (Turnbull blue) by potassium ferricyanide. Again, hydrochloric acid is used to split off the remaining protein moiety from the iron. The method is regarded as specific.

SCHMELTZER TECHNIQUE (Schmeltzer, 1933)

Notes

Schmeltzer utilized ammonium sulphide treatment to convert the ferric iron to ferrous iron, and then by subsequently carrying out the Tirmann reaction, simultaneously demonstrated both ferric and ferrous iron.

There seems to be considerable discrepancy in the literature as regards the concentrations of the hydrochloric acid and potassium ferricyanide of the reaction, also of the yellow ammonium sulphide to be used. This usually means that it is of little real significance in practice! Celloidinization of sections is advisable, mainly due to the action of the ammonium sulphide.

Solutions

Undiluted yellow ammonium sulphide solution (usually 10% of H_2S w/v).

20% aqueous potassium ferricyanide.

2% hydrochloric acid.

1% aqueous neutral red.

Technique

1. Take test and control sections to distilled water.
2. Treat with the ammonium sulphide solution for 1–3 h.
3. Wash well in several changes of distilled water over several minutes.
4. Mix equal parts of the hydrochloric acid and potassium ferricyanide solutions and filter on to the sections. Leave for 15–20 min.
5. Wash well in water for several minutes.
6. Stain with the neutral red solution for 5 min. Wash in water.
7. Dehydrate and differentiate in alcohol. Clear and mount in a DPX-type mountant.

Results

Ferric and ferrous iron	blue
Nuclei	red
Background	pale red

Note that any silver or lead salts present will be seen as black deposits.

CALCIUM

We are concerned here with the demonstration of insoluble inorganic salts normally found in bone and teeth. (See also crystals identification p. 245.) Calcium circulates in the blood in free ionic form, which is not demonstrable histochemically. It is found abnormally in areas of tissue necrosis associated with tuberculosis, infarction or atheromatous lesions of blood vessels.

DEMONSTRATION

Various types of calcium salt can be demonstrated but the most commonly occurring are calcium phosphate and calcium carbonate. There is a wide range of techniques available. Calcium salts are usually monorefringent (but see p. 246 concerning calcium oxalate demonstration).

H and E appearance

Calcium salts are often purple-blue in colour but may occasionally not stain at all. The haematoxylin staining is attributed to trace elements of iron in the calcium salts and is not, therefore, truly diagnostic for calcium as such.

Chemical test to differentiate between phosphate and carbonate radicals

In order to more positively identify a given calcium salt, two paraffin sections are taken to distilled water and a coverslip placed on each. A small drop of conc. hydrochloric acid is drawn under the coverslips and the effect noted microscopically. If the salt consists of calcium carbonate it will dissolve liberating bubbles of carbon dioxide. If the salt is that of calcium phosphate the salt will dissolve without effervescence.

Staining with dyes. Various dyes react with calcium salts in a variety of ways: for example alizarin, purpurin, naphthochrome green B and nuclear fast red act by forming chelate complexes with the metallic calcium; alcian blue stains by salt linkage with the phosphate radical. On the whole these methods stain only the larger deposits of calcium salts well, the smaller deposits staining only weakly. None of these stains is specific as such for calcium.

Von Kossa technique. The technique and principle of this method is given on page 244. Calcium salts as such are not demonstrated (only the phosphate or carbonate radicals). It gives good demonstration of both large and small deposits of calcium. Although not specific (melanin also tends

to blacken) it remains the method of choice. In place of the reduction of silver using light or ultraviolet rays, it is possible to use 0.5% aqueous hydroquinone for 5 min following silver nitrate treatment for 10–20 min in the dark (Gomori, 1952). Unfortunately, this variant tends to result in a rather granular background and is not widely used.

As a general rule, non-acidic fixation should be used such as formalin or alcohol.

ALIZARIN RED S METHOD FOR CALCIUM (McGee-Russell, 1958)

Notes

Calcium forms an orange-red dye lake with alizarin red S. The staining time is dependant upon the amount of calcium in the sections. The staining should be microscopically controlled, until the deposits are orange-red in colour but not too diffuse. The calcium deposits stained with alizarin red S are birefringent. The dye-lake is specific for calcium at pH 4.2.

Solution

2% alizarin red S (aqueous). pH adjusted to 4.2 with 10% ammonium hydroxide.

Technique

1. Sections to water.
2. Rinse in distilled water.
3. Transfer sections to alizarin red S solution for 1–5 min (see Notes).
4. Blot, rinse in acetone for 30 s.
5. Treat with acetone-xylene 1 : 1 for 15 s.
6. Rinse in fresh xylene and mount in DPX.

Results

Calcium deposits orange-red

PURPURIN TECHNIQUE (taken from Lillie, 1965)

Notes

Purpurin demonstrates only the larger aggregates of calcium salts and does so by forming a mordant lake with the metal. Counterstaining should be light as the purpurin staining is easily masked. The post-staining treatment with sodium chloride presumably acts to stabilize the stain compound formed.

Solutions

Saturated alcoholic purpurin (synonym: 1 : 2 : 4-trihydroxyanthraquinone).

0.75% aqueous sodium chloride.

Technique

1. Take paraffin sections to alcohol.
2. Place in a Coplin jar of the alcoholic purpurin solution for 10 min.
3. Treat with the sodium chloride solution for 3 min. Wash in water.
4. Counterstain, if desired, with Mayer's haematoxylin solution for $1\frac{1}{2}$ min. Wash in water and blue.
5. Wash in water. Dehydrate, clear and mount as desired.

Results

Calcium	red
Nuclei	blue

CALCIUM-PRUSSIAN BLUE TECHNIQUE
(Hurst, et al, 1951)

Notes

Calcium ammonium ferrocyanide is precipitated by the reaction of calcium salts with a potassium ferrocyanide-ammonium acetate solution. This precipitate, when treated with ferric chloride, forms Prussian blue.

This is an ingenious method for demonstrating calcium salts in tissue but, unfortunately, only the larger deposits react well.

Following treatment with the ferrocyanide-ammonium acetate the section is rinsed in 40% alcohol. This rinsing must be minimal or the reaction will be weakened. The final colour product is not particularly strong so that counterstaining should be light.

Any magnesium salts present in the tissue will also react but this is unlikely, in practice to cause confusion.

Solutions

Ferrocyanide-ammonium acetate
Dissolve 10 g ammonium acetate in 100 ml of 40% alcohol, add 1 g potassium ferrocyanide. Dissolve by placing in the 56° C oven. Cool before use.

10% aqueous ferric chloride.

Technique

1. Take sections to alcohol and rinse in 40% alcohol.
2. Treat with the ferrocyanide-ammonium acetate solution for 30 s.
3. Rinse quickly in two baths of 40% alcohol, then in distilled water.
4. Treat with the ferric chloride solution for 5 min.
5. Wash in water and, if desired, stain lightly with 0.5% aqueous neutral red.
6. Dehydrate, clear and mount in a DPX-type mountant.

Results

Calcium salts	blue
Background	pale blue or colourless

FLUORESCENT MORIN TECHNIQUE (taken from Pearse, 1960)

Notes

A number of metallic salts are demonstrated by this method. Like many fluorescence techniques there is a gradual loss of fluorescent staining on storage of the sections.

A control section treated with hydrochloric acid should also be taken through; any dissolved morin-positive crystals can be regarded as being calcium salts.

Solutions

1% hydrochloric acid.

0.2 g morin (synonym: pentahydroxyflavone)

dissolved in a solution consisting of 0.5% acetic acid in 85% alcohol.

Technique

1. Take two duplicate sections to distilled water. Treat only one with the hydrochloric acid solution for 10 min.
2. Wash well in water. Wash sections in alcohol.
3. Treat both sections with the morin reagent for 3 min.
4. Wash and dehydrate in alcohol, clear in xylene, mount in a DPX-type mountant.

Results

Using a fluorescence microscope with a mercury vapour lamp and a BG 12 exciter and K 530 (yellow) barrier filter:

Calcium, aluminium, barium, zirconium (also red blood cells) bright yellow-green

Background dull green

Calcium salts will not be stained in the extracted section.

COPPER

Copper is a normal constituent of many tissues. There are no histochemical methods sensitive enough to demonstrate it at normal body levels. In Wilson's disease the level of copper is increased, especially in the liver and brain. In primary biliary cirrhosis and sometimes in alcoholic cirrhosis and α_1-antitrypsin disease copper can be demonstrated in liver (Beresford et al, 1980).

DEMONSTRATION

There are four main methods available for showing copper. The dye-lake method of Mallory & Parker (1939) using non-ripened alkaline haematoxylin, the DMABR method of Howell (1959), the Rhodanine technique (Jain et al, 1978) and the standard method of Uzman (1956) utilizing rubeanic acid which is described below.

RUBEANIC ACID TECHNIQUE (from Okamoto & Utamura, 1938)

Notes

Rubeanic acid (dithio-oxamide) forms a coloured copper rubeanate compound with copper. The technique, whilst not particularly sensitive gives clear-cut results and is the method of choice. Fixation is important, for whilst formalin may be used, fixatives such as mercuric chloride are contra-indicated.

A section of positive control material should always be taken through with the test sections.

Solution

0.1% rubeanic acid in absolute alcohol 5 ml to which is added 10% aqueous sodium acetate 100 ml.

Technique

1. Take sections to distilled water.
2. Place in a Coplin jar filled with the rubeanic-acetate solution for 8–16 h at 37° C.
3. Wash briefly in distilled water and blot dry. Counterstain briefly in 0.5% aqueous neutral red.
4. Dehydrate, clear and mount as desired.

Results

Copper rubeanate greenish black
Nuclei red

EXOGENOUS PIGMENTS AND MINERALS

These pigments are usually found in the body due to industrial exposure. Their most likely sites are the lungs and skin (Table 11.6).

CARBON

Found in the lungs except the newborn, and in lymph nodes. It is an inert and unreactive element

Table 11.6 Exogenous pigments

Pigment	Usual site	Method
Carbon	Lungs; lymph nodes	None available
Silica	Lungs	None available but birefringent
Asbestos	Lungs	Perls'; birefringent if recent (and therefore uncoated)
Lead	Kidney; bone	Rhodizonate method, see Bancroft & Stevens (1982)
Beryllium	Lungs; skin	See below
Aluminium	Lungs; skin	See below
Silver	Skin; nasal mucosa	Rhodanine method, see Bancroft & Stevens (1982)

and has no methods for its demonstration. Resistant to bleaching and to strong acids. Easily identified because of its blackness, localization and irregular shape.

SILICA

Tiny particles are found abnormally in fibrous tissue of the lungs and lymph nodes. Again an inert substance for which there is no definitive technique; the particles show birefringence.

ASBESTOS

This is seen in the form of long beaded fibres which cause a fibrous reaction. Prolonged exposure leads to the disease asbestosis. Initially the fibres show birefringence; after the fibrous reaction the fibres become coated in protein and develop their characteristic morphology. The protein sheath contains haemosiderin, giving a positive reaction with Perls' method. The asbestos fibre with its coated protein sheath is known as an asbestos body. They are easily seen in an H and E stain as well as the Perls' reaction.

ALUMINIUM AND BERYLLIUM

Tissue deposition of aluminium and beryllium chiefly occurs in industrial disease and most commonly affect the lungs. In addition, workers in industries involving aluminium salts may present with skin nodules.

The appearance of the aluminium in an H and E preparation varies from a fine brown granule to small crystalline plates staining a pale pink colour. In addition to the technique described, aluminium will exhibit a secondary fluorescence in the Morin technique (see p. 154). Beryllium deposits are usually seen in lung tissue and often present as calcified conchoidal (shell-like) bodies which are typical of, but not specific to beryllium. These beryllium conchoidal bodies usually give positive reactions for haemosiderin (Perls' technique, see p. 151). The naphthochrome green B method can also be employed but is less selective than the solochrome azurine as other metallic dye-lakes may be formed.

SOLOCHROME AZURINE TECHNIQUE
(Pearse, 1957)

Notes

Beryllium and aluminium will form a deep blue complex with the chelating agent solochrome azurine. The technique is simple to do and can be carried out on conventionally fixed, paraffin processed material. Both aluminium and beryllium will stain with the solochrome azurine in aqueous solution, but at an alkaline pH aluminium will fail to react. We have found the method to work well.

Positive control sections should always be taken through if these are available.

PIGMENTS 157

Solutions

Solution A

0.2% aqueous solochrome azurine (syn. Pure blue B).

Solution B

0.2% solochrome azurine in molar sodium hydroxide.

Technique

1. Take two duplicate sections to distilled water.
2. Stain one section in solution A and one in solution B for 20 min.
3. Wash in water. Counterstain in 1% aqueous neutral red for 3–5 min.
4. Wash in water. Dehydrate, clear and mount in a DPX-type mountant.

Results

Solution A: aluminium and beryllium	blue
Solution B: beryllium only	blue-black
Nuclei	red

LEAD AND SILVER

These are not often seen in tissue sections.

A useful bleaching technique for silver granules in tissue is to treat sections for up to 5 min with a solution consisting of 5% aqueous sodium thiosulphate — 32 ml and 0.5% aqueous potassium ferricyanide — 8 ml. (This is conveniently done in a Coplin jar.)

REFERENCES

Beresford P A, Sunter J P, Harrison V, Lesna M 1980 Histological demonstration and frequency of intrahepatocytic copper in patients suffering from alcoholic liver disease. Histopathology 4: 637
Bunting H 1949 Histochemical detection of iron in tissues. Stain Technology 24: 109
Corrodi H, Hillarp N A, Jonsson G 1964 Fluorescence methods for the demonstration of monoamines. 3. Sodium borohydride reduction of the fluorescent compounds as a specificity test. Journal of Histochemistry & Cytochemistry 12: 582
Cripps D J, MacEachern W N 1971 Hepatic and erythropoietic protoporphyria. Archives of Pathology 91: 497
Cripps D J, Scheuer 1965 Hepatobiliary changes in erythropoietic protoporphyria. Archives of Pathology 80: 500
Dunn R C 1951 Hemoglobin stain for histologic use based on cyanol-hemoglobin reaction. Archives of Pathology 41: 476
Dunn R C, Thompson 1946 A simplified stain for haemoglobin in tissue and smears using patent blue. Stain Technology 21: 65
Drury R A B, Wallington E A 1980 Carleton's histological technique 5th ed. Oxford University Press
Eranko O 1955 Distribution of adrenaline and noradrenaline in the adrenal medulla. Nature 175: 88
Fontana A 1912 Verfahren zur intensiven und raschen Farbung des Treponema pallidum und anderer Spirochäten Dermatologische Wochenschrift 55: 1003
Fouchet A 1917 Methode nouvelle de recherche et de dosage des pigments biliares dans le serum sanguin. Comptes Rendus de Seances de la Societe de Biologie et de ses Filiales

Glenner G 1957 Simultaneous demonstration of bilirubin, hemosiderin and lipofuschin pigments in tissue sections. American Journal of Clinical Pathology 27: 1
Golodetz L, Unna P C 1909 Zur chemie der Haut III. Das Reduktionsvermögen der histologischen Elemente der Haut. Mh. Prakt. Dermatogie 48: 149
Gomori G 1952 Microscopic histochemistry. Chicago University Press
Howell J S 1959 Histochemical demonstration of copper in copper fed rats and in the hepatolenticular degeneration. Journal of Pathology & Bacteriology 77: 423
Hoyt R F, Sorokin S P, Bartlett 1979 A simple fluorescence method for serotonin-containing endocrine cells in plastic embedded lung, gut and thyroid gland. Journal of Histochemistry & Cytochemistry 27: 721
Hurst V, Hutton W E, Nycholls J 1951 A new histochemical reaction for calcium. Journal of Dental Research 30: 489
Jain S, Scheuer P J, Archer B, Newman S P, Sherlock S 1978 Histological demonstration of copper and copper associated protein in chronic liver diseases. Journal of Clinical Pathology 31: 784
Lendrum A C 1949 Staining of crythrocytes in tissue sections; a new method and observations on some of the modified Mallory connective tissue stains. Journal of Pathology & Bacteriology 61: 443
Lillie R D 1954 Histopathologic technique and practical histochemistry. McGraw-Hill, New York
Lillie R D 1965 Histopathologic technique and practical histochemistry 3rd ed. McGraw-Hill, New York
Lison L 1938 Zur Frage der Ausscheidung und Speicherung des Hämoglobins in der Amphibienniere. Beitrage zur Pathologichen Anatomie und zur Allgemeinen Pathologie 101: 94

McGee-Russell S M 1958 Histochemical methods for calcium. Journal of Histochemistry & Cytochemistry 6: 22

Mallory F B, Paiker F 1939 Fixing and staining methods for lead and copper in tissues. American Journal Pathology 16: 517

Masson P 1914 La glande endocrine de l'intestine chez l'homme. Comptes Rendus Hebdomadaires des Seances de l'Academie des Sciences 158: 59

Okamoto K, Utamura M 1938 Biologische Untersuchen des Kupfers uber die histochemische Kupfernachweiss Methode. Acta Scholae Medicinalis Universitatis Imperialis in Kisto 20: 573

Pearse A G E 1957 Solochrome dyes in histochemistry with particular reference to nuclear staining. Acta Histochemica 4: 95

Pearse A G E 1960 Histochemistry, theoretical and applied, 2nd Churchill, London

Perls M 1867 Nachweis von Eisenoxyd in geweissen Pigmentation. Virchow's Archive fur Pathologische Anatomie und Physiologie und fur Klinische Medizin 39: 42

Pucht er H, Sweat F 1962 Amido black as a stain for hemoglobin. Archives of Pathology 73: 245

Quincke H I 1880 Zur Pathologie des Blutes. Dtsch. Archive Klin. Medicine 25: 567

Schmeltzer W 1933 Der mikrochemische Nachweis von Eissen in Gewebselementenmitels Rhodenwasserstoffsaure und die Konservierung der Reaktion in Paroffinol. Zeitschrift fur Wissenschaftliche Mikroscopie 50: 99

Stein J 1935 Reaction histochemique stable de detection de la bilirubine. Comptes rendus de seances de la Societe de Biologie et de ses Filiales 120: 1136

Tiedemann F, Gmelin P J 1826 Die Verdauung nach Versuchen, Vol 1. Heidelberg & Leipzig, K. Gross

Tirmann J 1898 Ueber den Uebergang des Eisens in die Milch. Gorbersdorfer Veroffentt 2: 101

Uzman L L 1956 Histochemical localisation of copper with rubeanic acid. Laboratory Investigation 5: 299

12

The diffuse neuroendocrine (APUD) system

The APUD system is the concept applied to groups of cells that contain cytoplasmic neurosecretory granules. The title 'APUD' was coined by Pearse (1968) because of the biochemical ability of the cells. They have a high amine content and are able to take up and decarboxylate amine precursors hence '*Amine Precursor Uptake and Decarboxylation*.'

The APUD cell system was thought by Pearse to have originated with Nonidez (1932), who demonstrated that thyroid parafollicular cells contained argyophil granules, and were involved in an endocrine secretion. Later after work by many people it was demonstrated that calcitonin was produced by these cells. The hormone is involved in controlling blood calcium levels in the body. As a result Pearse and his co-workers called the thyroid parafollicular cells 'C'. The cytochemistry and electron microscopy of these and similar amine-containing cells was thoroughly investigated by these workers between 1964 and 1970. In the 1968 concept, three sets of characteristics were discussed. The cytochemical, the morphological, and the origins of the cells. In this chapter we are only concerned with the first two.

CYTOCHEMICAL FEATURES

Pearse considered the cytochemical characteristics as the principal criteria for including a cell in the APUD system. The main findings are that the cells:-

1. Contain an amine or can secondarily take it up.
2. Contain an amino acid decarboxylase.
3. Contain α-glycerophosphate dehydrogenase.

4. Contain nonspecific esterase and/or cholinesterase.
5. Contain sufficient concentration of side chain carboxyl groups to enable them to be seen by masked metachromasia.

MORPHOLOGICAL FEATURES

1. Electron-dense, fixation-labile mitochondria.
2. High content of free ribosomes.
3. High levels of smooth endoplasmic reticulum.
4. Low levels of rough endoplasmic reticulin.
5. Secretory vesicles.
6. Prominent microtubules and centrosomes.

The ultrastructural characteristics are not as specific as the cytochemical ones. According to Gould (1978) most protein secreting cells exhibit the features discussed above to some degree. Following the work on the 'C' cells it has been shown that other polypeptide hormone producing cells have the same cytochemical and ultrastructural characteristics. These other cells together with the 'C' cells form the system to date. In some sites such as the pancreatic islets, adrenal medulla and the anterior pituitary, the polypeptide hormone producing cells are clumped together to form a recognisable endocrine gland. Elsewhere, and particularly in the gastro-intestinal tract where they are scattered throughout the mucosa, they form a diffuse system.

Table 12.1 indicates the major groups of cells of the APUD system. It is not intended to be complete; and additions are constantly being made. The table is drawn from Pearse (1968), Dawson (1976, 1982) and Gould (1978).

Table 12.1 The APUD cell system. *Key*: 5 HT, 5 hydroxytryptamine; A, adrenaline; NA, noradrenaline; EC, enterochromaffin; GIP, gastrin inhibitory polypeptide; VIP, vasoactive intestinal peptide.

Source of cells	Name of cells	Polypeptide secreted	Amine stored
Thyroid	C	Calcitonin	5 HT
Pituitary	Corticotroph	ACTH	
	Melanotroph	MSH	
	Somatotroph	ST	Tryptophan
	Mammotroph	Prolactin	
Pancreatic islets	A (α2)	Glucagon	5 HT or Dopamine
	B (β)	Insulin	5HT or Dopamine
	D (α1)	Somatostatin	
Duodenum and small bowel	S	Secretin	
	D	G.I.P.	
	EG	Enteroglucagon	5 HT
	EC	—	
	H	VIP	
	D	Somatostatin	
Stomach	G	Gastrin	5 HT or Dopamine
	A	Enteroglucagon	
	D	Somatostatin	
	EC	Serotonin	5 HT
G.I. tract	EC (Kultschitsky)		5 HT
Adrenal medulla	A	—	Adrenaline
	NA	—	Noradrenaline

APUDOMAS

It is possible for any of the cells in the APUD series to give rise to a tumour. The first described was by Szijj et al (1969) who introduced the term 'apudoma' to describe a tumour arising from C cells of the thyroid. These tumours are frequently termed apudoma, followed by the peptide hormone they are secreting (e.g.) an apudoma secreting insulin (Pearse, 1974). A list of the more common tumours is given in Table 12.2.

CARCINOID TUMOURS (ENDOCRINE CELL TUMOUR; APUDOMA)

The terminology carcinoid is applied to a tumour that arises from argentaffin or argyrophil and related endocrine cells. The term 'carcinoid' was used to distinguish it from a carcinoma and the appellation argentaffin and argyrophil to their histological reactivity (q.v.). The carcinoid tumour when developing from argentaffin cells can also be called an argentaffinoma. The majority of carcinoids are seen in the gastro-intestinal tract, in the appendix and small intestine, also to a much lesser extent in the stomach. The second most common site is the lung, where the carcinoids may be malignant or occur as adenomas. Occasionally carcinoids can be seen in the ovary, and carcinoid tumours of the pancreas, urinary bladder and liver have been reported.

Carcinoids that develop from argentaffin cells usually appear yellowish macroscopically following fixation in formaldehyde. The tumours from non-argentaffin endocrine cells do not display this yellow colouration. Histologically carcinoids consist of nests and islands of tightly arranged cells of similar appearance surrounded by stroma. Following formalin fixation acidophilic granules can be seen in the cytoplasm of the cells. The carcinoids of the appendix and small intestine are invariably argentaffinomas showing the argentaffin and argyrophil reactions. Autolysis causes the argentaffin cells to lose their reducing properties reasonably quickly, so rapid fixation is required. The argyrophil reaction is not lost as rapidly, but then it must be remembered that not all carcinoids will show the argentaffin reaction. Azo coupling is a specific method of demonstration for argentaffin carcinoids, other suitable methods being the ferric ferricyanide (Schmorl) and the Gibbs reaction.

Table 12.2 Examples of tumours developing from cells of the APUD system

Tumour	Site
Medullary carcinoma	Thyroid
Acidophil adenoma Carcinoma	Pituitary
Islet cell adenoma Islet cell carcinoma	Pancreas
Gastrinoma	Stomach
Carcinoid	G.I. tract; lung
Phaeochromocytoma	Adrenal

DEMONSTRATION OF APUD CELLS

It is important that aldehyde fixation is used for the cells of the APUD system that store an amine. The reaction between the amine and the aldehyde produces, in the case of 5HT, a carboline derivative and this reduces the various reagents used in the demonstration of the cells.

In H and E stained sections the majority of APUD cells have the same characteristics: they are oblong or triangular in shape with a broad base abutting the basement membrane and the underlying vascular supply (Dawson, 1982). The variable number of secretory granules they contain are difficult to see without using specialized techniques. The different types of methods for the demonstration of APUD cells are listed below. It is worth noting that the β cells of the pancreas do not conform to the guidelines laid down for APUD cells with histochemical techniques. They are usually identified by their sulphur amino acid content, e.g. with aldehyde fuchsin.

Chromaffin cells

These cells are associated with the sympathetic nervous system. They are found in the adrenal medulla, sympathetic ganglia and paraganglia. In the adrenal medulla the cells are divided into A cells, which produce adrenaline and NA cells, which secrete noradrenaline. These substances will precipitate chrome salts resulting in the chromaffin reaction. Chromate oxidation rapidly produces the brown pigment seen in adrenaline and noradrenaline containing cells. Iodates can also be used as an oxidizing agent and are employed to distinguish between the two substances as they oxidize noradrenaline far more rapidly than adrenaline. Chromaffin granules will reduce ammoniacal silver and ferricyanide showing the argentaffin reaction (see below) and a positive Schmorl's reaction respectively.

Enterochromaffin cells (*Kultschitzky cells*)

Scattered cells in the gastric mucosa of various animals were identified as yellow cells following fixation in dichromate (Heidenhain, 1870). Kultschitzky (1897) described them as containing fine oxyphil granules. Schmidt (1905) recognized them in the human duodenum and called them chromaffin cells. Ciaccio (1907) attributed their chromaffin reaction to adrenalin and called the 'chromaffin cells' found in gastric mucosa, enterochromaffin cells (EC). Masson (1914) showed that the cells produced the argentaffin reaction (see below). Erspamer & Asero (1952) identified the amine as 5-hydroxytryptamine (5HT). The cells that are scattered throughout the intestinal tract comprise the major part of the 'diffuse' endocrine system and today the term enterochromaffin is unsuitable for all these cells as only a few of the cells will demonstrate the chromaffin reaction. A far better title is endocrine cells of the gastro-intestinal tract which then can be divided into suitable subgroups depending upon the hormone they secrete. The subgrouping of cells in relation to their staining reactions is still viable and a brief description of these is given below.

Argentaffin cells

These cells can be found in almost all areas of the gastro-intestinal tract. They also occur in the pancreas, gall-bladder and genito-urinary tract. There are many argentaffin cells in the duodenum, ileum, appendix in the crypts of Lieberkuhn. Few are seen in the stomach as these are mainly argyrophil cells. Argentaffin cells are usually pear-shaped and they have an eosinophilic cytoplasm. The granules they contain lie between the nucleus and the basement membrane. Following formalin fixation these granules will directly reduce silver (argentaffin reaction), couple with diazonium salts and reduce ferric ferricyanide (Schmorl). They exhibit a bright autofluorescence. They have an affinity for osmic acid and will show the argyrophilic reaction. Argentaffin cells will show the chromaffin reaction but differ from the adrenal medulla cells showing the reaction after formaldehyde fixation. The concensus of opinion is that they produce 5-hydroxytryptamine (5HT).

Argyrophil cells

These are found in the gastro-intestinal mucosa in similar locations as argentaffin cells but in much larger numbers. Many are found in stomach mucosa, a rare site for argentaffin cells. They can also be located in the pancreas. Argyrophil cells can be impregnated with silver but a reducing agent is required to produce the deposit of metallic silver. The main difference between argentaffin and argyrophil cells is probably the amount of reducing substance to be found in the argentaffin cells.

The argyrophil cells can be demonstrated in general by the Bodian silver, and lead haematoxylin methods; specific argyrophil cells such as α_1 and α_2 cells of the pancreas are best demonstrated by the Grimelius and Hellerström and Hellman methods respectively.

Argentaffin reaction

Cells that have the ability to directly reduce silver solutions producing an insoluble black metallic silver precipitate are termed argentaffin cells. Aldehyde fixation is mandatory for this reaction in order that beta-carboline type of reducing groups are formed.

Argyrophil reaction

These cell granules will also react with silver solutions. They differ from argentaffin cells because argyrophilic cells require an additional reducing agent (usually hydroquinone or formalin) before they can reduce silver solution to metallic silver. There are many more of them than argentaffin cells. It is necessary to remember that all argentaffin cells will show argyrophilia, but the argentaffin reaction will not be seen in argyrophilic cells.

Table 12.4 Recommended staining methods. (All argyrophil methods will also demonstrate argentaffin cells.)

Chromaffin cells	Chromaffin reaction
	Iodate reaction (NA cells)
	Formalin induced fluorescence
	Giemsa
	Schmorl
	Masson-Fontana
	Lead haematoxylin
APUD argentaffin cells	Alkaline diazo
	Schmorl
	Singh
	Lead haematoxylin
	Masson-Fontana
	Gibbs reaction
APUD argyrophil cells	Bodian
	Grimelius (α_2 cells of pancreas)
	Pascual
	Hellerstrom and Hellman (α_1 cells of pancreas)
	Lead haematoxylin

Table 12.3 Effects of fixation

Cells	Fixation	Result
Chromaffin cells	Dichromate	Brown granules
Chromaffin cells	Formaldehyde	Unstained granules
Chromaffin cells	Formaldehyde postfixed in dichromate	Weak yellow-brown
Argentaffin cells	Formaldehyde	FIF; silver reduction
Argentaffin cells	Formaldehyde postfixed in dichromate	Weak chromaffin reaction
Argentaffin cells	Dichromate	Variable chromaffin reaction

TYPES OF TECHNIQUE

1. Basic dyes including metachromatic dyes.
2. Argyrophilic silver methods.
3. Amine identification.
4. Polypeptide identification.
5. Electron microscopy.

BASIC DYES

Cationic dyes will react with carboxyl groups in polypeptides. They are not specific as they are unable to demonstrate hormones. Metachromatic dyes are frequently used with prior acid hydrolysis in 0.2 M HCl. This unmasks further side chain carboxyls (Solcia et al, 1968). In our opinion and those of Dawson (1982) better results are obtained by using haematoxylin combined with stabilized lead solution. The staining mechanism is the same; the lead imparting a stronger colouration to the APUD cells. Both methods are given below.

METACHROMATIC DYES AFTER ACID HYDROLYSIS (after Solcia et al, 1968)

Notes

Cationic dyes react with carboxyl, sulphate and phosphate groups of polypeptides. The result can be improved by prior hydrolysis which removes the reactive groups in nucleotides and unmasks protein side chain carboxyls.

Solutions

Azure solution

0.005% azure A in distilled water.

Toluidine blue solution

0.01% toluidine blue in distilled water, buffered to pH 5 with McIlvaine's buffer

Acid solution for hydrolysis

0.2 M hydrochloric acid.

Technique

1. Paraffin sections to water.
2. Place in acid hydrolysis solution (0.2 M HCl) for 3–4 h at 60–65° C (formalin, paraformaldehyde, Bouin fixed), or 12 h at 60–65° C (glutaraldehyde or Helly fixed).
3. Wash well in water.
4. Stain in either:
   a. Azure A solution for 6 h.
   b. Toluidine blue solution for 6 h.
5. Either rinse in water and mount in glycerine

Table 12.5 Histochemical features of normal endocrine cells of pancreas and G.I. tract. (Compiled from Dawson, 1976.)

| Cell type | Secretion | 5HT | | Argyrophilia | | | Metachromasia | | | Others | | |
		Argen-taffin	Diazo	D + H.H.	Grim-elius	Bodian	Tol. Blue	Acid hydrol	Lead H	PTAH	DMAB nitrite	Alde-hyde fuchsin
Pancreas												
A₂	Glucagon	−	−	−	+	+	±	+	+	+	+	−
B	Insulin	−	−	−	−	−	−	−	−	−	−	+
D(A₁)	Somatostatin	−	−	+	+	+	+	+	+	+	+	−
G.I. tract												
EC	5HT	+	+	+	+	+	+	+	+	0	0	0
EG	Enteroglucagon	−	−	+	+	+	±	+	+	0	0	0
G	Gastrin	−	−	±	±	−	−	±	+	0	0	0
S	Secretin	−	−	0	±	0	0	0	+	0	+	0
VIP	VIP	−	−	0	0	0	0	0	±	±	0	0
GIP	GIP	−	−	0	+	0	0	0	+	0	0	0

Key: +, positive staining; ±, doubtful or faint staining; −, no staining; 0, no reliable observations available jelly, *or* blot dry, soak in absolute isopropanol for 1 min, clear in xylol and mount in DPX.

Results

APUD granules   purple-red

LEAD HAEMATOXYLIN TECHNIQUE
(Solcia, et al, 1969)

Note

It is thought there is a carboxyl linkage with lead haematoxylin. An optional satisfactory counter-stain is tartrazine in Cellosolve.

Solutions

Stabilized lead solution

5% aqueous lead nitrate	50 ml
Saturated aqueous ammonium acetate	50 ml

Filter, then add 2 ml of 40% formaldehyde.
The saturation point of ammonium acetate in water is approximately 120%.

Lead haematoxylin staining solution

Stabilized lead solution	10 ml
0.2 g haematoxylin in 1.4 ml 95% ethanol	1.5 ml
Distilled water	10 ml

Mix in the above order with repeated stirring. The mixture is allowed to stand for 30 min, filtered, and the filtrate made up to 75 ml with distilled water.

Technique

1. Dewax in xylol, hydrate through graded alcohols to water.
2. Stain in lead haematoxylin staining solution for 2–3 h at 37° C *or* 1–2 h at 45° C.
3. Wash in distilled water, dehydrate, clear and mount.

Results

Carcinoid tumours, endocrine and APUD cell granules	dark blue-black

(Note that other structures, e.g. muscle, nerves, nuclei, also stain blue-black.)

ARGYROPHILIC SILVER METHODS

Silver methods that employ a reducing agent (argyrophilic) will demonstrate some APUD cells. These methods according to Dawson (1982) are semispecific and are of value for screening purposes. In fact, by using the methods given below it is possible to identify and separate A (α2) cells and D (α1) cells of the pancreas.

GRIMELIUS SILVER METHOD FOR ARGYROPHIL CELLS, ESPECIALLY A (α2) CELLS OF THE PANCREAS (Grimelius, 1968)

Notes

A silver reduction method, for which Bouin fixed material gives best results. To increase the impregnation following reduction, wash well in distilled water and return to the silver bath at 60° C for 5–10 min. Drain the slide and repeat the reduction step.

Solutions

Silver solution

Acetate buffer (pH 5.6)	10 ml
Redistilled water	87 ml
1% silver nitrate (aqueous), fresh	3 ml

Reducing solution

Hydroquinone	1 g
Sodium sulphite (cryst)	5 g
Distilled water	100 ml

Freshly prepared.

Technique

1. Sections down to distilled water.

2. Transfer sections to silver solution at 60° C for 3 h.
3. Drain silver solution from slides.
4. Place sections in freshly prepared reducing solution at 45° C for 1 min.
5. Rinse sections in distilled water.
6. Counterstain if required.
7. Wash in tap water.
8. Dehydrate in graded alcohols.
9. Clear in xylene and mount in DPX or Canada balsam.

Results

Carcinoid tumours, argyrophil islet cells (A cells)	positive (brown-black)
B and D cells	negative
Many other argyrophil cells	positive (brown-black)

ALCOHOLIC SILVER NITRATE METHOD FOR ARGYROPHIL CELLS, ESPECIALLY D (α1) CELLS OF THE PANCREAS (Hellerstrom & Hellman, 1960)

Note

This is an alcoholic silver reduction method. Bouin fixation is necessary, either as a primary or secondary step.

Solutions

Silver solution

Silver nitrate	10 g
Distilled water	10 ml
95% alcohol	90 ml
M nitric acid	0.1 ml

Before use the pH of the solution is adjusted to 5.0 with conc. ammonium hydroxide.

Developing solution

Pyrogallic acid	5 g
95% alcohol	95 ml
Formaldehyde (40%)	5 ml

Technique

1. Sections down to tap water, 1 h.
2. Dehydrate to 95% alcohol.
3. Place sections in silver solution at 37° C overnight and protect from light.
4. Rinse rapidly in 95% alcohol — no longer than 10 s.
5. Transfer sections to developing solution for 1 min.
6. Rinse in three changes of 95% alcohol for 1 min.
7. Rinse in absolute alcohol for 1 min each.
8. Mount in DPX.

Results

D cell granules of the pancreas (α1)	positive (brown-black)
A and B cells	negative
Some other argyrophil cells	positive

BODIAN PROTARGOL TECHNIQUE (Bodian, 1936)

Notes

The protargol method gives strong argyrophilic demonstration of a number of tissue entities, nerve fibres, melanin, α cells of the pancreas and argyrophil cells. Sections are treated with protargol (a compound formed of gelatine and silver nitrate) in the presence of metallic copper. Regarding the function of copper it is suggested that nitric acid is formed, leading to a fall in pH of the solution producing a slowing down of the reaction, with consequent lessened risk of overimpregnation.

Following copper-protargol treatment, the sections are progressively reduced in a hydroquinone-gold chloride-oxalic treatment. Background precipitation is not uncommon in this technique, and thorough washing between the various treatments will reduce this.

A number of sources of protargol have been found to be unsatisfactory for this technique. We would recommend the supply of Messrs. Roques of Paris.

Solutions

Copper-protargol solution

Prepare fresh 50 ml of 1% aqueous protargol to which are added (in a Coplin jar) 2 g of clean copper foil cut into small pieces.

Primary reducer

Hydroquinone 1 g; sodium sulphite 5 g; in 100 ml distilled water. Prepare fresh (the sodium sulphite acts as a stabiliser allowing the solution to be kept for up to 2 days at 4° C).

Technique

1. Take sections to distilled water.
2. Treat with the copper-protargol solution overnight at 37° C (exact time is not critical but do not leave for more than 48 h).
3. Wash in several changes of distilled water and reduce in the hydroquinone solution for 10 min.
4. Wash well in distilled water. Thorough washing at this stage is most important, rinse first in distilled water, then in tap water for several minutes and finally in distilled water again.
5. Treat with 1% aqueous yellow gold chloride for 5 min.
6. Wash well in several changes of distilled water.
7. Treat with 2% aqueous oxalic acid for 5 min (only at this stage should silver blackening be evident).
8. Fix in 5% hypo.
9. Wash well in distilled water.
10. Rinse in tap water.
11. Counterstain in 1% neutral red.
12. Rinse in tap water.
13. Dehydrate, clear and mount in a synthetic resin.

Results

α cells of the pancreas (A & D)	black
Argyrophil cells	black

REDUCING SILVER METHOD FOR ARGYROPHIL CELLS (Pascual, 1976)

Notes

Silver methods using a reducing agent will blacken argyrophil and argentaffin cells. The Bodian (1936) method using protargol with hydroquinone reduction has been widely used and a number of silver techniques, such as that of Grimelius (1968) for argyrophil cells, have been developed for the identification of different argyrophil cells of the APUD system. The double silver impregnation modification of Pascual (1976) gives good contrast of the argyrophil cells without background impregnation. As indicated, argentaffin cells also stain. For comparison a direct silver reduction method should also be used.

Solution

Bodian's reducing solution

Anhydrous sodium sulphite	5 g
Hydroquinone	1 g
Distilled water	100 ml

Technique

1. Sections to water.
2. Place in freshly prepared 0.5% silver nitrate in distilled water for 2 h at 60° C or overnight at room temperature.
3. Rinse in distilled water.
4. Transfer sections to freshly prepared Bodian's reducing solution, heated to 60° C, for 5 min.
5. Wash in tap water for 3 min and rinse in distilled water.
6. Re-impregnate in the same silver solution at 60° C for 10 min.
7. Rinse in distilled water.
8. Repeat the reducing solution as in steps 4 and 5.
9. Counterstain neutral red for 3 min.
10. Rinse in tap water, dehydrate, clear and mount in synthetic resin.

Results

Argyrophil cells	black
Nuclei	red

AMINE DETECTION

The capacity of APUD cells to produce and store amines by taking up their precursor substance is their most important feature. Some also take up dihydroxyphenylalanine (DOPA) and decarboxylate it to its respective amine. Amines combine with aldehydes to produce specific fluorescent compounds. The majority of amines diffuse rapidly from their cells, so for their demonstration the technique of freeze drying and formaldehyde vapour is needed to demonstrate them (Bancroft, 1975, 1982). As can be seen from Table 12.1 5-hydroxytryptamine (5HT) and dopamine are the most important amines and these diffuse slowly from their granules. They combine with paraformaldehyde and aqueous formaldehyde to produce a yellow fluorescence. This is known as formaldehyde induced fluorescence (FIF) and is a good method for demonstrating 5HT (see p. 150). The combination of 5HT and formaldehyde produces β carboline and as well as being fluorescent it is a reducing agent. It is capable of reducing silver salts to metallic silver (argentaffin): ferricyanide to ferrocyanide (Schmorl reaction) and to couple with a diazonium salt (Fast red B) to produce an insoluble coloured azo dye. Two standard methods are given below, the Singh silver reduction method and the alkaline diazo method of Gomori; both methods are commonly used to identify carcinoid tumours.

SINGH'S MODIFICATION OF THE MASSON-HAMPERL ARGENTAFFIN TECHNIQUE (Singh, 1964)

Notes

This is a direct silver reduction method. Some workers prefer to leave the sections overnight in the silver solution at room temperature in a light-tight container.

Solution

To 10% silver nitrate add ammonia (0.880) until the precipitate formed just dissolves. To this clear solution add 10% silver nitrate drop by drop until a fine persistent opalescence is obtained. To each 1 ml of silver solution add 9 ml of distilled water.

Technique

1. Sections to water.
2. Wash well in several changes of distilled water.
3. Place in prewarmed silver solution at 60° C for 15–30 min.
4. Rinse in distilled water.
5. Fix in 1% sodium thiosulphate for 1 min.
6. Wash in distilled water.
7. Dehydrate through graded alcohols to xylene.
8. Mount in DPX.

Results

Argentaffin cells	contain black discrete
Argentaffin carcinoid tumours	granules

ALKALINE DIAZO TECHNIQUE (Gomori, 1952)

Notes

The argentaffin cells reduce the diazonium salt to produce an insoluble coloured azo dye. Fresh tissue fixed in formaldehyde is best. The method rarely works on postmortem material. Should the reaction not work well on well-fixed tissue it is often profitable to obtain different sources of the diazonium salt. There appears to be a variation in batches sold. The salts also have a limited shelf life.

Solution

1% fast red B	5 ml
Saturated lithium carbonate (aqueous)	2 ml

Keep solutions at 4° C before mixing, then use immediately.

Technique

1. Sections to water.

2. Transfer sections to incubating solution at 4° C for 1–4 min.
3. Wash well in tap water.
4. Lightly stain nuclei in haematoxylin.
5. Wash well in tap water.
6. Dehydrate through graded alcohols to xylene.
7. Mount in DPX.

Results

Argentaffin cell granules	orange
Nuclei	blue
Background	yellow

GIBBS' METHOD FOR ARGENTAFFIN GRANULES (Gibbs, 1926; Gomori, 1952)

Notes

This method depends upon the formation of a brownish or black indophenol dye when a phenol in alkaline solution reacts with Gibbs' reagent (2 : 6-dichloroquinone-chloroimide).

Solution

Dissolve 50 mg of 2:6-dichloroquinone-chloro-imide in 5–10 ml of alcohol; add 50 ml of distilled water and a few drops of a saturated solution of borax.

Technique

1. Take sections to water.
2. Immerse in the staining solution at room temperature for 10–15 min.
3. Wash well in running water.
4. Counterstain nuclei with 1% neutral red.
5. Dehydrate rapidly with alcohol and clear in xylene.
6. Mount in a synthetic resin mountant.

Results

Argentaffin granules	grey-black. The granules of carcinoid tumours may be brownish.
Nuclei	red

POLYPEPTIDE HORMONE IDENTIFICATION

The demonstration of the secreting hormone is carried out by immunocytochemical methods. These techniques require a specific antigen against which an antibody can be raised. The sites of these antigen-antibody reactions are demonstrated by fluorescent dyes (immunofluorescent methods) or enzymes, using peroxidase (immunoperoxidase techniques). An introduction to the practical and theoretical aspects of immunochemistry is given in Chapter 14.

ELECTRON MICROSCOPY

Tissue processed for electron microscopy will show the presence of intracellular neurosecretary granules. The immunoperoxidase technique mentioned above can be adapted for immunoelectron cytochemistry.

CHROMAFFIN REACTION

Notes

Originally the chromaffin reaction was used to identify the adrenal medulla. It has long been known that if the adrenal was fixed in chrome salts then medullary cells could be seen by their brown colour. Other chromaffin cells in the gastro-intestinal tract and some enterochromaffin cells will show the reaction. The adrenaline and noradrenaline produced by these cells are oxidized by chrome salts to produce a melanoid pigment. Iodate oxidation is thought to demonstrate NA (noradrenaline) producing cells more intensely than A (adrenaline) cells. It was reported by Coupland & Hopwood (1966) that initial fixation of the adrenal medulla in glutaraldehyde (pH 7.4) followed by fixation in chrome salts produced a strong chromaffin reaction in the NA cells, but the A cells (adrenaline storing) were negative.

The chromaffin reaction can be applied to either frozen sections or material processed for paraffin. The following fixatives give acceptable results, Orth's, Muller's or Regaud's.

Method

1. Fix for 2 days.
2. Wash in tap water.
3. Process tissue and embed in paraffin wax.
4. Section (5 μm) and dewax.
5. Mount sections in DPX.

Results

Chromaffin cells   yellow-brown

THE IODATE METHOD FOR NORADRENALINE (Hillarp & Hökfelt, 1955)

Notes

This depends upon the more rapid oxidation by iodate of noradrenaline than adrenaline.

Technique

1. Place thin (0.5 mm) blocks of fresh adrenal in 10% aqueous potassium iodate. Leave for 16 h at room temperature. Do not exceed the time.
2. Place in 10% formalin for 2 h.
3. Cut frozen sections 10–20 μm thick.
4. Wash in distilled water.
5. Sections may be counterstained and then dehydrated, cleared and mounted.

Results

Noradrenaline   brown

MODIFIED GIEMSA FOR CHROMAFFIN CELL GRANULES

Notes

The best results with this method are obtained if fixation is carried out in a dichromate-containing fixative. If this is not possible then secondary fixation, either tissue or section, in dichromate gives an acceptable result. Sections should be as thin as possible.

Solution

Standard Giemsa stain	2 ml
Buffered distilled water	48 ml

p63

Technique

1. Sections to water.
2. Rinse in distilled water.
3. Stain in the dilute Giemsa stain overnight.
4. Rinse in distilled water.
5. Wash in 0.5% acetic acid until the section becomes pink (about 2 min).
6. Wash in tap water.
7. Dehydrate rapidly through graded alcohols to xylene.
8. Mount in synthetic resin.

Results

Chromaffin cell granules greenish-yellow or bottle green, depending upon primary fixation.

REFERENCES

Bodian D 1936 A new method for staining nerve fibres and nerve endings in mounted paraffin sections. Anatomy Records 65: 89

Ciaccio 1907 Sopra speciali cellule granulose della mucosa intestinale. Archives Ital. Anat. Embriol, 6: 482

Coupland R E, Hopwood D 1966 The mechanism of the differential staining reaction for adrenaline and noradrenaline storing granules in tissue fixed in glutaraldehyde. Journal of Anatomy (London) 100: 227

Dawson I M P 1976 The endocrine cells of the gastro-intestinal tract and the neoplasms which arise from them. Current Topics in Pathology 63: 221

Dawson I M P 1982 In: Bancroft J D, Stevens A (eds) Theory and practice of histological techniques. Churchill Livingstone, Edinburgh

Erspamer V, Asero B 1952 Identification of Enteramine, the specific hormone of the enterochromaffin cell system as 5-hydroxytryptamine. Nature (London) 169: 800

Gibbs H D 1926 Chemical Review 3: 291

Gomori G 1952 Microscopic histochemistry. Chicago University Press, Chicago

Gould R P 1978 In: Anthony P P, Woolf N (eds) Recent advances in histopathology. Churchill Livingstone, Edinburgh

Grimelius L 1968 A silver nitrate stain for $\alpha2$ cells in human pancreatic islets. Acta Societa Medica Uppsala 73: 243

Heidenhain R 1870 Untersuchungen über den Bau der Labdrüsen. Archives Mikrosk Anatomica 6: 368

Hellerstrom C, Hellman B 1960 Some aspects of silver impregnation of the islets of Langerhans in the rat. Acta Endocrinologica 35: 518

Hillarp N A, Hökfelt B 1955 Histochemical demonstration of noradrenaline and adrenaline in the adrenal medulla. Journal of Histochemistry & Cytochemistry 3: 1

Kultschitsky N 1897 Zur Frage über den Bau des Darmkanals. Archives Mikrosk Anatomy 49: 7

Masson P 1914 La glande endocrine de i'intestine chez l'homme. C. R. Acad. Sciences, Paris 158: 159

Nonidez J F 1932 The origin of the parafollicular cell, a second epithelial component of the thyroid gland of the dog. American Journal of Anatomy 49: 479

Pascual J S F 1976 A new method for easy demonstration of argyrophil cells. Stain Technology 51: 231

Pearse A G E 1968 Common cytochemical and ultrastructural characteristics of cells producing polypeptide hormones (the APUD series) and their relevance to thyroid and ultimobranchial C cells and calcitonin. Proceedings of the Royal Society B. 170: 71

Pearse A G E 1974 In: Summers S (ed) Pathology annual. Appleton Century Crofts, New York

Schmidt J E 1905 Beiträge zur normalen und pathologischen Histologie einiger Zellarten der Schleimhaut des menschlichen Darmkanales. Archives Mikrosk Anatome 66: 12

Singh I 1964 A modification of the Masson-Hamperl method for staining argentaffin cells. Anatomische Anzeiger 115: 81

Solcia E, Vassallo G, Capella C 1968 Selective staining of endocrine cells by basic dyes after acid hydrolysis. Stain Technology 43: 267

Szijj I, Csapó Z, Lasló F A, Kovacs K 1969 Medullary cancer of the thyroid gland associated with hypercorticism. Cancer 24: 167

13

Enzyme histochemistry

Before a histological diagnosis can be made, suitable preparation of the tissue is necessary. The way the tissue is handled and the subsequent sections produced, depends upon the type of information required from the preparation. Surgical specimens have specialized handling and processing. Muscle biopsies may require enzyme histochemistry and most of the methods are applied to unfixed sections.

It is necessary to be aware of the different techniques available, particularly those that produce the maximum information from a specimen to allow a diagnosis to be made. There is little point in attempting to carry out enzyme methods on paraffin embedded tissue. It is on receipt of the specimen that the decision has to be made. What information is going to be required from this specimen? And which methods will produce the results required?

Whatever methods are going to be employed the first step on receiving the specimen is its preservation. The choice of methods of preservation at our disposal is considerable, but one basic decision that has to be made is; is the tissue to be fixed? Or, is it to be frozen? Tissues frozen to $-70°C$ or below are well preserved and there seems little loss of enzyme activity, and the tissue can be stored for some time. The other choice of preservation, is to employ a fixative and the choice of fixative is governed by the subsequent method. Freezing as a means of preservation is employed where fixation or subsequent processing will affect the results of the demonstrating method, as with the ATPase methods in muscle biopsy specimens. The majority of specimens are fixed on arrival in the laboratory: formaldehyde based fixatives are suitable for most techniques.

The drawbacks of routine processing on tissue constituents are shown in Table 13.1, modified from Bancroft (1975).

Table 13.1 Effects of tissue processing

Fixation at room temperature Most fixatives	Loss of enzyme activity Denatured proteins (depending upon fixative and length of fixation) Diffusion of enzymes Loss of some carbohydrates Diffusion of other carbohydrates
Dehydration in alcohol (room temperature)	Loss of enzyme activity General diffusion of enzymes Loss of lipids Shrinking, hardening
Clearing in either xylene, chloroform, toluene, etc.	Loss of enzyme activity Loss of lipids Shrinkage, hardening of tissue block (depending upon clearing agent)
Wax embedding Paraffin wax, 56–60° C	Loss of enzyme activity Loss of lipids Shrinkage and hardening of tissue

FROZEN SECTIONS

The rapid development of the cryostat over the last 30 years or so has been due to the expansion of histochemistry and the need to increase the quality of sections produced as 'urgent frozen sections.' The use of the cryostat has all but taken over as a means of cutting frozen tissue. Compared with the freezing microtome it is possible to produce

171

thin sections down to 2–3 µm and in a much shorter time. The principle involved is simple in comparison with paraffin wax embedding. The water in the tissue is frozen and in the form of ice produces a firm block of tissue, the ice acting as the embedding medium. The consistency of frozen blocks is affected by two factors, firstly as in paraffin sections by the nature of the tissue and also by the amount of water to be found in the tissue. Tissues that have a low water content section better at lower temperatures, those with a higher content being harder due to more ice crystals, section better at higher temperatures. It is possible then to improve sectioning of frozen blocks in the cryostat by adjusting the temperature of the block of tissue (Table 13.2).

Table 13.2 Suitable cutting temperatures of unfixed frozen tissue

Tissue	Best sectioning temperatures
Brain	−12° C
Lymph node	−15° C
Liver	−16° C
Kidney	−16° C
Spleen	−16° C
Skin	−25° C
Breast	−25° C
Muscle	−20° C
Thyroid	−20° C
Breast with fat	−30° C or below
Adipose tissue	−30° C or below

The cutting of fixed tissue whatever its nature, is best done at −5 to −10° C.

FREEZING UNFIXED TISSUE

In general the more rapid the tissue is frozen the better its appearance under the microscope. In the freezing of muscle biopsies it is imperative that a solution such as isopentane, super-cooled by liquid nitrogen is used to avoid ice crystal artefact being produced. Other tissue can normally be frozen by carbon dioxide gas.

FREEZING FIXED TISSUE

Due to the increased amount of water in the tissue it is advisable to freeze the tissue slowly to avoid disruption of the tissue. In the majority of instances it is probably best to place the tissue in the cryostat and allow it to freeze.

FIXATION BEFORE FREEZING

For the demonstration of many hydrolytic enzymes (alkaline phosphatase, acid phosphatase, etc.) it is better to use controlled fixation before freezing and sectioning. Without prior fixation diffusion of the reaction product will occur. A suitable method of fixation is given on page 176.

PRINCIPLES OF ENZYME HISTOCHEMISTRY

Histochemistry is expanding rapidly; it is no longer to be considered an insignificant part of histopathology but a subject in its own right with roots in both histology and biochemistry.

The expansion of the subject has been most marked in the demonstration of enzymes (Table 13.3). Enzymes are protein catalysts for the chemical reactions that occur in biological systems. They are necessary for the normal metabolic processes within the tissues.

Table 13.3 Commonly Demonstrated Enzymes

Oxidoreductases	Hydrolases
Oxidative (transfer of electrons)	Hydrolytic (addition or removal of water)
Examples:	Examples:
Dehydrogenases	Specific phosphatases
succinate	AT Pase
malate	Glucose-6-phosphatase
isocitrate	alkaline phosphatase
	acid phosphatase
	esterases

Enzymes have long been assayed biochemically; when Pearse (1953) published the first edition of his histochemistry book, he stated that methods existed for at least 18 enzymes to be demonstrated histochemically. In the last 30 years or so this number has increased to over 100. Many of the early methods demonstrated hydrolytic enzymes, enzymes that hydrolyze the substrate. The largest expansion in recent years has been in the demonstration of the group of enzymes known as oxidative, i.e. enzymes which oxidize the substrate.

APPLICATIONS

Enzyme methods are not applied to routine surgical material due to the partial or total loss of activity after paraffin processing. A few enzymes are still identifiable, such as chloroacetate esterase and this is used to demonstrate mast cells and white blood cells. In the main, cryostat sections of frozen material are required for the majority of enzyme methods and retrospective investigations are not usually feasible. If good communications exist between clinician and pathologist then a number of enzyme techniques can be applied to freshly received tissue. The current uses of enzyme histochemistry in surgical laboratories are:

1. Muscle biopsies using mainly oxidative enzymes to demonstrate muscle fibre sizes.
2. Demonstration of white blood cells of the myeloid series, using chloroacetate esterase.
3. Detection of ganglia in Hirschprung's disease using nonspecific esterase.
4. Prostatic carcinoma using acid phosphatase.
5. Jejunal biopsy using acid and alkaline phosphatase in cases of gluten enteropathy.
6. In lymphoma diagnosis (i.e. identity of histiocytic entities).
7. As immunohistochemical markers.

PRESERVATION

Due to the labile nature of enzymes their preservation is a problem. Enzymes react in various ways to outside influences; mitochondria, which contain many of the oxidative enzymes, are damaged rapidly when denied a supply of blood. The membranes become damaged and a loss of enzyme activity occurs, so as little time as possible must be wasted in preparing tissue for this type of histochemical technique. Lysosomes which contain many of the hydrolytic enzymes, are damaged by the freezing and thawing of tissue blocks and

sections, and the enzymes diffuse from the damaged organelles. This is the main cause of the gross diffusion artefact seen in post-fixed sections of acid phosphatase. Careful fixation of the tissue, and treatment in gum sucrose before incubation will help to retard this diffusion. The fixative will localize the enzyme and protect it from the effects of freezing and thawing. A small loss of enzyme takes place but this is reduced by employing the fixative at 4° C.

Most mitochondrial enzymes are removed or destroyed by normal histological fixation, but are much less sensitive to the effects of freezing and thawing, since the freezing and thawing appears not to rupture the mitochondrial membrane. A loss of enzyme activity occurs when tissue is left at room temperature, so in enzyme histochemistry the rapid handling of tissue is important. The damage caused to some of the mitochondrial enzymes can be avoided by the use of hypertonic protection media such as polyvinyl pyrrolidone (PVP) first described by Novikoff (1956), now used with sucrose. The different enzymes react in varying degrees to the damaging agents discussed. Some of them are more resistant than others to damage; alkaline phosphatase is more able to withstand the effects of fixation than acid phosphatase. Often a choice has to be made in the case of hydrolytic enzymes as to whether fixation, leading to some enzyme loss but better localization, is to be preferred to post-fixation or no fixation, with little or no loss of enzyme activity but considerable enzyme diffusion. The dehydrogenases have to be demonstrated on unfixed sections but a choice remains as to whether a protection solution is used.

FACTORS AFFECTING ENZYME ACTIVITY

Temperature

The optimal temperature for the majority of enzyme reactions is 37°C. At higher temperatures enzymes are rapidly denatured due to their protein content. Lower temperatures between 4 and 30°C can be usefully employed in histochemistry for the rate of the enzymic reaction is slowed and, in the case of active enzymes, a better localization demonstrated.

pH

The majority of enzymes have a pH at which the rate of the reaction is optimal. For a large number of enzymes this is pH 7.0–7.2. Alkaline phosphatase at pH 9.2 and acid phosphatase at pH 5.0 are examples of exceptions to this rule.

Inhibitors

Enzyme activity in sections can be destroyed by using chemical substances known as inhibitors. There are three main types of inhibitor:

1. Specific inhibitors, e.g. eserine for the cholinesterases.
2. Nonspecific inhibitors, e.g. heat for all enzymes.
3. Competitive inhibitors, e.g. chemicals which compete with the substrate for active enzyme sites.

The specific inhibitor affects the reactive site of the enzyme molecule. Nonspecific inhibitors destroy the enzyme reaction by denaturing the protein enzyme. The competitive inhibitors are chemicals like eserine which compete with the substrate for active enzyme sites.

Activators

These are chemicals that are used to promote enzyme activity. An example is magnesium ions, used in the Gomori metal precipitation technique for alkaline phosphatase.

TECHNIQUES OF DEMONSTRATION

The basic principle in most enzyme histochemistry techniques is that enzyme in the tissue is presented with its own specific substrate in the incubating medium and a reaction takes place. Unfortunately, the immediate product of this reaction, the primary reaction product (PRP), is frequently invisible and must therefore be allowed to couple with another substance so that an insoluble and visible final reaction product (FRP) is produced at the site of the enzyme activity. The coupling substance used varies, for example, diazonium salts in the demonstration of the phosphatases ('azo-dye methods'), tetrazolium salts in the demonstration of dehydrogenases, and inorganic chemicals like ammonium sulphide in the metal precipitation techniques.

Four basic techniques are available for the demonstration of enzymes:

1. Metal precipitation techniques.
2. Simultaneous coupling using diazonium salts.
3. Post-incubation coupling using diazonium salts.
4. Self-coloured substrate.

Metal precipitation

This technique is commonly applied to the demonstration of phosphatases (see later). The phosphate ions released as a result of enzyme activity on the substrate combine with a suitable metallic cation to produce an insoluble precipitate of metal phosphate. The phosphates so produced are usually invisible but can be rendered visible by converting them to black sulphides by treatment with ammonium sulphide. The metallic cations frequently used for combining with the released phosphate are calcium and lead. This technique may be regarded as a type of simultaneous coupling, but using metallic ions instead of diazonium salts.

Simultaneous coupling using diazonium salts

This occurs when an incubation mixture containing a substrate and a diazonium salt are applied to suitable sections in a buffered solution. The enzyme present in the section hydrolyzes the substrate to form an invisible primary reaction product. This complex is immediately coupled with the diazonium salt to produce the final reaction product which is seen as a visible, often coloured, deposit under the microscope. This type of method (Fig. 13.1) is exemplified by the azo dye methods for phosphatases.

The PRP is colourless whereas the FRP is coloured. The substrate must be soluble in water or in the buffer medium to an extent that there is

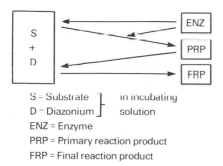

S = Substrate ⎱ in incubating
D = Diazonium ⎰ solution
ENZ = Enzyme
PRP = Primary reaction product
FRP = Final reaction product

Fig. 13.1 Azo dye method for phosphatases

sufficient substrate available in solution for the enzyme to hydrolyze. The histochemical method must be performed at a pH at which the enzyme shows maximal activity, for a large number of enzymes this is pH 7.0, and the substrate adequate solubility. The diazonium salt also has an optimal pH for its most efficient rate of coupling, and this must be considered when the pH at which the method is to be performed is chosen. The PRP must be fairly insoluble; if it is too soluble then not all of it will couple with the diazonium salt. The quantity of the substrate and diazonium salt in the incubating medium is also important; too much of either will cause inhibition of the rate of hydrolysis of the substrate on one hand, and inhibition of the formation of the FRP on the other.

Post-incubation coupling using diazonium salts

In this procedure the enzyme hydrolyzes the substrate and produces a reasonably insoluble PRP. The subsequent coupling is carried out in a separate solution. This type of method relies upon the PRP remaining at the initial site of the hydrolysis. It is important that diffusion of the PRP does not occur during the coupling process. Post-incubation coupling has many theoretical advantages. The optimal pH for the initial substrate enzyme reaction can be attained in the first incubation, say pH 7.0, and a possibly different optimal pH for the coupling can be produced in the second (coupling) stage, e.g. pH 9.1. The method avoids the deleterious effects that diazonium salts may have upon the initial reaction, and also avoids the effects of these diazonium salts when the incuba-

tion time is long, for many workers consider that these salts tend to inactivate enzymes or interfere with hydrolysis. Long exposure of tissue to diazonium salts in acid or alkaline solutions produces nonspecific staining. The serious drawback to this type of method results from the solubility of the PRP leading to excessive diffusion between the two stages. Localization may be poor unless the PRP is extremely insoluble.

Self-coloured substrate

There are few methods using this type of procedure. The substrate is a coloured but soluble substance, and the effect of the enzyme to be demonstrated is to remove the solubilizing group without interfering with the colour. The PRP is therefore coloured and insoluble, and no coupling stage is necessary. The insoluble coloured reaction product is precipitated at the site of enzyme activity.

DIAZONIUM SALTS

Diazonium salts are prepared by treating primary aromatic amines with an acid solution of sodium nitrate. The resulting salt, generally a chloride, will react readily with phenols or with aryl amines to produce the corresponding intensely coloured insoluble azo dye. There are about 30 stabilized diazonium salts in current usage.

Diazonium salts cannot be kept indefinitely; they must be stored in a cool dark place and renewed at 6-monthly intervals. During incubation it is important to choose conditions carefully so that combination of the reactants takes place as rapidly as possible, and the product so formed remains insoluble through subsequent processing. Failure in either of these respects reduces the accuracy of localization of the enzyme activity.

The rate of coupling of diazonium salt depends not only on the chemical nature of the diazonium salt used, but also on the pH of the incubating medium, and the optimal pH for enzyme activity therefore determines to a large extent the choice of diazonium salt. Precision in locating the sites of enzyme activity also depends upon the concentration of diazonium salt used. There is an average optimal concentration for diazonium salts in the incubating solution. If the concentration is less than optimal, diffusion of the PRP may be a problem. If the concentration is much greater than optimal then inhibition of enzyme activity may occur and the risk of nonspecific background staining becomes increased.

THE USE OF CONTROLS

Controls are a necessary part of enzyme histochemistry. Substrates, diazonium salts and other chemical solutions used will deteriorate with time, leading to the possible failure of the method; occasionally false positives may be produced. A positive control should be carried through when incubating test sections, to show that all the chemical solutions are working.

Omission of the substrate from the incubating medium and the inclusion of specific enzyme inhibitors (if available) afford adequate control measures. If further controls are deemed necessary, competitive inhibitors may be added to the incubating solution. Sections may also be pretreated by immersing them in boiling water for a few minutes, and then processing through the rest of the method, or by 'incubating' in distilled water. In each case, the absence of reaction product indicates that the positive results obtained with the authentic techniques are yielding useful information about the distribution of the enzyme. Non specific background staining is also excluded as a possible source of error if control sections give negative results. Any activity in control sections must be regarded as a false result.

FIXATION OF TISSUE FOR ENZYME DEMONSTRATION

Solutions

4% formal calcium
40% formaldehyde	4 ml
Distilled water	96 ml
Calcium chloride	1 g

Further calcium chloride is added if necessary until pH reaches 7.0.

Gum sucrose
Gum acacia	2 g
Sucrose	60 g
Distilled water	200 ml

Allow to dissolve and store at 4° C.

Formaldehyde-gelatin mixture
| 1% gelatin | 25 ml |
| 2% formalin | 25 ml |

Technique

1. Cut small block of fresh tissue.
2. Place in formal calcium solution precooled to 4° C overnight.
3. Blot dry, wash in tap water for 2 min, blot dry.
4. Place in gum sucrose solution at 4°C for 24 h.
5. Blot dry.
6. Attach blocks to cryostat holder and freeze by standing in the cryostat.
7. Section at 8–10 μm at −10° C.
8. Pick sections up on slides or coverslips precoated with formaldehyde-gelatin mixture; allow to dry before incubating.

PHOSPHATASES

Phosphatases are present in a wide variety of animal and plant tissues. They are responsible for the hydrolysis of organic phosphate esters. Some phosphatases act specifically on a single substrate and are known as specific phosphatases. Of these, a number can be demonstrated by reliable histochemical techniques. An example of a specific phosphatase is adenosine triphosphatase which specifically hydrolyzes adenosine triphosphate. The remainder, whose substrate specificity is less limited, are divided into two groups: those exhibiting optimal activity at high pH values (alkaline phosphatases) and those exhibiting optimal activity at low pH values (acid phosphatases).

Reliable histochemical methods are available for the demonstration of the following five phosphatases:

Alkaline phosphatases (see below).
Acid phosphatases (see p. 180).
5′-Nucleotidase
Glucose-6-phosphatase.
Adenosine triphosphatase (see p. 183).

The hydrolysis of organic phosphate esters during incubation provides the basis for histochemical reactions. The released phosphate ions or the remaining organic residue is made visible by a variety of means. Phosphate ions are precipitated as insoluble salts, i.e. lead or calcium phosphate and then converted to coloured sulphides which are visible under the microscope. This is the basis of the many Gomori-type metal precipitation techniques. Alternatively, the alcoholic residue of the substrate, after enzymatic hydrolysis, reacts with a diazonium salt to produce a highly coloured insoluble azo dye. Phosphate esters of α-naphthol or its derivatives are the most commonly used substrates in the azo dye techniques.

Coupling may take place during incubation (simultaneous coupling) or after incubation (post-coupling). The relative merits of each method have been discussed earlier.

In the demonstration of phosphatases Pearse (1960) states that the average optimal concentration of the diazonium salt is 1 mg per 1 ml of incubating solution. If the concentration is less, diffusion of the primary reaction product, α-naphthol may occur. On the other hand if the concentration is much greater, say 5 mg per ml of incubating medium, inhibition of PRP formation occurs, and nonspecific background staining seen.

Adequate controls should be used to eliminate the possibility of failure of the method, and of producing false positives. In phosphatase histochemistry the general points made on page 176 should be considered. In addition, false positive reactions can be obtained if calcium or iron is present in the tissues.

The pH of the final incubating solution is critical, acid phosphatases and alkaline phosphatases exhibit optimal activity at pH 5.0 and pH 9.2 respectively. The optimal pH values for glucose-6-phosphatase and 5′-nucleotidase occur at pH 6.5 and pH 7.5–8.5 respectively. Adenosine triphosphatase has an optimal pH of 7.2. The importance of pH in determining the choice of diazonium salt has been emphasised earlier.

ALKALINE PHOSPHATASES

These enzymes exhibit optimum activity at alkaline pH in the region of 9.0–9.6 and are widely distributed throughout many tissues, kidney making an ideal control. They are activated by magnesium, manganese and cobalt ions. Cyanide and cysteine inhibit alkaline phosphatase activity and may be incorporated in the incubating medium to provide a control.

There are two types of histochemical methods available for the demonstration of alkaline phosphatases. They are:

Gomori calcium phosphate method (metal substitution).
Azo-dye coupling methods, using either simultaneous coupling or post-coupling.

GOMORI CALCIUM PHOSPHATE METHOD (GOMORI, 1952)

Notes

The original method for the demonstration of alkaline phosphatases was described by two people, quite independently, in 1939. Gomori and Takamatsu provided the incentive for further study with the publication of their methods. A variation of the original Gomori technique published in 1952 is still in common use today. The incubating medium includes sodium β-glycerophosphate, calcium nitrate and magnesium chloride.

If a section is placed in an incubating solution containing a substrate (i.e. sodium β-glycerophosphate) and calcium ions (i.e. calcium nitrate), plus an activator for the phosphatase (i.e. magnesium chloride), a precipitate of calcium phosphate is formed at the sites of enzyme activity. The alkaline phosphatase liberates phosphate from the sodium β-glycerophosphate and then combines with calcium ions to form calcium phosphate. This precipitate is treated with cobalt nitrate to produce cobalt phosphate, which is then treated with dilute ammonium sulphide to form cobalt sulphide. This is visible as a black deposit. The reactions can be summarized in the following flow diagram.

Sodium β-glycerophosphate $\xrightarrow{\text{Alkaline phosphatase}}$ Phosphate ions

Phosphate ions + calcium ions $\longrightarrow$ Calcium phosphate

Calcium phosphate + cobalt ions $\longrightarrow$ Cobalt phosphate

Cobalt phosphate + sulphide ions $\longrightarrow$
Cobalt sulphide (black fine precipitate)

The incubating medium does not keep and it is advisable to make up fresh solutions immediately before use. The final pH of the solution is critical. If pH values less than 9.0 are employed, enzyme activity is impaired and the intensity of the final reaction product is reduced. Furthermore, localization is adversely affected owing to the solubility of calcium phosphate at lower pH.

Incubation is carried out at 37° C. The duration of incubation must be determined by experiment, and varies with the type of tissue used. Unnecessarily long incubation times should be avoided, as this favours diffusion of the enzyme, especially in unfixed sections. In general, shorter times are necessary for cryostat sections, and the longest for fixed and paraffin processed material.

Solution

2% sodium β-glycerophosphate	2.5 ml
2% sodium veronal	2.5 ml
2% calcium nitrate	5.0 ml
1% magnesium chloride	0.25 ml
Distilled water	1.25 ml

The final pH of the incubating medium should be between 9.0 and 9.4.

Technique

1. After suitable fixation, bring sections to water, incubate at 37°C for 45 min to 6 h.
2. Wash well in distilled water.
3. Repeat wash.
4. Treat section with 2% cobalt nitrate (3 min).
5. Wash well in distilled water.
6. Repeat wash.
7. Immerse sections in 1% ammonium sulphide, 2 min.

8. Wash well in distilled water.
9. Counterstain in 2% methyl green (chloroform extracted).
10. Wash well in running tap water.
11. Mount in glycerin jelly.

Results

Alkaline phosphatase activity	brownish black
Nuclei	green

AZO-DYE METHODS

1. SIMULTANEOUS COUPLING METHOD

This method was first described by Menton et al (1944). The original technique has been modified and improved upon by a number of people, notably by Gomori (1951). The method employs sodium α-naphthyl phosphate as the substrate, together with a suitable diazonium salt. The incubating medium is buffered to pH 9.2. The enzyme liberates α-naphthol from the substrate. This is subsequently coupled to a diazonium salt to produce an insoluble azo-dye at the sites of enzyme activity.

Best results are obtained when coupling between the α-naphthol and the diazonium salt occurs as rapidly as possible. This depends to a great extent on the choice of diazonium salt and upon the pH of the incubating solution.

Sodium α-naphthyl phosphate $\xrightarrow{\text{Alkaline phosphatase}}$ Primary reaction product (α-naphthol)

(PRP) α-naphthol + diazonium salt $\longrightarrow$
Final reaction product coloured precipitate

2. SIMULTANEOUS COUPLING METHOD USING SUBSTITUTED NAPHTHOLS

The introduction of substituted naphthols for use in the demonstration of alkaline phosphatases is due to Gomori (1952a) and further developmental work was carried out by Burstone (1958, 1961).

He studied three substituted naphthol esters: naphthol AS-BI phosphate, naphthol AS-CL phosphate and naphthol AS-TR phosphate. These esters are hydrolyzed rapidly by alkaline phosphatases yielding extremely insoluble naphthol derivatives. These are then made to react with a diazonium salt to produce an insoluble azo-dye at the site of activity.

Many workers agree that the localization with substituted naphthols is superior to that obtained using alternative methods.

Substituted naphthols will also couple with diazonium salts over wider pH ranges. Against these advantages must be mentioned the higher cost of the substituted naphthol substrates. Stock solutions of substituted naphthol phosphates may be made by dissolving the compound in dimethylformamide (DMF) and adding distilled water and buffer to pH 8.3. These solutions will keep in a refrigerator for several months. To carry out the reaction it is simply necessary to add a suitable diazonium salt (e.g. Fast red TR, Fast blue RR) to the required amount of incubating solution in the ratio of 1 mg/ml. The incubating solution should be prepared immediately before use. Incubation is carried out for 30 min at 37°C.

ALKALINE PHOSPHATASE: AZO-DYE COUPLING METHOD (SIMULTANEOUS COUPLING)

Solution

Sodium α-naphthyl phosphate	10 mg
0.1 M tris buffer (stock solution), pH 10.0	10 ml
Diazonium salt (Fast red TR)	10 mg

The final pH of the incubating medium should be between 9.0 and 9.4. The sodium α-naphthyl phosphate is dissolved in the buffer, and the diazonium salt is added and the solution well mixed. The solution is then filtered and used immediately.

Technique

1. After fixation, bring sections to water, incubate at room temperature for 10–60 min.
2. Wash in distilled water.
3. Counterstain in 2% methyl green (chloroform extracted).
4. Wash in running tap water.
5. Mount in glycerin jelly.

Results

Alkaline phosphatase activity	reddish brown
Nuclei	green

ALKALINE PHOSPHATASE: NAPHTHOL AS-BI METHOD (SIMULTANEOUS COUPLING WITH SUBSTITUTED NAPHTHOLS)

Solution

Naphthol AS-BI phosphate	25 mg
N:N'-dimethyl formamide	10 ml
Distilled water	10 ml
Molar sodium carbonate	2–6 drops

The reagents are added in the above order, sufficient molar sodium carbonate being added until the pH is 8.0 then add:

Distilled water	300 ml
0.2 M tris buffer, pH 8.3	180 ml

The solution, which is faintly opalescent, is stable for many months.

Incubating solution

Stock naphthol AS-BI solution	10 ml
Fast red TR	10 mg

Shake well, filter and use immediately.

Technique

1. After fixation and bringing sections to water, incubate at room temperature for 5–15 min.
2. Wash in water.
3. Counterstain in 2% methyl green (chloroform extracted).
4. Wash well in running tap water.
5. Mount in glycerin jelly.

Results

Alkaline phosphatase activity	red
Nuclei	green

ACID PHOSPHATASES

These enzymes received less attention originally than alkaline phosphatases. This is doubtless connected with the fact that only in recent years have the methods for their demonstration become reliable. The problem is the relatively high solubility of acid phosphatases, and the difficulty of obtaining accurate localization of the final reaction product. Simultaneous coupling azo-dye methods are also beset by the difficulty of finding diazonium salts that couple efficiently under the acid conditions necessary for optimal enzyme activity.

The enzymes are distributed widely throughout the body; kidney, liver and spleen being particularly rich. Fluoride ions inhibit these enzymes, and the inclusion of sodium fluoride in the incubating medium affords a reliable control measure.

As with the alkaline phosphatases, there are two reliable techniques for the demonstration of these enzymes: the Gomori lead phosphate method, and the azo-dye coupling methods using simultaneous coupling.

GOMORI LEAD PHOSPHATE METHOD

Notes

This method was first introduced by Gomori (1941) and resembles his method for alkaline phosphatases.

Calcium phosphate, which is formed at the site of activity in the alkaline phosphatase technique (see p. 177), cannot be used in this instance because of its solubility at acid pH levels. Lead nitrate is therefore used to precipitate the phosphate ions.

The section is incubated in a medium containing sodium-β-glycerophosphate as the substrate and lead nitrate; no activator is required. The enzyme splits phosphate ions from the substrate and these form an insoluble precipitate of lead phosphate at the site of enzyme activity. The sections are treated with a dilute solution of ammonium sulphide and the precipitate converted to lead sulphide. This is visible under the microscope as a dense brown deposit. The deposit is granular,

and if the optimal conditions for the method have been fulfilled, the granules should be small.

$$\text{Sodium-β-glycerophosphate} \xrightarrow{\text{Acid phosphatase}} \text{Phosphate ions}$$

$$\text{Phosphate ions + lead ions} \longrightarrow \text{Lead phosphate (precipitate)}$$

$$\text{Lead phosphate + sulphide ions} \longrightarrow \text{Lead sulphide (fine brown black precipitate)}$$

The incubating medium must be made up fresh for each batch of sections to be incubated. It is convenient, however, to keep the individual reagents in stock solutions and stored at 4°C. The preparation of the incubating solution is important. It is necessary to use reagents of a high grade to obtain satisfactory results.

The pH of the final incubating solution is also important. The method works best at a pH of 4.8–5.0. If the pH is increased much above 5.5, it is possible to demonstrate phosphatases other than acid phosphatases. Incubation is carried out at 37°C for 30 min to 6 h, depending on the method of preparation of the material and the tissue used.

Solution

0.5 M veronal acetate buffer, pH 5.0	10 ml
Sodium-β-glycerophosphate	32 mg
Lead nitrate	20 mg

The lead nitrate must be dissolved in the buffer before the β-glycerophosphate is added. The pH of the incubating medium should be approximately 5.0.

Technique

1. Place sections in incubating medium at 37°C for ½–2 h.
2. Wash in distilled water.
3. Immerse in 1% ammonium sulphide (fresh), 2 min.
4. Wash well in distilled water.
5. Counterstain in either 2% methyl green, or Mayer's Carmalum.
6. Wash in tap water.
7. Mount in glycerine jelly.

Results

Acid phosphatase activity	black
Nuclei	green or blue

AZO-DYE METHODS

1. AZO-DYE SIMULTANEOUS COUPLING METHOD

The principle employed in the corresponding technique for alkaline phosphatase is again used for the demonstration of acid phosphatase. The substrate used is sodium α-naphthyl phosphate (1-naphthyl phosphoric acid) dissolved in 0.1 M veronal acetate buffer at pH 5.0. α-Naphthol is released at the site of enzyme activity and coupled with a suitable diazonium salt.

The problem with azo-dye methods for the demonstration of acid phosphatases is to find a diazonium salt that will couple satisfactorily at a low pH. Grogg & Pearse (1952) carried out a comprehensive study of different diazonium salts and their performance when used in the acid phosphatase technique. They concluded that Fast Garnet GBC gave the best results, and recommended that the salt be used with this method. The localization is considerably inferior however to that resulting from using a substituted naphthol as substrate and hexazonium pararosanilin as coupler.

2. SIMULTANEOUS AZO-DYE COUPLING METHOD USING SUBSTITUTED NAPHTHOLS

This method is also applicable to the demonstration of acid phosphatases, and was explored by Burstone (1958). All the substituted naphthols he studied coupled efficiently at an acid pH, but he recommended naphthol AS-BI phosphate as the substrate of choice for the acid phosphatase technique due to the extreme insolubility of the reaction product.

Barka (1960) recommended the use of hexazonium pararosanilin as the diazonium salt in the simultaneous coupling method for acid phospha-

tase. This salt was first used by Davis & Ornstein (1959) for the demonstration of alkaline phosphatases and esterases. According to Barka, hexazonium pararosanilin does not inhibit the enzyme at an acid pH, and he attributed the improved localization obtained using this salt to the extreme insolubility and substantivity of the azo-dye produced. The combination of hexazonium pararosanilin and naphthol AS-BI phosphate allows accurate localization of the reaction product and is recommended.

The diazonium salt is prepared in two stages. In the first, pararosanilin hydrochloride is dissolved in distilled water and acidified with concentrated hydrochloric acid. The solution is filtered and stored at room temperature where it is stable for several months. Diazotization is achieved by the addition of 4% sodium nitrite in distilled water. It is important that the solution is freshly prepared.

Incubation is carried out at room temperature for periods of 30 min to 2 h, or at 37° C for 10–30 min. A bright red colour indicates the site of enzyme activity. Methyl green (chloroform extracted) is an ideal counterstain for this method. It provides selective staining of the nuclei without affecting the colour of the final reaction product. The sections may be dehydrated rapidly through graded alcohols to xylene, and mounted in DPX. This causes very little loss in staining reaction and allows permanent preparations to be made.

ACID PHOSPHATASE: AZO-DYE COUPLING METHOD (SIMULTANEOUS COUPLING)

Solution

Sodium α-naphthyl phosphate	10 mg
0.1 M acetate buffer, pH 5.9	10 ml
Fast Garnet GBC	10 mg

The sodium α-naphthyl phosphate is dissolved in the buffer and the diazonium salt added. The solution is then filtered and used immediately.

Technique

1. Incubate at 37°C for 15–60 min.
2. Wash in distilled water.

3. Counterstain in 2% methyl green (chloroform extracted).
4. Wash in running tap water.
5. Mount in glycerin jelly.

Results

Acid phosphatase activity	red
Nuclei	green

ACID PHOSPHATASE: THE NAPHTHOL AS-BI PHOSPHATE METHOD (BURSTONE, 1958; MODIFIED BY BARKA, 1960) (SIMULTANEOUS COUPLING WITH SUBSTITUTED NAPHTHOLS)

Solutions

1. Substrate solution

Naphthol AS-BI phosphate	50 mg
Dimethyl formamide	5 ml

2. Buffer solution
Veronal acetate buffer stock A (see p. 261).

3. Sodium nitrite

Sodium nitrite	400 mg
Distilled water	10 ml

4. Pararosanilin stock, see below.

5. Distilled water

Preparation of incubating solution

Solution (1)   0.5 ml
Solution (2)   2.5 ml
Solution (3) ⎫
                ⎬ 0.8 ml { 0.4 ml of solutions (3) and (4) mixed before adding to incubating solution
Solution (4) ⎭
Solution (5)   6.5 ml

It is necessary for the success of the technique that equal parts of solutions (3) and (4) are mixed together and allowed to stand for 2 min before being added to the incubating medium.

The final pH should be between 4.7–5.0; it is adjusted if necessary with 0.1 M NaOH.

Technique

1. Incubate sections at 37°C for 15–60 min.
2. Wash in distilled water.
3. Counterstain in 2% methyl green (chloroform extracted).
4. Wash in running water.
5. Either (a) mount in glycerin jelly; or
            (b) dehydrate rapidly through fresh alcohols to xylene and mount in DPX.

Results

Acid phosphatase activity	red
Nuclei	green

PREPARATION OF HEXAZOTIZED PARAROSANILIN (DAVIS & ORNSTEIN, 1959)

Solution 1

Pararosanilin hydrochloride	1 g
Distilled water	20 ml
Hydrochloric acid (conc)	5 ml

The pararosanilin is dissolved in the distilled water and the hydrochloric acid is added. The solution is heated gently, cooled, filtered and stored in a refrigerator.

Solution 2

Sodium nitrite	2 g
Distilled water	50 ml

This solution will keep overnight at 4° C.

Solution for use

Solutions (1) and (2) in equal parts, allow to stand for 30 s until the solution becomes amber.

ADENOSINE TRIPHOSPHATASE

This specific phosphatase has a surgical application in the diagnosis of skeletal muscle biopsies. By applying the technique at different pH levels it is possible to demonstrate muscle fibre types and the changes in the number, size and relative proportions of the fibres. The method can only be applied to fresh unfixed cryostat sections. Prefixation will destroy the enzyme activity.

ATPase acts on the substrate adenosine triphosphat to produce phosphate. This is combined with calcium ions. The use of ammonium sulphide converts these ions into a brown precipitate of calcium sulphide at the site of enzyme activity.

Note

The method can employ lead or calcium to combine with the released phosphate. Calcium is preferred when the method is used on muscle biopsies.

Solutions

a. pH 9.4 buffer (veronal acetate)

0.1M sodium barbitone solution	2 ml
0.18M calcium chloride solution	2 ml
Distilled water	6 ml

Adjust pH to 9.4 with 0.1M NaOH.

b. pH 4.6 buffer (veronal acetate) — as (a) but adjust pH to 4.6 with 0.1 MHCl

c. pH 4.2 buffer (veronal acetate) — as (a) but adjust pH to 4.2 with 0.1 MHCl

Incubating medium

0.1M sodium barbitone	2 ml
0.18M calcium chloride	1 ml
Distilled water	7 ml
ATP (disodium salt)	25 mg

Adjust pH to 9.4

Technique at pH 9.4

1. Incubate section in solution (a) for 15 min at room temperature.
2. Incubate in solution (d) for 45 min at room temperature.
3. Wash in three changes of 1% calcium chloride for a total of 10 min.
4. Transfer to 2% cobalt chloride for 3 min.
5. Wash well in six changes of 0.01M sodium barbitone.
6. Wash in tap water for 30 s.
7. Place in 1% yellow ammonium sulphide solution for 20–30 s.
8. Rinse well in tap water.
9. Dehydrate through alcohols, clear in xylene and mount in Permount.

METHOD (WITH PRE-INCUBATION AT pH 4.6 AND pH 4.2)

As above but replace step (1) by incubation in solution (b) (for pH 4.6 method) or solution (c) (for pH 4.2 method). Both incubations are for 5 min at room temperature and should be followed by a rinse in solution (a) for 30 s. Then resume above method at step (2).

Result

ATPase activity in muscle fibres: brown-black as follows:

At pH 9.4

Type 1	+
Type 2 ABC	+++

At pH 4.2

Type 1	+++
Type 2 AB	−
Type 2 C	++

At pH 4.6

Type 1	+++
Type 2 A	−
Type 2 BC	+++

ESTERASES

Esterases are enzymes which are capable of hydrolyzing esters. Therefore by definition the phosphatases dealt with earlier are strictly esterases, since they hydrolyze phosphate esters. This section is devoted to those esterases which hydrolyze esters of carboxylic acids. Within this group there are many types of esterases, acting upon a number of substrates. Unfortunately, there is considerable overlap between the different types of esterases, since many of them are capable of hydrolyzing the same substrate. This makes a classification of esterases difficult to define. Any subdivision of esterases depends upon the application of enzyme inhibitors to the various enzyme methods. The most useful classification is based upon differential inhibition.

NONSPECIFIC ESTERASES

If the substrate is a simple ester such as α-naphthyl acetate the hydrolyzing enzyme is called nonspecific esterase. However, because of the considerable overlap in activity previously mentioned the more specific esterases such as cholinesterase are capable of hydrolyzing these simple esters. Nonspecific esterases can be further subdivided into several different groups, according to the particular type of ester they hydrolyze most efficiently and according to the effect of organophosphate inhibitors.

The subdivision of nonspecific esterases based on their most suitable substrate is:

1. Carboxyl esterases
2. Aryl esterases
3. Acetyl esterases.

Fortunately this approximate classification coincides neatly with the classification based on the effects of organophosphate inhibitors.

SPECIFIC ESTERASES

The most important specific esterases histochemically are the cholinesterases; these are of two types, acetyl cholinesterase ('true') and cholinesterase ('pseudo'). Acetyl cholinesterases are capable of hydrolyzing acetyl thiocholine, whereas cholinesterases will hydrolyze esters of choline other than acetyl thiocholine more rapidly. Both these enzymes are capable of hydrolyzing simple esters. Cholinesterases are differentiated from the nonspecific esterases by their capacity to hydrolyze choline esters and by the fact that this capacity is destroyed by the action of the specific inhibitor eserine (10^{-5} M). Nonspecific esterases are not inhibited by eserine.

LIPASES

The term is generally applied to those esterases which have a facility for hydrolyzing long chain esters (i.e. those esters containing fatty acids with more than seven carbon atoms in the chain). There is, however, considerable overlap between the lipases and nonspecific esterases since both are capable of hydrolyzing simple esters.

INHIBITORS

The application of esterase inhibitors to the histochemical reactions has permitted a more accurate identification of various enzymes. The use of the specific inhibitor, eserine, in the identification of the cholinesterases and acetyl cholinesterases has already been mentioned. The most useful esterase inhibitors are the organophosphorus compounds such as di-isopropyl fluorophosphate (DFP) and diethyl p-nitrophenyl phosphate (E600). The esterases have been subdivided into so-called A, B and C esterases as described by Pearse (1972). The A esterases are resistant to a concentration of 1 mM of E600 but sensitive to other inhibitors, whereas B esterases are sensitive to E600 in a concentration as low as 10 mM. The C esterases are resistant to most esterase inhibitors. The A, B and C esterase are resistant to the effects of eserine, but since the specific cholinesterases are also sensitive to low concentrations of E600 some authorities arbitrarily group them with the B esterases. The carboxyl esterases are B-type esterases, the aryl esterases are A-type esterases and the acetyl esterases are C-type esterases.

DEMONSTRATION OF ESTERASES

Because of the wide range of activity of the various types of esterases, substrates such as α-naphthyl acetate, indoxyl acetates and substituted naphthol acetates can be used in the demonstration of A, B and C esterases as well as cholinesterases.

NONSPECIFIC ESTERASES

α-NAPHTHYL ACETATE METHOD FOR NONSPECIFIC ESTERASE

This method will probably demonstrate all types of esterase activity. It is normally carried out at a pH of 7.4. It is an azo-dye simultaneous coupling method which was first described by Nachlas & Seligman (1949). The authors suggested the use of β-naphthyl acetate as a substrate, and Diazo blue B as a coupling agent. Gomori (1950) substituted α-naphthyl acetate for β-naphthyl acetate, pointing out that the azo-dye produced with the latter was soluble in water, but that produced with α-naphthyl acetate was not. Localization of the enzyme is therefore more precise. The method can be carried out employing the diazonium salt Fast blue B as the coupling agent, or by using the hexazonium pararosanilin technique as suggested by Davis & Ornstein (1959).

METHOD WITH FAST BLUE B

Notes

The incubating medium contains α-naphthyl acetate dissolved in acetone and buffered to pH 7.4 with phosphate buffer. The diazonium salt, fast blue B, is included in the incubating medium in the concentration of 3 mg/ml, as the coupler. The esterase activity in the section splits the α-naphthyl acetate, releasing α-naphthol. This combines rapidly with the fast blue B salt to produce an insoluble azo-dye at the site of enzyme activity.

The reaction product marks the site of all types of esterase activity, including cholinesterases; the latter can be inhibited by eserine (10^{-5} M) and a comparison made between the two sections.

Solution

α-naphthyl acetate	5 mg
Acetone	0.1 ml
0.2 M phosphate buffer, pH 7.4	10 ml
Fast blue B	30 mg

The α-naphthyl acetate is dissolved in the acetone and the phosphate buffer added and thoroughly mixed. The Fast blue B is added and the solution filtered, and used immediately.

Technique

1. After suitable fixation, bring section down to water.
2. Place in incubating medium for 30 s to 15 min at room temperature.
3. Wash in running tap water (3 min).
4. Counterstain in Mayer's carmalum (5 min).
5. Wash in running tap water (3 min).
6. Mount in glycerine jelly.

Results

Esterase activity	reddish brown
Nuclei	red

METHOD WITH PARAROSANILIN HYDROCHLORIDE

Notes

The histochemical reaction is as previously described except that the coupling agent is hexazonium pararosanilin, instead of fast blue B. This was first used for the demonstration of esterases by Davis & Ornstein (1959). The results obtained should be similar to the above technique except that the localization of the final reaction product is improved. An advantage in using hexazonium pararosanilin coupling is that sections may be dehydrated through alcohol to xylene and mounted in a synthetic mounting medium (DPX).

Solution

1. Substrate solution

α-Naphthyl acetate	50 g
Acetone	5 ml

2. Buffer solution
0.2 M phosphate buffer, stock solution A (see Appendix 3)

3. Sodium nitrite

Sodium nitrite	400 mg
Distilled water	10 ml

4. Pararosanilin-HCl stock

Pararosanilin hydrochloride	2 g
2 M-hydrochloric acid	50 ml

Heat gently, cool to room temperature and filter.

5. Distilled water.

Preparation of incubating medium

Solution (1)	0.25 ml	
Solution (2)	7.25 ml	
Solution (3)		0.4 ml of solution (3)
Solution (4)	0.8 ml	and (4) are mixed before adding to
		incubating solution
Solution (5)	2.5 ml	

It is important that equal parts of solutions (3) and (4) are mixed together before adding to the incubating medium. Adjust pH to 7.4 if necessary with solution (2).

Technique

1. After suitable fixation bring sections to water.
2. Incubate at 37° C for 2–20 min.
3. Wash in running water.
4. Counterstain in 2% methyl green (chloroform extracted).
5. Wash well in tap water.
6. Dehydrate rapidly through fresh alcohol to xylene and mount.

Results

Esterase	reddish brown
Nuclei	green

INDOXYL ACETATE METHOD (HOLT, 1954)

Notes

This method will also demonstrate nonspecific esterases, and is a simultaneous method with potassium ferricyanide as coupler. The technique was first introduced by Barrnett & Seligman (1951), and Holt & Withers (1952). It is probably the most accurate for the localization of nonspecific esterase. The substrate suggested in these two initial papers was indoxyl acetate. Holt (1954) introduced 4-chloro-5-bromo-indoxyl acetate as a substrate and this gives superior results to the earlier substrate.

The incubating medium consists of 4-chloro-5-bromo-indoxyl acetate, potassium ferrocyanide, potassium ferricyanide, calcium chloride and tris buffer, pH 7.2. The esterase in the section hydrolyzes the 5-bromo-indoxyl acetate to produce 5-bromo-indoxyl. This is a soluble product which is then oxidized by the potassium ferricyanide to an insoluble indigo dye. The potassium ferrocyanide in equimolar solution with the ferricyanide prevents over-oxidation of the indigo. The calcium chloride in the medium acts as an enzyme activator.

Solution

5-bromo-4-chloro-indoxyl acetate	1 mg
Ethanol	0.1 ml
Tris buffer (0.2M), pH 7.2 (see p. 261)	2 ml
Potassium ferricyanide (0.05M) (1.6%)	17 mg
Potassium ferrocyanide (0.05M) (2.1%)	21 mg
Calcium chloride (0.1M) (2.1%)	11 mg
Distilled water	7.9 ml

The 5-bromo-4-chloro-indoxyl acetate is dissolved in the ethanol and the buffer is then added. The remaining chemicals are dissolved in the distilled water and the solution is mixed. It is important that the solution is freshly prepared.

Technique

1. After suitable fixation, bring sections to water.
2. Incubate at 37° C for 15–60 min.
3. Rinse in tap water.
4. Counterstain in Mayer's carmalum for 5 min.
5. Rinse in tap water.
6. Mount in glycerin jelly or
7. Dehydrate through graded alcohols to xylene.
8. Mount in DPX.

Results

Esterase activity	blue
Nuclei	red

CHOLINESTERASES

These are specific esterases, two types can be demonstrated, acetyl cholinesterase (true cholinesterase) and cholinesterase (pseudocholinesterase). Acetyl cholinesterase is found in the nervous system and muscle. It hydrolyzes the substrate acetyl thiocholine. Pseudocholinesterase will hydrolyze other esters of choline more rapidly than true cholinesterase. It is found in parafollicular cells of the thyroid and other endocrine glands.

The enzyme will hydrolyze the acetyl thiocholine to produce thiocholine, which combines with copper ions. The copper thiocholine is treated with dilute ammonium sulphide to form a brown precipitate at the site of enzyme activity.

THIOCHOLINE TECHNIQUE (GEREBTZOFF, 1959)

Note

Both enzymes will be demonstrated by the technique. If differentiation between the two enzymes is required, then duplicate sections and two substrates are required, e.g. acetyl and butyryl thiocholine iodide.

Solutions

Solution (a)
   0.1M acetate buffer, pH 5.0 or 6.2 (see Appendix 3)

Solution (b)

Acetylthiocholine iodide	15 mg
Cupric sulphate	7 mg
Distilled water	1.4 ml

This solution is centrifuged at 4000 r/min for 15 min and the supernatant used.

Solution (c)

Glycine	375 mg
Distilled water	10 ml

Solution (d)

Cupric sulphate	250 mg
Distilled water	10 ml

Solution (e)
   Distilled water

Preparation of incubating medium

Solution (a)	5 ml
Solution (b)	0.8 ml
Solution (c)	0.2 ml
Solution (d)	0.2 ml
Solution (e)	3.8 ml

The pH of the incubating medium is varied according to the tissue and the amount of activity expected in the tissue. Gerebtzoff (1959) states that 'tissues with high cholinesterase activity are incubated at pH 5.0 and other tissues at 6.2.'

Technique

1. Incubate sections at 37° C for 10–90 min.
2. Rinse in two changes of distilled water.
3. Treat sections with 2% ammonium sulphide for 2 min.
4. Wash well in distilled water.

5. Counterstain if required.
6. Wash in tap water.
7. Mount in glycerin jelly.

Results

Cholinesterase activity	brown

LIPASE

Lipase is the terminology applied to a group of enzymes which have the ability to hydrolyze long chain esters, particularly those containing saturated fatty acids. The enzymes are located in the pancreas and in smaller amounts in the liver and adrenals.

There is overlap in the demonstration of lipases and nonspecific esterases as both will hydrolyze the same substrate. The method depends upon the enzyme hydrolyzing the substrate Tween 60, to produce fatty acids. These are then combined with calcium ions to form relatively insoluble calcium soaps which are treated with lead ions and converted by ammonium sulphide to form a dark brown deposit at the site of enzyme activity.

TWEEN METHOD

Notes

It is necessary to employ a control section. It is passed through the technique but the incubating medium lacks the substrate. Comparisons are made between test and control sections. No staining should be seen in the control. Formalin fixed frozen sections work well and acetone fixed paraffin sections give acceptable results. Pancreas is the most suitable control tissue.

Solutions

Solution (a)
  Tris buffer, pH 7.2

Solution (b)

Tween 60	5 g
Tris buffer, pH 7.2	100 ml
Thymol	1 crystal

Solution (c)

Calcium chloride	200 mg
Distilled water	10 ml

Incubating medium

Solution (a)	9 ml
Solution (b)	0.6 ml
Solution (c)	0.3 ml

Technique

1. After suitable fixation, bring sections to water. water.
2. Incubate at 37° C for 2–8 h. If paraffin sections, leave for 24 h.
3. Rinse sections in three changes of distilled water.
4. Place section in preheated 1% lead nitrate at 55° C for 10 min.
5. Rinse sections in distilled water for 2 min.
6. Wash in tap water for 10 min.
7. Place sections in 1% ammonium sulphide for 3 min.
8. Rinse in distilled water.
9. Wash in tap water.
10. Counterstain in Mayer's carmalum for 5 min.
11. Wash in tap water for 1 min.
12. Mount in glycerin jelly.

Results

Lipase activity	yellow to brown-black
Nuclei	red

CHLOROACETATE ESTERASE

This esterase is capable of resisting the effects of paraffin processing and can be demonstrated in paraffin sections. The technique is used to demonstrate mast cells and white cells of the myeloid series.

Notes

The pH of the incubating medium must be below 7.1. The incubation time varies according to the type of sections used; frozen sections show strong activity after 5 min while paraffin sections will require a longer time. Mast cells will stain rapidly while myeloid cells, if in paraffin sections, may take several hours. The temperature of the water-bath should be kept below 37° C. If the method given below fails to work on paraffin sections an alternative method is given by Moloney et al (1960). Stevens (1983) has shown that a positive result can be obtained on bony fragments after a short decalcification in EDTA.

Solution

Naphthol AS-D acetate (dissolved in 0.5 ml dimethylformamide)	5 mg
Distilled water	25 ml
0.2M Tris buffer (pH 7.1)	25 ml
Fast blue RR salt	30 mg

Mix reagents in order given, shake well and filter. Check that pH is below 7.1.

Technique

1. Paraffin sections to water.
2. Incubate sections in freshly filtered incubating medium at room temperature 5 min to several hours.
3. Rinse in water.
4. Counterstain nuclei in Mayer's carmalum (10–15 min).
5. Wash in water and mount in glycerin jelly.

Result

Esterase activity	shades of blue (intense in mast cells, variable in myeloid cells).
Nuclei	red

DEHYDROGENASES

The dehydrogenases are enzymes which have the ability to remove hydrogen from the substrate and transfer it to another substance. The substance which acts as a hydrogen acceptor is either nicotinamide adenine dinucleotide (NAD), or nicotinamide adenine dinucleotide phosphate (NADP), or a flavoprotein. NAD and NADP are also known as co-enzymes 1 and 2 respectively (Table 13.4). When they have accepted the hydrogen released by the action of the dehydrogenase they are known as reduced NAD and NADP, signified as NADH and NADPH.

Table 13.4 Co-enzymes

Chemical name	Standard abbreviations
Nicotinamide adenine dinucleotide	NAD
Nicotinamide adenine dinucleotide reduced	NADH
Nicotinamide adenine dinucleotide phosphate	NADP
Nicotinamide adenine dinucleotide phosphate reduced	NADPH

In some instances the dehydrogenase itself can act as a hydrogen acceptor, and is then reduced by flavoproteins in a subsequent reaction.

Because of the ability of dehydrogenases to remove hydrogen from the substrate, they are regarded as oxidative enzymes.

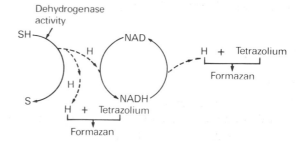

Fig. 13.2 Reduction pathway for tetrazolium salts

Some of the dehydrogenases which can be demonstrated histochemically, with the reactions which they catalyze are listed in Table 13.5.

The 'diaphorases' are dehydrogenases which catalyze the dehydrogenation of the reduced forms of NAD and NADP, i.e. they catalyze the reactions.

$$NADH \rightarrow NAD^+ + H$$
$$NADPH \rightarrow NADP^+ + H$$

The dehydrogenases are mitochondrial enzymes and will be removed by standard fixation techniques.

Table 13.5 Dehydrogenase reactions

Dehydrogenase	Reaction catalyzed
Succinate dehydrogenase	Succinate → fumarate
Lactate dehydrogenase	Lactate → pyruvate
Malate dehydrogenase	Malate → oxaloacetate
Isocitrate dehydrogenase	Isocitrate → oxalosuccinate
Glutamate dehydrogenase	Glutamate → ketoglutarate
Glucose-6-phosphate dehydrogenase	Glucose-6-phosphate → 6 phosphogluconolactone
Alcohol dehydrogenase	Ethanol → acetaldehyde
NAD diaphorase	NADH → NAD$^+$
NADP diaphorase	NADPH → NADP$^+$

RATIONALE OF DEMONSTRATION OF DEHYDROGENASES

Dehydrogenase activity is demonstrated histochemically using tetrazolium salts. These salts, which are almost colourless and are water-soluble, are able to accept the hydrogen released from the substrate by the enzyme action. Tetrazolium salts which have been reduced in this way produce an insoluble, highly coloured, microcrystalline deposit of a formazan compound. In histochemical reactions the conditions of the method have to be carefully controlled for the successful production and accurate localization of the formazan deposit.

An unfixed frozen section is incubated in a medium containing the specific substrate, the tetrazolium salt, buffer, the co-enzyme (if required), and any activators or chelators necessary.

Types of tetrazolium salts

In the development of histochemistry many types of tetrazolium salts have been tried for a number of techniques. They are used in the field of oxidase and dehydrogenase histochemistry. Two main types are used, the monotetrazolium salts and the ditetrazolium salts. A great deal of work has been devoted to tetrazolium salts to make them suitable for histochemical procedures. At the present time, salts from each of the two groups are in routine use for dehydrogenase methods.

Ditetrazolium chloride-nitro-BT (NBT) was introduced into dehydrogenase histochemistry by Nachlas et al (1957) for the demonstration of succinic dehydrogenase. The formazan produced with this salt is highly coloured, microcrystalline and insoluble in lipid; thus deposits of formazan may be seen in areas of lipid.

The salt of the monotetrazolium group is 3(4:5-dimethyl thiazolyl-2): 5-diphenyl tetrazolium bromide (MTT). This monotetrazole was introduced by Pearse (1957). The formazan produced with this salt is immediately chelated to cobalt ions, which are present in the incubating medium. The final formazan deposit is deeply coloured and finely granular. It is soluble in fat deposits. Using this tetrazolium salt, Scarpelli et al (1958), Hess et al (1958) and Pearse (1972) described methods for a number of dehydrogenase enzymes.

HISTOCHEMICAL METHODS

Succinate dehydrogenases: MTT technique

Succinate dehydrogenase in the section releases hydrogen from the substrate (sodium succinate). The hydrogen reduces the tetrazolium salt to form a formazan which is then chelated with cobalt ions to form a coloured insoluble granular deposit. For the histochemical demonstration of succinate dehydrogenase no co-enzyme is required since the enzyme itself acts as a hydrogen acceptor.

Succinate dehydrogenase: NBT technique

Succinate dehydrogenase in the section releases hydrogen from the succinate. This reduces the nitro-BT to form a water-insoluble coloured formazan. Again no co-enzyme is required.

Lactate dehydrogenase: NBT or MTT techniques

Lactate dehydrogenase in the section releases hydrogen from the lactate in the incubating medium. NAD is required as a hydrogen acceptor before the tetrazolium salt can be converted into a formazan.

Other dehydrogenases

Other dehydrogenase methods work on the principles outlined above.

NAD and NADP diaphorases: MTT technique

The NAD and NADP diaphorases oxidize NADH and NADPH to NAD and NADP respectively. The hydrogen passes to the tetrazolium salt which then chelates with the cobalt to form a formazan deposit at the site of activity.

PREPARATION OF SECTIONS AND INCUBATING METHODS FOR DEHYDROGENASE TECHNIQUES

Sections for the demonstration of dehydrogenase enzymes should be prepared from fresh unfixed material. Fixation of any sort will destroy dehydrogenase activity except for a small amount of enzyme firmly bound in the cytoplasm. Cryostat sections are recommended. The material should be frozen by one of the techniques described earlier. Sections are incubated unfixed at 37° C for 30–40 min. After incubation, the sections are transferred to formal saline to stop the reaction and to fix the section. They are then counterstained in 2% methyl green (chloroform-washed) or Mayer's Carmalum.

Preparation of tetrazolium stock solution

MTT* (1 mg per 1 ml distilled water)	2.5 ml
Tris buffer, pH 7.4	2.5 ml
0.5 M cobalt chloride	0.5 ml
0.05 M magnesium chloride	1.0 ml
Distilled water	2.5 ml

The pH is checked and adjusted to 7.0; if necessary, using either stock tris buffer or M-hydrochloric acid. The stock solution is kept frozen and is stable for many months if stored in this manner.

The co-enzymes are added just before use. The pH should be checked and adjusted to 7.0–7.1.

Note that in the methods for the diaphorases, the respective co-enzymes are the substrates for the reaction.

PRACTICAL DEMONSTRATION OF DEHYDROGENASES

The method detailed below illustrates the techniques of dehydrogenase histochemistry. The same technique can be applied to the dehydrogenases listed in Table 13.7 by simply applying the specific substrate solutions, with the addition or substitution of the correct co-enzyme if needed.

Solutions

1. Stock substrate solution (see Table 13.6).
2. Stock MTT tetrazolium solution.

Incubating medium as shown in (Table 13.7).

Technique

1. Cover sections with incubating medium at 37° C (30 min–1 h).
2. Transfer sections to formal saline (10–15 min).
3. Wash well in tap water (2 min).

Table 13.6 Preparation of stock substrate solutions with pH adjusted to 7.0

Substrate	Chemical	Conc. (M)	Amount of substance	Vol. of water (ml)	Neutralization	Final vol. (ml)
Succinate	Sodium succinate	2.5	6.75 g	8	0.05 ml M-HCl approx.	10
Malate	Sodium hydrogen	1	1.55 g	8	0.9 ml 40% NaOH	10
Glucose-6 phosphate	Glucose-6-phosphate (Disodium salt)	1	0.30 g	0.8	0.06 ml M-HCl	1.0
Isocitrate	DL-isocitric acid (trisodium salt)	1	0.27 g	0.8	0.1 ml 1 M-HCl approx.	1.0
Glutamate	L-glutamic acid (Na salt) Monohydrate	1	1.87 g	8	0.05 ml M-HCl	10

*3(4:5-Dimethyl thiazolyl-2)5-diphenyl tetrazolium bromide.

Table 13.7 Dehydrogenase working solutions

Enzyme to be demonstrated	Vol. of stock tetrazolium soln (ml)	Vol. of substrate stock soln (ml)	Vol. of distilled water (ml)	Co-enzyme 2 mg
NAD Diaphorase	0.9	Nil	0.1	NADH
NADP Diaphorase	0.9	Nil	0.1	NADPH
Succinic dehydrogenase	0.9	0.1	Nil	Nil
Malate dehydrogenase	0.9	0.1	Nil	NAD
Glucose-6-phosphate dehydrogenase	0.9	0.1	Nil	NADP
Isocitrate dehydrogenase	0.9	0.1	Nil	NAD
Glutamic dehydrogenase	0.9	0.1	Nil	NAD

4. Counterstain in 2% methyl green (chloroform washed) (5 min).
5. Rinse in tap water.
6. Mount in glycerin jelly.

Result

Succinate dehydrogenase	black formazan deposit
Nuclei	green

DOPA-OXIDASE

Melanin is thought to be produced from tyrosine by the action of an enzyme complex called tyrosinase (syn. DOPA-oxidase). The tyrosinase localized within the cells will oxidize DOPA to form an insoluble pigment. It is possible to demonstrate the sites of tyrosinase activity. The technique is most suitable when applied to post-fixed cryostat sections. The method was originally designed for blocks of tissue and both methods are given below.

Melanin producing cells are shown by treating the tissue with dihydroxyphenylalanine (DOPA). The enzyme within the cells will oxidize the DOPA to form insoluble brownish granules.

TISSUE BLOCK METHOD (Bloch, 1917; Rodrigues & McGavian, 1969)

Notes

Any melanin producing tissue should act as a suitable control. A negative control should always be employed.

Solutions

pH buffer 7.4
Dissolve 42.8 g sodium cacodylate and 9.6 ml M hydrochloric acid in 1 litre distilled water.

Primary fixative
10% formalin in the pH 7.4 buffer (v/v) plus 0.44 M sucrose.

Reactant
0.1% DOPA in the pH 7.4 buffer.

Technique

1. Fix two thin (2 mm) pieces of the test material in the primary fixative for 3 h at 4° C.
2. Rinse in cold (4° C) pH 7.4 buffer for 5 min.
3. Incubate one piece of tissue in the buffered DOPA solution for 16–20 h at 37° C. Change the solution for fresh buffered DOPA at least once during this time. The remaining tissue block is treated with buffer only at 37° C during this period.
4. Wash both blocks in distilled water for 5 min. Fix in a conventional 10% formalin solution for 1–2 days.
5. Paraffin process in the usual way. Cut 10 μm-sections and mount using plasma as an adhesive.

Results

Newly-formed melanin will be present in the DOPA-treated block only.

DOPA-OXIDASE IN SECTIONS
TECHNIQUE (BLOCH, 1917; LAIDLAW & BLACKBERG, 1932)

Notes

For this variant of the above reaction, use either fresh-frozen sections or frozen sections cut from tissue fixed in formalin for no longer than 2–3 h. Again, it is essential to take through a negative control, in this instance a duplicate section incubated in buffer only.

Solutions

pH buffer 7.4

Dissolve 42.8 g sodium cacodylate and 9.6 ml M hydrochloric acid in 1 litre distilled water.

Primary fixative

10% formalin in the pH 7.4 buffer (v/v) plus 0.44 M sucrose.

Reactant

0.1% DOPA in the pH 7.4 buffer.

Technique

1. Place sections in distilled water for a few seconds only.
2. Treat with DOPA solution for 30 min at 37° C. A duplicate section should be placed in pH 7.4 buffer only at 37° C and left there for a period corresponding to that received by the test section in DOPA.
3. Change with fresh solution and inspect the section microscopically every 30 min or so. In 2–3 h the solution will turn a reddish colour and in 3–4 h a sepia brown. By this stage the reaction should be complete.
4. Wash in several changes of distilled water. Counterstain with Mayer's haematoxylin solution for 1–2 min. Blue, wash, dehydrate, clear and mount as desired.

Results

DOPA-oxidase	brown
Nuclei	blue

REFERENCES

Bancroft J D 1975 Histochemical techniques, 2nd ed. Butterworth, London

Barka T 1960 A simple azo dye method for histochemical demonstration of acid phosphatases. Nature 187: 248

Barrnett R J, Seligman A M 1951 Histochemical demonstration of esterases by production of indigo. Science 114: 579

Bloch B 1917 Des problem de pigmentbildung in der haut. Archives of Dermato-Syphiligraphiques 124: 129

Burstone M S 1958 Histochemical demonstration of acid phosphatases with Naphthol AS-phosphates. Journal of National Cancer Institute 21: 523

Burstone M S 1961 Histochemical demonstration of phosphatases in frozen sections with naphthol AS-phosphates. Journal of Histochemistry & Cytochemistry 9: 146

Davis B J, Ornstein L 1959 High resolution enzyme location with a new diazo reagent hexazonium pararosanalin. Journal of Histochemistry & Cytochemistry 7: 297

Dubowitz V, Brooks M H 1973 Muscle biopsy a modern approach. W B Saunders, London

Gerebtzoff M A 1959 Cholinesterases. Pergammon, Oxford

Gomori G 1941 Distribution of acid phosphatase in the tissues under normal and pathologic conditions. Archives of Pathology 32: 189

Gomori G 1950 An improved histochemical technique for acid phosphatase. Stain Technology 25: 81

Gomori G 1951 Alkaline phosphatase of cell nuclei. Journal of Laboratory & Clinical Medicine 37: 526

Grogg E, Pearse A G E 1952 Coupling azo dye methods for Review of Cytology 1: 323

Grogg E, Pearse A G E 1952 Coupling azo dye methods for histochemical demonstration of alkaline phosphatase. Nature, London 170: 578

Hess R, Scarpelli D G, Pearse A G E 1958 Cytochemical localisation of pyridine nucleotide linked dehydrogenases. Nature, London 181: 1531

Holt S J 1954 A new approach to the cytochemical localisation of enzymes. Proceedings of Royal Society Series B 142: 160

Holt S J, Withers R F J 1952 Cytochemical localisation of esterases using indoxyl derivatives. Nature 170: 1012

Laidlaw G F, Blackberg S N 1932 Melanoma studies; DOPA reaction in normal histology. American Journal of Pathology 8: 491

Menton M L, Junge J, Green M H 1944 Coupling azo dye

test for alkaline phosphatase in the kidney. Journal of Histochemistry & Cytochemistry 5: 420

Moloney W C, McPherson K, Fliegelman L 1960 Esterase activity in leukocytes demonstrated by the use of Naphthol AS-D chloro-acetate substrate. Journal of Histochemistry & Cytochemistry 8: 200

Nachlas M M, Seligman A M 1949 The histochemical demonstration of esterase. Journal of the National Cancer Institute 9: 415

Nachlas M M, Tsou K C, Sousa E, Cheng C S, Seligman A M L 1957 Cytochemical demonstration of succinic dehydrogenase by the use of a new p-nitrophenyl substituted ditetrazole. Journal of Histochemistry & Cytochemistry 5: 420

Novikoff A B 1956 Preservation of the fine structure of isolated liver cell particulates with polyvinylpyrollidone sucrose. Journal of Biophysical, Biochemical Cytology 2: 65

Pearse A G E 1953 Histochemistry theoretical and applied. Churchill, London.

Pearse A G E 1957 Intracellular localisation of dehydrogenase systems using monotetrazolium salts and metal chelation of their formazans. Journal of Histochemistry & Cytochemistry 5: 515

Pearse A G E 1960 Histochemistry theoretical and applied, 2nd ed. Churchill, London

Pearse A G E 1972 Histochemistry theoretical and applied, 3rd ed, Vol. 2. Churchill Livingstone, Edinburgh

Rodriguez N A, McGavan M H 1969 A modified DOPA reaction for the diagnosis and investigation of pigment cells. American Journal of Clinical Pathology 52: 219

Scarpelli D G, Hess R, Pearse A G E 1958 The cytochemical localisation of oxidative enzymes (1) Diphosphopyridine nucleotide diaphorase and triphosphopyridine nucleotide diaphorase. Journal of Biophysics, Biochemistry & Cytology 4: 747

Stevens A 1983 Personal Communication

14

Immunohistochemistry

The most rapidly developing aspect of histology has changed in recent years from enzyme histochemistry to immunochemistry. The science of immunochemistry is applied to the relationship between tissue structure and the chemical activities of the immunoglobulin molecule (Table 14.1). It is necessary at this stage to give some definitions to allow the reader, possibly new to the subject, to understand what follows.

Antigen (Ag) (immunogens) This is the term applied to a substance which causes the formation of antibodies. They are substances of different chemical types (usually protein) capable of stimulating the immune system of an animal to produce a response specifically directed at the inducing substance and not other related substances. The antigen produces a mutual specificity with the antibody it causes (Weir, 1973).

Antibodies (Ab) are complex protein molecules produced by plasma cells and certain lymphocytes. The producing cells can be found in the germinal centres of lymph nodes, follicles of the spleen and other sites. The antibodies are produced in response to an antigen stimulus, and are known as immunoglobulins.

Immunoglobulins (Ig) share a similar basic structure. They are glycoproteins consisting of two heavy and two light polypeptide chains linked by disulphide bonds. Splitting produces two univalent fragments capable of binding antigen (Fab) and a third fragment without this capacity (Fc). There are five classes of human immunoglobulins, referred to as IgG, IgM, IgA, IgE and IgD.

IgG is the immunoglobulin of internal body fluids. It crosses the placental barrier and is the major immunoglobulin in the neonate. It combats micro-organisms and their toxins and forms approximately 80% of the total immunoglobulins.

IgM is largely restricted to plasma. It is a very effective agglutinator, produced early in the immune response. It is the first line of defence forming 6% of the total immunoglobulins.

IgA is the main immunoglobulin in sero-mucous secretions in respiratory and gastro-intestinal tracts, where it defends surfaces by inhibiting adhesion of organisms to the epithelium. It is 13% of the total immunoglobulins.

IgE is raised in parasitic infections. It attaches to skin and mast cells, and is about 0.002% of the total immunoglobulins.

IgD is thought to be present on lymphocyte surfaces. It is 1% of the total immunoglobulins.

Antiserum is a solution containing several different antibodies all of which are directed against the same antigenic molecule.

Monoclonal antiserum is a solution containing a

Table 14.1 Uses of immunohistochemistry

1. Demonstration of immunoglobulins of lymphoreticular origin	Multiple myeloma Hodgkins disease Lymphomas, etc.
2. Skin diseases (bullous disorders) a. Pemphigus b. Pemphigoid	IgG on prickle cell junctions IgG on basement membranes
3. Identification of hormone containing cells and tumours	Gastrin Calcitonin Testosterone, etc.
4. Tumour and cell markers	α-1-antitrypsin α-fetoprotein Carcino-embryonic antigen Factor VIII, etc.
5. Identification of organisms	Hepatitis B, antigen Herpes simplex, etc.
6. Localization of enzymes	Most common enzymes

single antibody which is directed against a specific antigenic determinant.

Labelled antiserum is available from commercial sources. It can be fluorescein, rhodamine peroxidase conjugated.

It is possible to demonstrate specific antigens and antibodies in tissue sections and in many instances to localize the site of antigen-antibody reactions (Table 14.2). The reaction sites are too small to be seen by the light microscope alone, so a suitable marker is used. The first antibody techniques were introduced by Coons et al (1942). They introduced the immunofluorescent method, which utilizes the fact that it is possible to conjugate antibodies with a fluorescent dye and at the same time not affect the capacity of the antibodies to react with an antigen. Coons and his workers using frozen sections combined the antibodies with fluorescein isocyanate producing a fluorescent antibody solution. There are many difficulties with immunofluorescent techniques, despite the use today of dyes that emit stronger fluorescence and are easier to prepare, such as fluorescein and rhodamine B isothiocyanates. Recently there has been a move to use enzymes instead of fluorescence as markers in immunochemical methods. These latter techniques allow the use of formalin fixed paraffin sections; a great advantage for a routine laboratory. The technique of immunohistochemistry is a combination of immunocytochemistry, where the tracer is attached to the specific antigen within the section, and enzyme histochemistry which allows us to see the tracer at the light or electron microscope level. During the development of the technique several enzymes were tried as markers, notably acid and alkaline phos-

phatase and glucose oxidase. The best results however were obtained using horseradish peroxidase, hence the term 'immunoperoxidase' methods. A considerable advantage of this type of technique over the immunofluorescence is the use of counterstains allowing for the tracer to be precisely located. The disadvantages of the immunofluorescent technique were clearly spelled out by Drury & Wallington (1980) and are listed below in slightly modified form:

1. Fresh tissue required.
2. Fixed tissue and paraffin embedded tissue unsuitable.
3. Impermanent, results fade.
4. Comparative studies difficult.
5. Expensive equipment necessary.
6. Photography necessary and difficult to do.
7. Not suitable for electron microscopy.
8. Expensive.

Not withstanding these drawbacks immunofluorescence still has a lot to offer for the detection of chemically specific materials, because of its greater sensitivity. A technique that is being used increasingly in routine laboratories is the identification of auto-antibodies in sera. The technique is used to detect antinuclear factor and antibodies to various structures. The indirect sandwich technique is used in which the test serum is applied to unfixed cryostat sections of rat tissues and a human tissue. After washing, the sections are treated with fluorescein labelled antihuman globulin. This will react with antibodies from the serum that initially reacted with an antigen in the tissue section. The sections are then viewed by a fluorescence microscope. The immunoperoxidase method can be employed in a similar manner. The immunofluorescence method is given below.

In the immunoperoxidase technique the fluorochrome is replaced by peroxidase and the peroxidase labelled antigen-antibody complex is demonstrated by histochemical means of a coloured reaction product at the site of peroxidase activity. The most suitable substrate to date is 3,3′ diamino-benzidine (DAB). There has been considerable concern about the chemical due to its possible carcinogenicity and some workers have used alternative substrates such as 3-amino-9-ethylcarbazole.

Table 14.2 Autoimmune disease

Examples of disease	Predominant antigen
Hashimoto's	Thyroglobulin
Chronic active hepatitis	Smooth muscle
Rheumatoid arthritis	IgG and nuclear antigens
Goodpasture's syndrome	Basement membranes
Primary biliary cirrhosis	Thyroid and kidney mitochondria
Systemic lupus erythematosus	DNA: nuclear proteins
Pernicious anaemia	Gastric parietal cells intrinsic factor

THE INDIRECT IMMUNOFLUORESCENT TECHNIQUE FOR AUTO-ANTIBODIES

Notes

1. Fresh cryostat sections are required from a composite block of rat tissues consisting of liver, kidney and stomach and separate cryostat sections of human thyroid.
2. Air dry the sections for 20 min at room temperature. An electric fan will assist the drying.
3. The sections must not be allowed to dry after Step 1 of the method.
4. Control sections must always be prepared at the same time as the test sections.
5. Parallel sections should be treated with known positive and negative sera as well as phosphate buffered saline in Step 3.
6. Positive sera are usually re-examined quantitatively using doubling dilutions of serum. The final titre is the last dilution showing positive fluorescence.
7. Antisera are pipetted into aliquots and stored at $-20°$ C or below.
8. Antisera is spun down hard to remove protein particles (e.g. 4500 r/min $\frac{1}{2}$–1 h) to reduce nonspecific background staining.
9. Ring the sections with a felt tip pen (a) to identify site of section and (b) to conserve the reagents.
10. Phosphate buffered saline, see below, is used in the washes and for the dilution of the serum.
11. The dilution of the test and control serum should be determined for each batch. Different supplier sera will show a variation in the optimal dilution.
12. A dilution of sera 1 : 5 with buffer is a good starting point.

Solutions

Test and control sera.

Phosphate buffered saline

Fluorescein labelled antihuman globulin
  This may be mono or polyvalent; the latter is normally used for routine serum investigation.

Technique

1. The test and control diluted sera are applied to the air dried cryostat sections in a covered moistened container for 20 min.
2. Wash well in phosphate buffered saline (two changes) for 15 min (mechanical agitation is recommended).
3. Remove excess saline.
4. Apply the diluted fluorescein labelled antihuman globulin to the sections in the container for 20 min.
5. Wash in phosphate buffered saline for 20 min with at least one change.
6. Mount sections in buffered glycerol.
7. Examine in fluorescence microscope.

Results

Autoimmune antibodies against tissue components will produce a bright yellow fluorescence at site. The colour of the resulting fluorescence can be varied by the choice of filters used in the microscope.

IMMUNOHISTOCHEMICAL METHODS

1. DIRECT TECHNIQUE (Fig. 14.1a)

In this technique, the primary antiserum directed against the antigen (rabbit antibody) is linked to horseradish peroxidase. This is the quickest method but the least sensitive, it requires a reasonable supply of antisera, to ensure that an adequate quantity of it is conjugated.

2. INDIRECT METHOD (Fig. 14.1b)

In this instance the sections are first incubated in the rabbit antibody which is unlabelled and directed against the antigen being demonstrated. The sections are then incubated with swine anti-rabbit sera which has been conjugated with peroxidase. This type of method is far more sensitive and requires less primary antisera. Furthermore, purified conjugated antisera are readily available from commercial sources.

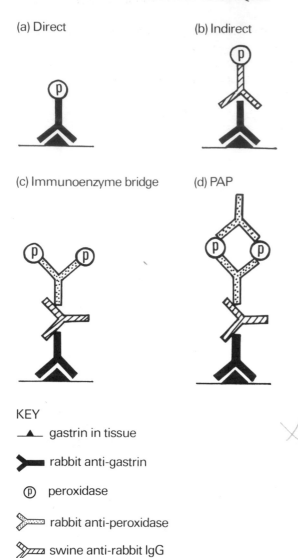

(a) Direct

(b) Indirect

(c) Immunoenzyme bridge

(d) PAP

KEY

▲ gastrin in tissue

➤ rabbit anti-gastrin

Ⓟ peroxidase

➤ rabbit anti-peroxidase

➤ swine anti-rabbit IgG

➤ peroxidase rabbit anti-peroxidase complex (PAP)

Fig. 14.1 Immunoperoxidase methods for the localization of antigens, e.g. gastrin

3. IMMUNOENZYME BRIDGE METHOD (Fig. 14.1c)

This method uses a bridging antibody to join the peroxidase to the antigen. The antigen is first incubated with an unlabelled rabbit antibody immunoglobulin and then bound to rabbit anti-

horseradish peroxidase by using the bridging unlabelled swine anti-rabbit immunoglobulin in excess

UNLABELLED ANTIBODY ENZYME METHOD USING PAP. (Fig. 14.1d)

Sternberger, et al (1970) modified the above method by adding a further stage. The rabbit antihorseradish peroxidase antibody is incubated with free horseradish peroxidase to form a soluble complex, peroxidase antiperoxidase (PAP) prior to incubation with the tissue section previously incubated with the rabbit antibody and the bridging swine immunoglobulin. This method produces a more intense colouration of the reaction product.

VISUALIZATION OF BOUND HORSERADISH PEROXIDASE

This is accomplished by the DAB reaction for peroxidase and is the end stage of the technique. The peroxidases catalyse the transfer of oxygen from the hydrogen peroxide. The DAB acts as a hydrogen donor. An insoluble coloured reaction product is formed.

FIXATION AND PRESERVATION

Fixation effects the activity of antigens. The choice of fixative depends upon the antigen or hormone to be detected. In general formaldehyde gives acceptable results and formaldehyde freshly generated from paraformaldehyde powder does not interfere with the immunoreactivity of many antigens (Robinson & Dawson, 1979). Acidic fixatives, formal-mercuric chloride, Bouin, Susa, Zenker and non-buffered formalin also give acceptable results. In the routine laboratory there is often little hope of having optimal fixation as most of the studies are retrospective. The standard embedding procedures have little effect on the reactivity of antigens and most methods work satisfactorily on routine embedded material. Depending upon the antigen, it is possible to demonstrate immunoperoxidase in resin embedded material (Robinson, 1982).

TREATMENT OF SECTIONS FOR ENDOGENOUS PEROXIDASES

It is usually necessary to treat sections prior to immunochemical staining to remove any endogenous peroxidases which will cause a pseudo reaction. These enzymes are present in many normal and pathological tissues. If not removed they will react with the substrate being used to localize the enzyme tracer, and produce false positives. The treatment of sections in methanol containing 0.3% hydrogen peroxide for 30 min at room temperature will remove this endogenous peroxidase activity without affecting the reactivity of the antigens.

UNMASKING OF REACTIVITY USING PROTEOLYTIC ENZYMES

One of the problems of immunoperoxidase techniques can be the variable results that are obtained with formalin fixed material — formaldehyde affecting some but not all of the antigens that we attempt to demonstrate. Mepham et al (1979) published work showing that enzymatic pretreatment reactivated the antigens as well as enhancing the staining reaction and improving the reliability of the immunoperoxidase methods. There are several factors that affect the pretreatment time with enzymes. Mepham et al (1979) compared the effects of different enzymes, concentration, temperature, and other factors. Their conclusions are shown in the trypsin method below; they warn that over-incubation will increase non-specific background staining. The method is not required when the tissues have been fixed and processed by a method which is known not to affect the reactivity of the antigen being demonstrated.

BACKGROUND STAINING

This can be seen in two forms: specific staining e.g. fibrinogen in blood vessels; or nonspecific,

involving the affinity of some tissue structures, notably reticulin and collagen for the immunoglobulin used in the staining methods. Normal swine serum is often used as a preliminary step in immunoperoxidase techniques to minimize this connective tissue staining. The complex subject of background staining is discussed by Robinson (1982).

STAINING METHODS

The practice of immunochemical staining is not difficult as it is a straightforward incubation and rinse, with no differentiation necessary. It is important that at no stage are any of the solutions allowed to evaporate off the sections. Equal care should be taken to ensure that the washing between stages is thorough.

DILUTIONS

To obtain optimal staining and to prevent a nonspecific precipitation of antibody onto the sections, it is necessary to use each antiserum at the correct dilution. Incorrect dilutions can produce false negatives. In the PAP technique the concentration of the primary specific antiserum is varied; the bridging molecule and PAP (see Fig. 14.1) are kept constant. In general a dilution of 1 : 20 is used for the bridging molecule and 1 : 60 for the PAP solution, but it is important to establish the optimal dilution for each new batch of antiserum.

WASHING

It is most important that adequate washing occurs between each stage of the technique. If this is not done a formation of antigen-antibody complexes will precipitate onto the sections. Between each stage a Tris buffered saline solution is used.

Given below is the method of preparing the DAB solution of Graham & Karnovsky (1966), the trypsin digestion method of Mepham et al (1979) for the unmasking of reactive sites, and examples of an indirect method and a peroxidase-antiperoxidase (PAP) technique all taken from Robinson (1982).

PREPARATION OF DAB (Graham & Karnovsky, 1966)

Solutions

Add 5 mg DAB to 10 ml 0.05 M Tris/HCl buffer, pH 7.6 (see Appendix 3) and stir until solid dissolves. Add 0.1 ml of freshly prepared 1% hydrogen peroxide.

This medium should be used immediately after preparation, and 5 min incubation at room temperature is generally sufficient. The reaction end product, which is brown in colour, resists alcohol dehydration and clearing in xylene. Due to the possible carcinogenic nature of the salt it is advisable to work in a fume cupboard, use disposable vessels for weighing and mixing, and to wear disposable rubber globes during preparation of the medium and incubation.

TRYPSIN DIGESTION METHOD (Mepham et al, 1979)

Notes

The trypsinization medium must be freshly prepared as its activity decreases with time.

As the time for treatment is not the same for all specimens, it is necessary to treat a series of slides for varying durations; for most tissues optimum digestion occurs within 15–30 min and, therefore, digestion times of 10, 20 and 30 min are recommended.

Solutions

Add 0.1 g trypsin (pancreatic type II, Sigma) to 100 ml 0.1% calcium chloride and mix thoroughly with a magnetic stirrer. With continuous stirring, add 0.1 M sodium hydroxide until pH is 7.8. Place working solution in a Coplin jar and equilibrate to 37° C in a waterbath before use.

Technique

1. Equilibrate temperature of section to 37° C by placing in distilled water at 37° C for 10 min.
2. Place in digestion solution for 10–30 min at 37° C.
3. Wash in running cold water for 15 min.

INDIRECT METHOD TO DEMONSTRATE HUMAN INSULIN

Notes

Both this and the PAP technique that follows are *examples* of suitable schemes for demonstrating a wide range of tissue antigens. The various steps of the techniques remain unchanged. It is the primary antiserum which will need to be appropriate to the antigen to be demonstrated (this will appear brown).

Solutions

0.3% hydrogen peroxide in absolute methanol.

3% normal swine serum in Tris saline.

Primary antiserum (rabbit antihuman insulin).

Peroxidase-conjugated swine antirabbit IgG.

DAB medium, see above.

Technique

1. Dewax sections and take to absolute alcohol.
2. Inhibit endogenous peroxidase activity by incubating in 0.3% hydrogen peroxide in absolute methanol for 30 min.
3. Hydrate sections by passing through graded alcohol series and wash in running water for 15 min.
4. Incubate sections in 3% normal swine serum diluted in Tris/saline for 15 min.
5. Drain off excess normal swine serum.
6. Incubate sections in primary antiserum diluted, 1 : 1000, 1 : 500, 1 : 250, 1 : 100, and 1 : 50 in 1% normal swine serum in Tris/saline for 30 min.
7. Jet wash off excess antiserum and then wash slides in Tris/saline for three 2 min changes.
8. Incubate in peroxidase-conjugated swine

antirabbit IgG diluted 1 : 20 in Tris/saline for 30 min.

9. Jet wash off excess antiserum and then wash slides in Tris/saline for three 2 min changes.
10. Incubate sections in DAB medium for 5 min.
11. Wash in running water for 10 min.
12. Counterstain in Harris' haematoxylin, dehydrate, clear and mount.

The following controls are recommended

1. Stain an untreated section with DAB to check for endogenous peroxidase activity and the effectiveness of the methanol/hydrogen peroxide treatment.
2. Omit the primary antiserum.
3. Pre-absorb the primary antiserum overnight with excess antigen.
4. Replace the primary antiserum with a rabbit antiserum directed against an unrelated antigen e.g. rabbit anti-gastrin serum.
5. Block the binding of the conjugated-antiserum by incubating for 30 min in unconjugated swine anti-rabbit IgG, diluted 1 : 20 with Tris/saline, after step (7) in the above sequence. Then wash in Tris/saline and proceed to step (8).
6. If available, include a known positive control.

PEROXIDASE-ANTI-PEROXIDASE (PAP) METHOD (e.g. to demonstrate IgM)

Solutions

0.3% hydrogen peroxide in absolute methanol.
3% normal swine serum in Tris/saline.
Primary antiserum (e.g. rabbit anti-human IgM).
Swine anti-rabbit IgG.
PAP complex.
DAB medium (see p. 200).

Technique

1. Dewax sections and take to absolute alcohol.
2. Block endogenous peroxidase activity by incubating in 0.3% hydrogen peroxide in absolute methanol for 30 min.

3. Hydrate sections by passing through graded ethanol series and wash in running water for 15 min.
4. Incubate sections in 3% normal swine serum diluted in Tris/saline for 15 min.
5. Drain off excess normal swine serum.
6. Incubate sections with primary antiserum diluted 1 : 2000, 1 : 1000, 1 : 500, 1 : 250 and 1 : 100 in 1% normal swine serum in Tris/saline for 30 min.
7. Jet wash off excess antiserum and then wash slides in Tris/saline for three 2 min changes.
8. Incubate sections in swine anti-rabbit IgG diluted 1 : 20 in Tris/saline for 30 min.
9. Jet wash off excess antiserum and then wash slides in Tris/saline for three 2 min changes.
10. Incubate sections in PAP complex diluted 1 : 60 in 1 % normal swine serum in Tris/saline for 30 min.
11. Jet wash off excess complex and wash in Tris/saline for three 2 min changes.
12. Incubate sections in DAB medium for 5 min.
13. Wash section in running water for 10 min.
14. Counterstain in Harris' haematoxylin, dehydrate, clear and mount.

The recommended controls are similar to those outlined with the indirect method, with the exception that the staining blocking control i.e. control (5) is undertaken with rabbit IgG for 30 min at a 1 : 20 dilution in Tris/saline after step (9) in the sequence above.

If either technique results in negative test and negative positive control sections, try less dilute primary antiserum. If the reaction continues to be negative, try controlled trypsin digestion (see p. 200); this is undertaken after step (3) in both schedules. If this fails, it will be necessary to systematically study the effect of various fixative solutions on the preservation of the antigen. If fixed tissues are still negative, it will be necessary to use fresh-frozen sections. It should be remembered, however, that there is likely to be extensive diffusion of some antigens in unfixed cryostat sections. If the technique does not work on these sections, recheck the specificity of all antisera.

REFERENCES

Coons A H, Creech H J, Jones R N, Berliner E 1942 The demonstration of pneumococcal antigen in tissues by the use of a fluorescent antibody. Journal of Immunology 45: 159

Drury R A B, Wallington E A 1980 Carleton's Histological technique, 5th edn. Oxford University Press, London

Graham R C, Karnovsky M J 1966 The early stages of absorption of injected horseradish peroxidase in the proximal tubules of mouse kidney. Ultrastructural cytochemistry by a new technique. Journal of Histochemistry and Cytochemistry 14: 291

Mepham B L, Frater W, Mitchell B S 1979 The use of proteolytic enzymes to improve immunoglobulin staining by the P.A.P. technique. Histochemical Journal 11: 345

Robinson G 1982 In: Bancroft J D, Stevens A (eds) Theory and practice of histological techniques, 2nd edn. Churchill Livingstone, Edinburgh

Robinson G, Dawson I M P 1979 A formalin fixative for immunochemical and ultrastructural studies on gastro-intestinal endocrine cells. Journal of Clinical Pathology 32: 40–5

Sternberger L A, Hardy P H, Cuculis J J, Meyer H G 1970 The unlabelled antibody enzyme method of immunohistochemistry: preparation and properties of a soluble antigen-antibody complex (horseradish peroxidase-antiperoxidase) and its use in identification of spirochaetes. Journal of Histochemistry and Cytochemistry 18: 315

Weir D M 1973 Immunology for undergraduates, 3rd edn. Churchill Livingstone, Edinburgh

15

Infective agents in tissue

ORGANISMS

There must be few laboratory workers who are not familiar with the method devised by Gram nearly a century ago. This, along with its numerous modifications, has remained the standard technique for the demonstration of organisms in pathology. Sometimes tissues will show a non-specific inflammatory reaction and by demonstrating micro-organisms, a definitive diagnosis can be made. This may well not have been possible if only the H and E preparation had been studied.

The principle of the method is that some blue cationic dyes are used to stain the nucleic acids of the organisms (the background tissue also stains); following this, the sections are treated with iodine and then differentiated in a suitable dye solvent: alcohol, aniline or acetone. The tissue background and some types of organism lose their blue staining but take up a cationic dye of contrasting (usually red) colour subsequently applied. The blue-stained organisms are termed 'Gram-positive' and those stained with the counterstain (red) are 'Gram-negative'. The net result is that not only are the organisms demonstrated, but different strains are shown in differing colours affording an arbitary division of organisms into two main groups aiding their identification.

The means by which some organisms retain the blue primary dye and others lose it upon differentiation is due to the action of iodine. The exact way in which the iodine influences dye fastness to differention is not at all clear. The traditional view is that the iodine combines with the dye and Gram-positive organisms as a type of mordant or trapping agent to form a solvent-resistant dye complex, but this viewpoint is undoubtedly oversimplified and one must consider the role played by iodine in dye penetration or isoelectric point deviation. Indeed, it has even been suggested that iodine, far from causing the Gram-positive organisms to retain the blue dye, is responsible for the Gram-negative organisms losing the blue primary dye. For example, if the iodine step is omitted, it will be found that differentiation needs to be prolonged. The tissue background is less easily differentiated and remains Gram-positive. Fibrin too, will remain largely Gram-positive in the absence of the iodine treatment. The potassium iodide in the iodine will facilitate solution of the relatively insoluble iodine in the aqueous solvent. As a general point in Gram staining it should be noted that non-viable Gram-positive organisms will often stain Gram-negative.

A few of the Gram variants will be presented, together with specialized techniques for organisms such as the mycobacteria, legionella and spirochaetes. Other techniques that will demonstrate organisms are Giemsa (see p. 63) and methyl green-pyronin (see p. 83).

Most organisms in clumps stain a weak blue colour in H and E preparations and can usually be seen fairly readily, but the individual organism can be visualized only with difficulty and therefore the special stains are necessary. Fixation is not an important factor either as choice of solution or initial freshness of tissue.

The use of positive controls when carrying out the various special stains is important, so should the test section be negative it is an indicator that the solutions and the skill of the operator are beyond reproach!

Bacteria may be found in tissue in conditions

such as gas gangrene, anthrax, bronchopneumonia, subacute endocarditis, septicaemic abscesses of kidney, lung and skin also in intestinal infections such as typhoid, bacillary dysentery and situations when tissue necrosis (infarction) is present. The more common organisms are shown in Table 15.1.

Table 15.1 Significant organisms and their Gram reactivity

Type	Form	Gram staining
Actinomyces	Filaments	Positive filament/negative clubs
Anthracis	Large straight bacilli	Positive
Bacteroides	Bacilli or cocco-bacilli	Negative
Clostridia	Large bacilli	Positive
Escherichia coli	Bacilli	Negative
Haemophilus	Cocco-bacilli	Negative
Klebsiella	Bacilli	Negative
Lactobacillus	Bacilli	Positive
Mycobacterium	Bacilli	Positive
Neisseria	Diplococci	Negative
Pneumococcus	Diplococci	Positive
Proteus	Bacilli	Negative
Pseudomonas	Bacilli	Negative
Salmonella	Bacilli	Negative
Shigella	Bacilli	Negative
Staphylococcus	Cocci (in clusters)	Positive

GRAM TECHNIQUE (from Gram, 1884)

Notes

Both Gram-positive and Gram-negative bacteria are demonstrated. Although overdifferentiation with the acetone is possible, it is the best method for obtaining consistently good results.

The technique for dealing with smears is similar in principle to that for sections. The main points to remember are that they should either be heat-dried on a hot-plate prior to staining, or wet-fixed for 20–30 min in 95% alcohol. Prior to staining it will not be necessary to take the smears through xylene and alcohols.

Solutions

Crystal violet
0.5% crystal violet in 25% alcohol (74 O.P. industrial methylated spirit is satisfactory).

Gram's and Lugol's iodine
Add 1 g iodine to 2 g potassium iodide plus a few ml of distilled water in a mortar. Grind until dissolved and make up to 300 ml volume for Gram's and 100 ml for Lugol's, with distilled water.

Technique

1. Take sections to water.
2. Stain with the crystal violet solution for 2 min.
3. Wash in water. Treat with the iodine solution for 2 min.
4. Wash in water and differentiate in acetone for 1 or 2 s only. Wash in water.
5. Counterstain with 1% aqueous neutral red for 3 min.
6. Wash, dehydrate quickly, clear and mount in a DPX-type mountant.

Results

Gram-positive organisms, fibrin, some fungi, Paneth cell granules, keratohyalin, keratin	blue
Gram-negative organisms, cell nuclei	red

MODIFIED GRAM TECHNIQUE (Weigert, 1887)

Notes

Although only Gram-positive organisms are demonstrated by this technique, exceptionally brilliant staining is afforded. Unfortunately the method is inclined to be capricious; it is not always possible to fully extract background crystal violet staining using the aniline-xylene differentiator. This is compensated to some degree by the fact that it is virtually impossible to overdifferentiate.

Solutions

5% aqueous eosin ws yellowish.

Crystal violet solution (see Gram's technique, above).

Gram's iodine solution (see Gram's technique, above).

Aniline-xylene mixture (equal parts).

Technique

1. Take sections to water.
2. Stain with the eosin solution for 5 min. Wash briefly in water.
3. Stain with the crystal violet solution for 2 min. Wash in water.
4. Treat with Gram's iodine solution for 2 min.
5. Wash briefly in water and blot dry.
6. After initial agitation leave in a Coplin jar of aniline-xylene for 5 min or so.
7. Rinse in xylene and mount in a DPX-type mountant.

Results

Gram-positive organisms,   blue
keratohyalin, keratin
Background   pink to red

GRAM-TWORT TECHNIQUE (Twort, 1924; Ollett, 1947)

Notes

This technique is relatively time-consuming and under- or overdifferentiation can occur. Even so a good preparation gives exceptional colour distinction of organisms from tissue background. Before differentiating, it is important that the slide is completely dry (warming over a lamp bulb for 10 min, following blotting, is often useful).

Solutions

Crystal violet solution (see Gram's technique, above).

Gram's iodine solution (see Gram's technique, above).

2% acetic acid in ethanol.

Stock neutral red-fast green stain
    0.2% neutral red in ethanol   90 ml
    0.2% fast green, FCF in ethanol   10 ml

Before use, dilute 1 part stock solution with 3 parts distilled water.

Technique

1. Take sections to water.
2. Stain with the crystal violet solution for 3 min. Wash in water.
3. Treat with the Gram's iodine solution for 3 min. Wash in water and blot dry (see notes).
4. Differentiate in preheated acetic-alcohol at 56° C until the section is a dirty-straw colour (15 min will usually suffice).
5. Wash briefly in distilled water.
6. Counterstain in neutral red-fast green stain solution for 5 min.
7. Wash in distilled water. Differentiate in acetic-alcohol at room temperature for approximately 10 s until no more red colour diffuses out.
8. Rinse in alcohol. Clear and mount in a DPX-type mountant.

Results

Gram-positive organisms, fibrin   blue
some fungi, keratohyalin, Paneth
cell granules, keratin
Gram-negative organisms,   red
cell nuclei
Cell cytoplasms, collagen,   green
red blood cells, etc.

ZIEHL-NEELSEN (ZN) TECHNIQUE FOR TUBERCLE BACILLI (Ziehl, 1882; Neelsen, 1883)

Notes

Tubercle bacilli have a lipid-rich cell wall which is capable of taking up strong phenol-dye solutions in such a way that they retain the dye upon subsequent differentiation in acid or alcohol, i.e. they are acid and alcohol fast. Most other organisms lose the dye and take up the counterstain.

It has been shown (Haroda, 1976) that the acid-fastness of mycobacteria stained with carbol fuchsin is due to the presence of carboxyl and hydroxyl groups on unsaturated lipids present in the bacterial cells.

The technique is not specific for tubercle bacilli as there is a tap water contaminant which stains similarly and is equally fast to the differentiators. Fortunately, the acid- and alcohol-fast organisms of tap water usually present as clumps sitting on the tissue, i.e. in a different focal plane, and are readily distinguishable. Whichever ZN variant is used, it is important to take through a positive control section as the carbol fuchsin solutions deteriorate with age (and newly prepared solutions may not work!).

The counterstaining should be kept light, otherwise the bacilli may be masked; some workers prefer to counterstain with one of the alum haematoxylin solutions as opposed to methylene blue. In our experience methylene blue does provide a slightly better contrast to the carbol fuchsin-stained organisms and is given in the following techniques.

The histological appearance in tuberculosis is usually (but not always) typical; even so, the demonstration of tubercle bacilli is a very useful confirmatory procedure. It should be appreciated that tissue which has the obvious histological characteristics of tuberculosis quite often will contain few or no stainable organisms. This may be traced to the fact that the patient had been treated with the usual antituberculous drugs, which results in non-staining organisms. Additionally, it must be said that tissue from unsuspected tuberculosis cases (i.e. untreated) may still contain only very few bacilli. For example, bone lesions usually contain far fewer organisms compared to lung. Basic fuchsin is the usual dye in the technique but other dyes, e.g. Victoria blue, may be used instead. The phenol in the staining solution probably acts as a surface tension depressant to allow the dye ions to enter the lipid envelope of the tubercle bacilli more easily.

Avoid decalcification of tissue in strong acids as acid-fastness may be lost; formic acid solutions are to be preferred (Wong & Wu 1979).

When heating the carbol fuchsin solution one should be aware of the hazards involved in the use of naked flames. An alternative course of action is to use a Coplin jar containing the dye in a 56° C incubator.

A Ziehl-Neelsen type method which employs a room temperature stain bath is that of Kinyouin and will be given.

Should potentially tuberculous unfixed material for cryostat sectioning be received, full aseptic procedures should be adopted, i.e. use of gloves, gowns etc. Following sectioning the slides should be fixed in 10% formalin for at least 10 min prior to staining. All equipment should be thoroughly sterilized in either formalin or Cidex including the cryostat interior. The 'Howie' 1978 Code of Practice handbook should be consulted for full details.

Solutions

Carbol fuchsin solution

Dissolve 1 g basic fuchsin (use the relatively coarse granule, not the more purified type specified for Schiff's reagent) in 10 ml ethanol. Dissolve 5 g of phenol in 100 ml of distilled water. Mix the two solutions together. Filter.

0.2% aqueous methylene blue.

Technique

1. Take sections to water.
2. Filter on the carbol fuchsin and heat three times until the 'steam rises' (over a period of 10 min), or heat in a Coplin jar at 56° C for 30 min.
3. Wash well in water. Differentiate in 1% acid-alcohol for 10 min. Wash in water for 5–10 min.
4. Counterstain with the methylene blue solution for 30 s. Wash in water.
5. Differentiate and dehydrate in alcohol until the sections are a weak blue. Clear and mount in a DPX-type mountant.

Results

Tubercle bacilli, hair shafts, and (to a lesser degree) red blood cells, clubs of actinomycotic filaments and spermatozoa heads	magenta
Background	weak blue

ALTERNATIVE ZN-TYPE TECHNIQUE
(Poltz et al, 1964).

Notes

With this variant of the ZN technique a combined differentiator and counterstain is used. This works quite well but the malachite green tends to fade, sometimes after a short time.

Solutions

Carbol fuchsin solution, see ZN technique above.

Differentiator-counterstain

2% aqueous malachite green	110 ml
Acetic acid	15 ml
Glycerol	25 ml

There is usually no need to filter the solution.

Technique

1. Take sections to water and stain with the heated carbol fuchsin (as for the ZN technique).
2. Wash in water.
3. Counterstain in a Coplin jar of the acidified malachite green solution for 4 min.
4. Wash, blot, dehydrate, clear and mount in a DPX-type mountant.

Results

Tubercle bacilli etc. (see results for standard ZN technique)	magenta
Background	pale blue-green

MODIFIED ZN TECHNIQUE (Kinyouins, 1915)

Notes

No heating of the carbol fuchsin is required in this technique which employs a stronger solution of the dye. The dye solution is an aqueous one, unlike the traditional solution and is difficult to prepare.

Our experience is that it is less reliable than other techniques.

Solutions

Carbol fuchsin solution

Dissolve, with the aid of heat, 4 g of basic fuchsin in 20 ml of distilled water. Melt some phenol crystals in a flask, under a hot tap and add 8 ml of the melted phenol to 100 ml of distilled water. Add the two solutions together, mix and filter.

0.2% aqueous methylene blue.

Technique

1. Take sections to water.
2. Filter on the carbol fuchsin solution for 4 min. Do not heat.
3. Wash. Differentiate in 1% acid-alcohol for 1 min.
4. Wash and counterstain as for the standard ZN technique.
5. Dehydrate, clear and mount in a DPX-type mountant.

Results

Tubercle bacilli etc. (see Results for standard ZN technique)	magenta
Background	pale blue

MODIFIED ZN TECHNIQUE FOR LEPROSY BACILLI (Faraco, 1938; Fite et al, 1947)

Notes

Compared with tubercle bacilli, the leprosy bacilli are much less acid- and alcohol-fast and their lipid envelope more easily affected by fat solvents, thus diminishing the staining reaction. Therefore, in this modification of the standard ZN technique, treatment with alcohol and acid is minimal. Initial dewaxing is accomplished in a mixture of vegetable oil and xylene.

It is most important not to overstain with the methylene blue, as it will not be possible to remove the excess dye in alcohol.

Solutions

As for standard ZN technique.

Technique

1. Warm the sections and deparaffinize by placing in a mixture of two parts xylene to one part vegetable oil (clove oil is suitable). Leave for at least 10 min.
2. Blot dry and wash in water. This step may be repeated, should any xylene-oil remain on the section.
3. Filter on the carbol fuchsin solution for 20 min. Do not heat.
4. Wash. Differentiate in 1% acid-alcohol for 1 min.
5. Wash well in water and counterstain in weak (0.2%) methylene blue for 5–10 s.
6. Wash, blot, dry and clear in xylene. Repeat the blotting-xylene treatment until the section is clear.
7. Mount in a DPX-type mountant.

Results

| Leprosy bacilli and (to a lesser degree) red blood cells | magenta |
| Background | pale blue |

FLUORESCENCE TECHNIQUE FOR TUBERCLE BACILLI AND LEPROSY BACILLI (Silver et al, 1966, taken from Matthaei, 1950)

Notes

It is a curious fact that most workers agree that the fluorescence demonstration of (particularly) the tubercle bacilli is superior to the ZN-type technique, and yet very few actually use it! (This may be due to the inherent problems of fluorescence microscopy, the relative impermanence of preparations, and also that a little expertise is necessary in order to initially visualize the section without too great a time consumption.) On the other hand, an important advantage is that screening of sections for tubercle bacilli is very much quicker as isolated bacilli are more easily seen.

Background tissue fluorescence is masked by the potassium permanganate treatment. To stain for leprosy bacilli, avoid alcohol dehydration at the conclusion of the technique and dewax initially in a vegetable oil-xylene mixture (see above).

Sections stained by the ZN technique can be destained by lengthy 1% acid-alcohol treatment if so wished, and restained using the following fluorescence technique. The converse gives unsatisfactory results.

Solutions

Auramine-rhodamine solution
Add 1.5 g of auramine O and 0.75 g rhodamine B to 50 ml of distilled water and 75 ml glycerol. Mix and add 10 ml phenol liquefied by melting at 56° C. This solution will keep for up to 2 months.

0.5% hydrochloric acid in alcohol (for tubercle bacilli) *or* 0.5% aqueous hydrochloric acid (for leprosy bacilli).

0.5% aqueous potassium permanganate.

Technique

1. Take sections to water.
2. Mix the auramine-rhodamine solution and filter onto the section for 10 min at 60° C (the stain should be preheated).
3. Wash in water for 2 min.
4. Differentiate in either of the hydrochloric acid solutions for 2–3 min.
5. Wash in water for 2 min.
6. Treat with the potassium permanganate solution for 1 min.
7. Wash in water for 2 min. Blot dry.
8. Dehydrate (omit for leprosy bacilli), clear and mount in a DPX-type mountant.

Results (using the fluorescence microscope with a yellow K530 barrier filter)

| Tubercle or leprosy bacilli | golden-yellow |
| Background tissue | dark green |

THE DEMONSTRATION OF LEGIONELLA PNEUMOPHILA

It was in 1976 that attention was focussed on a type of pneumonia having a high mortality, when at an American Legion convention in Philadelphia, USA, 182 cases were reported of which there were 29 deaths. In 1977 the causative organism was identified as a small Gram-negative coccobacillus and was named *Legionella pneumophila*.

From a purely histological point of view it is a difficult organism to demonstrate. It stains poorly by the Gram technique and in our hands is not stained by methyl green-pyronin, although it does stain weakly with the Giemsa technique. At present the most satisfactory means of demonstrating *L. pneumophila* seems to be the use of direct immunofluorescence on imprint smears or paraffin sections, employing a rabbit anti-*L. pneumophila* group 1 IgG conjugated with FITC (Cherry, 1978). The Dieterle silver technique, although originally described for the demonstration of spirochaetes, has proved to be a useful method for these organisms in routine histological sections and is described below.

DIETERLE TECHNIQUE FOR LEGIONELLA PNEUMOPHILA (Dieterle, 1927)

Notes

The gum mastic solution gives best results if used immediately after the 3 days needed for its preparation. It is important to ensure thorough solution of the gum mastic in the alcohol. It is also important for the reaction that the temperatures are strictly adhered to. Formalin fixed frozen and celloidin sections may be 'stained' as well as paraffin.

The uranyl nitrate step serves to prevent argy-cophilic background material such as nerve fibres from being impregnated, and the gum as a diffusion vehicle for the silver particles to give even impregnation. Otherwise the rationale is as for most silver techniques, i.e. reduction of bound silver nitrate to a black reduced silver salt. As with most silver techniques, the main disadvantages are that practice is required for consistent results, and that other background elements exhibit silver blackening to a varying degree, e.g. connective tissue fibres and various pigment granules.

It is important to note that the method is *not* specific for *L. pneumophila* as most other organisms are also blackened.

Solutions

0.5% uranyl nitrate in 70% alcohol.

10% gum mastic* in absolute alcohol (stand for 3 days before use).

1% aqueous silver nitrate.

Reducer

Hydroquinone	1.5 g
Sodium sulphite	0.25 g
Conc. formalin	10 ml
Acetone	10 ml
Pyridine	10 ml

Add distilled water to a final volume of 90 ml, mix and dissolve, then add 10 ml of the alcoholic gum mastic solution (the solution should now appear 'milky').

Technique

1. Take sections to distilled water.
2. Treat with uranyl nitrate solution for 30 min at 55° C.
3. Wash briefly in distilled water then in 95% alcohol.
4. Treat with gum mastic solution for 30 s.
5. Rinse in 95% alcohol for 1 s only then transfer to distilled water.
6. Treat with the silver nitrate solution for 1–6 h in the dark (take through several sections and remove at intervals until the optimal time is determined).
7. Wash in distilled water for 1 s only.
8. Place in reducer for 8 min.

*Gum mastic may be obtained from: J. Flach & Sons, 140 Falkland Road, Harringay, London.

9. Wash in distilled water for 1 s then 96% alcohol followed by acetone.
10. Clear and mount as desired.

Results

Organisms including L. *pneumophila* and melanin	black
Background	yellow

SPIROCHAETES

In tissue the most common spirochaete is *Treponema pallidum*, the causative organism of syphilis. Another less commonly seen spirochaete is a leptospira found in Weil's disease and which may be transmitted from rats. These organisms are not seen in routine preparations and special techniques are necessary. The Giemsa technique will stain the spirochaetes purple-red but visualization is not easy. The most successful methods employ silver impregnation and these will be described. Formalin fixation gives the best results.

BLOCK IMPREGNATION TECHNIQUE
(Bertarelli & Volpino, 1906)

Notes

This is a modification of the Levaditi method and gives, in our experience superior results. Block impregnation techniques tend on the whole to be less erratic than those designed for sections, but naturally suffer from the drawback of needing unprocessed tissue which may well not be available.

For reasons that are not clear, the reducing solution should be at least 3 months old, so that it is advisable to keep some ready for use on the shelf.

The addition of acetic acid, and a lower pH silver solution seems to give a clearer background than the Levaditi method.

Solutions

Silver solution
1.5 g silver nitrate in 50 ml ethanol and 50 ml distilled water.

Reducer

Tannic acid	3 g
Pyrogallic acid	5 g
Anhydrous sodium acetate	10 g
Distilled water	350 ml

The solution should be at least 3 months old before use.

Technique

1. Take a thin (2 mm) piece of formalin-fixed tissue and, if available, a similar block of positive control material, and wash well in several changes of distilled water over 1–3 h.
2. Place in the silver solution for 24 h at 37° C in the dark.
3. Add 0.25 ml glacial acetic acid for every 100 ml volume of the silver solution and leave for a further 4 days at 37° C in the dark.
4. Wash in several changes of distilled water over 1–3 h.
5. Reduce for 2–3 days at room temperature in the dark.
6. Wash in several changes of distilled water over 3 h.
7. Paraffin process and cut sections. It is wise to cut one section from the periphery of the block and one nearer the centre and thus obtain different degrees of silver impregnation. Mount on slides, dry, deparaffinize in xylene and mount as desired.

Results

Spirochaetes (plus some organisms and fungi)	black
Background	yellow

PARAFFIN SECTION TECHNIQUE (Warthin & Starry, 1920)

Notes

This is the standard silver technique for spirochaetes in paraffin sections. A certain degree of expertise is needed in order to obtain a reasonable result due to the variation in development of the silver; overdevelopment yields heavily impregnated spirochaetes against a dark and granular background, whilst underdevelopment shows weak impregnated spirochaetes against a pale background. The technique is time consuming. The temperature of the developer is all-important for successful results. In place of Scotch glue, gelatin can be used.

Solutions

Prepare a litre or so of pH 3.6 buffer and use in the preparation of all the following solutions (the Walpole acetate-acetic buffer is suitable, but *not* the acetate-hydrochloric acid variant, see Buffer Tables)

Silver solution

1% silver nitrate in pH 3.6 buffer.

Developer

Add 0.3 g hydroquinone to 10 ml of buffer. Take 1 ml of this solution and add 15 ml of warmed 5% Scotch glue; mix and maintain at 40° C. Take 3 ml of a 2% silver nitrate in pH 3.6 buffer and maintain at 55° C. The two solutions are mixed immediately prior to use.

Technique

1. Take sections to water and rinse in pH 3.6 buffer, (celloidinize the section to minimize background precipitation).
2. Stain with the preheated silver solution for 1½–1¾ h at 55–60° C. During this period prepare the developer, which should also be preheated (use water bath).
3. Treat with the developer for 3½ min at 55° C (the sections should turn a golden-brown).
4. Pour off the developer and rinse in tap water for several minutes at 55–60° C then in room temperature buffer. Tone if desired in 0.2% gold chloride.
5. Dehydrate, clear and mount as desired.

Results

Spirochaetes   black
Background   yellow-brown

MODIFIED DIETERLE TECHNIQUE FOR SPIROCHAETES (Burns, 1982)

This modified technique seems to give better results than the Warthin and Starry method for spirochaetes in paraffin sections. Because a somewhat 'dirty' background is given we have found this modified technique — though better than the original for demonstrating spirochaetes — less satisfactory for demonstrating *L. pneumophila*.

The temperatures specified for the various solutions are important and should be adhered to for good results.

Solutions

5% uranyl nitrate in 70% alcohol.

The other solutions are exactly as for the non-modified technique (see p. 209).

Technique

1. Take sections to distilled water.
2. Treat with preheated uranyl nitrate solution for 1 h at 60° C.
3. Treat with the gum mastic solution for 3 min.
4. Rinse in 95% alcohol.
5. Rinse in distilled water for 1 min and allow to drain until almost dry (approximately 10 min).
6. Place in preheated silver nitrate solution overnight at 40° C.
7. Rinse in distilled water.
8. Place in reducer for 3–5 min (until pale yellow to tan).
9. Rinse in distilled water, then in 95% alcohol followed by acetone.
10. Clear and mount as desired.

Results

Spirochaetes   black
Background   yellow-brown

FUNGI

The usual fungi to be encountered in tissue are those such as *Aspergillus fumigatus*, *Candida albi-*

Table 15.2 Reproduced from Coombs (1967) by courtesy of the author.

Organism	HE	Gram	PAS	CAS†	Gridley	Reticulin	Grocott	Alcian blue	Mucic-carmine	Best's carmine
Candida albicans	±	++	+	+	+	–	+	±	–	+
Aspergillus fumigatus (pulm.)	+	–	+	++	±	+	++	–	–	±
A. fumigatus (plug)	±	–	±	+	+	+	+	–	–	–
Cryptococcus neoformans	–	±	+	+	+	+	++	++	++	++
Histoplasma capsulatum	–	–	+	+	+	+	++	±	±	++
Sporotrichum schencki	–	+	+	+	+	+	+	+	–	+
Blastomyes dermatidis	–	–	+	+	+	+	++	–	–	+
Epidermaphyton floccosum	–	–	±	±	±	±	+	–	–	+
Trichophyton rubrum	–	–	±	±	±	+	++	–	–	+
T. verrucosum	–	–	+	+	+	+	++	–	–	+
*Actinomyces bovis**	–	+	±	+	+	+	+	–	–	±

*Not a true fungus
†CAS, chromic acid Schiff (Bauer technique)

cans and, less commonly, *Cryptococcus neoformans* and *Histoplasma capsulatum*. The latter two fungi are found as muco-encapsulated yeasts, whilst the former two exhibit both yeast forms and mycelia. Fungal mycelia, if plentiful, can often be seen in H and E preparations but the yeast forms with difficulty. Special stains are of undoubted value for fungal demonstration and there is a reasonably wide choice of techniques. These include PAS (see p. 102), Gram (see p. 204), Best's carmine (see p. 122), Southgate's mucicarmine (see p. 105), alcian blue (see p. 109); also two to be described below, the Grocott variant of Gomori's hexamine silver and the Gridley technique. It should be noted that when demonstrating cryptococci by the PAS or Grocott techniques the organism itself is coloured, whereas using the Southgate mucicarmine or alcian blue technique only the capsule is stained. It will be seen from Table 15.2 there are significant differences in results for fungi using staining techniques. Formalin fixation is usually recommended for fungi demonstration.

GROCOTT HEXAMINE-SILVER VARIATION (Gomori, 1946; Grocott, 1955)

Notes

This is the method of choice for demonstrating all fungi. Chromic acid-formed aldehydes from certain structures reduce a hexamine-silver mixture at an alkaline pH, and are selectively blackened. The method is not specific for fungi and is rather time consuming, but rarely fails to demonstrate any fungi present in tissue. A control should always be taken though to establish the efficacy of the reagents employed.

Overimpregnation will result in connective tissues being blackened and this will make fungal indentification more difficult. One should terminate treatment with the hexamine-silver when the fungi appear a dark brown colour and the background is still clear, i.e. aim at slightly under-impregnating.

The inclusion of the borate gives a final pH of approximately 8.0.

Solutions

5% aqueous chromium trioxide (chromic acid).

1% aqueous sodium metabisulphite.

Stock hexamine-silver solution
To 100 ml of 3% aqueous hexamine add 5 ml of 5% aqueous silver nitrate. A white precipitate will form which dissolves on shaking. This solution will keep for 1–2 months at 4° C.

Working solution
Dilute 2 ml of freshly prepared 5% aqueous soidum tetraborate solution with 25 ml of distilled water. Mix and add 25 ml of stock hexamine-silver. Mix.

Technique

1. Take test and control sections to water.
2. Treat with the chromic acid solution for 1 h. Wash in water.
3. Bleach in the metabisulphite solution for 1 min.
4. Wash in tap water 5–10 min, then in several changes of distilled water.
5. The working hexamine solution should have been preheated to 56° C using a Coplin jar in a water bath. Treat the section in this solution at 56° C and examine after 10–20 min and thereafter at 3 min intervals until the fungi are blackened (see Notes) but the background is clear.
6. Wash in 3 changes of distilled water and tone in 0.1% aqueous gold chloride for 3 min.
7. Wash in water, fix in 5% sodium thiosulphate (hypo) for 5 min. Wash again.

8. Counterstain in 0.2% light green in 0.2% acetic acid for ½–1 min. Wash in water.
9. Dehydrate, clear and mount as desired.

Results

Cellulose, *P. carinii*, fungi, chitin, some mucins, melanin, glycogen, starch	black
Background	green

GRIDLEY'S TECHNIQUE (Gridley, 1953)

Notes

This technique is basically the Bauer-Schiff and aldehyde fuchsin techniques in combination. Whilst some workers feel that the Gridley technique reveals more of the internal structure of fungi than other methods, it should be noted that the types of fungus demonstrated are paralleled by the much simpler PAS technique. Another point to bear in mind in that elastic fibres and some connective tissue mucins stain purple, making fungus demonstration more difficult in tissues such as skin.

Solutions

4% aqueous chromium trioxide (chromic acid).

Schiff's reagent, see page 102.

Aldehyde fuchsin solution, see page 55.

Saturated tartrazine in Cellosolve.

Sulphurous acid rinse
10% aqueous sodium metabisulphite	6 ml
Molar hydrochloric acid	5 ml
Distilled water to	100 ml

Technique

1. Take sections to water.
2. Treat with the chromic acid solution for 1 h. Wash well in tap water, then in distilled water.

3. Treat with Schiff's reagent for 15 min.
4. Treat with the sulphurous acid solution for 3 changes over 6 min.
5. Wash in water for 10 min.
6. Treat with the aldehyde fuchsin solution for 20–30 min.
7. Wash in 50% alcohol then in water.
8. Wash in absolute alcohol and stain with the tartrazine solution for $\frac{1}{2}$–1 min.
9. Wash and dehydrate in alcohol, clear and mount in a DPX-type mountant.

Results

Fungi, elastin, some mucins	purple
Background	yellow

VIRUSES AND THEIR INCLUSION BODIES

With the exception of the hepatitis B surface antigen, viruses are not easily identified or visualized by light microscopy with or without the use of special stains. In certain viral conditions intracellular aggregates form and these can be demonstrated in conventional tissue sections; they are known as virus inclusion bodies. They are invariably globular in shape and vary, not only in size, but in their location in that they may be intranuclear (e.g. cytomegalovirus and Herpes simplex), intracytoplasmic (e.g. rabies and measles) or both (e.g. viral warts of skin). The inclusion bodies vary greatly in their composition and can contain DNA or RNA.

The presence of either of the nucleic acids means that techniques such as the Feulgen for DNA (see p. 81) or methyl green-pyronin for RNA (see p. 83) can be successfully employed. The protein moiety imparts acidophila to virus inclusion bodies, enabling them to be seen to a lesser or greater extent in routine H and E preparations. Special stains are of a definite advantage in showing these structures although much depends on the type of virus inclusion present as to which method is of greater value. For example,

herpes and cytomegalic virus inclusion bodies are readily seen in conventional H and E preparations also Papanicolaou stained material, whilst those of rabies, measles and rickettsia stain better using techniques such as Giemsa (see p. 63), Mann's methyl blue-eosin (see p. 70) or phloxine-tartrazine (see p. 64). It should be noted that the latter method may stain Negri bodies of rabies brilliantly but inconsistently. Virus inclusions of the skin condition molluscum contagiosum are often only well shown by the Macchievello technique, and those of rabies (Negri bodies) by the phosphotungstic acid-eosin techniques. Both specialized virus inclusion techniques will be described, together with a modified orcein technique for virus hepatitis antigen

Whilst formalin fixation is perfectly adequate for these techniques, better results are given for virus inclusion bodies if mercuric chloride or potassium dichromate-containing solutions are used.

MACCHIAVELLO TECHNIQUE FOR VIRUS INCLUSION BODIES (Macchiavello, 1937)

Notes

This technique which is like a modified ZN stain, will demonstrate most inclusion bodies. Negri bodies are sometimes seen with this simple technique which requires some expertise to obtain a good result. The Mallory bleach stage is optional, and our experience with the method leads us to suspect that it is superfluous.

Solutions

0.5% basic fuchsin in pH 7.2 phosphate buffer. See Buffer Tables Appendix 3.

0.5% aqueous citric acid.

0.2% aqueous methylene blue.

Acidified potassium permanganate solution, see page 49.

Technique

1. Take sections to water.
2. Treat with the acidified potassium

permanganate solution for 5 min. Wash and bleach with 5% aqueous oxalic acid (see Notes). Wash well in water.
3. Stain with Macchiavello's solution for 5 min. Wash in water.
4. Differentiate in citric acid until only the virus inclusion bodies are left stained (3–6 min). Wash in water.
5. Counterstain lightly in the methylene blue solution for 10–20 s.
6. Wash, dehydrate, clear and mount as desired.

Results

Virus inclusion bodies	magenta
Background	pale blue

PHOSPHOTUNGSTIC-EOSIN TECHNIQUE FOR NEGRI BODIES (Massignani & Malferrari, 1961)

Notes

Whilst techniques such as Giemsa, Mann's or Macchiavello's purport to stain the typical formation of rabies, first described by Negri in 1903, they do not always give clear cut demonstrations. Indeed, an H and E preparation will often be as informative. As mentioned earlier, the phloxine-tartrazine method can yield very good results, but can prove unhelpful. The phosphotungstic acid-eosin technique is undoubtedly the best technique currently available. The solution is rather time-consuming to prepare but the results are consistently good.

According to the authors, the role of the phosphotungstic acid with eosin is that of dye-mordant formation rather than one of lowering the pH to give an acid eosin. An alternative mechanism to be considered is that the phosphotungstic acid, acting as a colourless dye, enters most of the tissue pores (intermicellar spaces), excepting those of fine porosity such as the virus inclusion bodies and red blood cells. The eosin is thus largely excluded from all but these two entities.

When staining the nuclei with haematoxylin, it is important to differentiate well so that the background is left unstained.

Solution

Grind together 1 g eosin ws yellowish and 0.7 g phosphotungstic acid. Add 10 ml of distilled water and mix. Bring the total volume to 200 ml with ethanol. Add two drops of saturated aqueous lithium carbonate and stir continuously for 10 min (an electric mixer is ideal for this purpose). Restore to the original 200 ml volume with ethanol and filter.

The solution keeps well under room temperature storage conditions.

Technique

1. Take sections to water.
2. Stain the nuclei with one of the alum haematoxylin solutions. Differentiate well and blue. Wash in water then in ethanol.
3. Stain in the phosphotungstic — eosin solution for 8 min.
4. Wash in water briefly then differentiate by giving short dips in 50%, 70%, 80% and 90% alcohol and longer dips in 95% and absolute alcohol. (Give two or more changes of absolute alcohol of 4 min each.)
5. Clear in xylene and mount in a DPX-type mountant.

Results

Negri bodies	bright pink
Red blood cells	pink
Background	pale pink or colourless
Nuclei	blue

MODIFIED ORCEIN TECHNIQUE FOR HEPATITIS B SURFACE ANTIGEN (Shikata, 1974)

Notes

In this type of viral hepatitis the affected hepatocytes show a typical ground glass appearance, and the contained HBs (Australia) antigen can be demonstrated by orcein and prior oxidation with potassium permanganate. The rationale is that of sulphur-containing proteins being oxidized to form reactive sulphonate residues which react with orcein. In a similar way, using a pre-oxidation step both aldehyde fuchsin and alcian blue will stain the HBs antigen. Although the definitive demonstration of HBs antigen must be the use of immuno-histochemistry[*], the Shikata orcein technique is still popular in many routine laboratories, together with the oxidation-aldehyde fuchsin technique. It must be appreciated that the non-immunohistochemical techniques are not specific for HBs antigen and although elastic fibres are easily distinguishable from the viral antigen deposits, a potential source of error is if copper-associated protein is present in the hepatocytes. The success or failure of the technique devolves around the batch of orcein employed. Most workers employ synthetic orcein and some advocate the need for freshly prepared solutions (Kilpatrick, 1982) but in our experience the important point is to obtain initially a batch of orcein that works and if it doesn't, try other batches or other dye suppliers (we currently use that of Raymond A. Lamb). It is important to take through a positive control slide in sequence with the test slides.

Solutions

Acidified potassium permanganate

0.25% aqueous potassium permanganate	95 ml
3% aqueous sulphuric acid	5 ml

[*]Immunoperoxidase technique for Hepatitis B surface antigen. We have had good results with the Dako PAP Kit obtainable from Mercia Brocades Limited.

Orcein solution

Orcein (synthetic)	1 g
70% ethanol	100 ml
Conc. hydrochloric acid	1 ml

Saturated tartrazine in Cellosolve (2-ethoxyethanol).

Technique

1. Take sections to water.
2. Treat with acidified potassium permanganate for 5 min.
3. Wash briefly in water.
4. Bleach sections with 1% oxalic acid for $\frac{1}{2}$ to 1 min.
5. Wash well in water (5 min or so).
6. Rinse in 70% alcohol.
7. Stain in preheated orcein for $1\frac{1}{2}$ h at 37° C (use Coplin jar).
8. Rinse in 70% alcohol and examine microscopically. and if the positive control is stained satisfactorily, proceed.
9. Rinse in Cellosolve, and stain with tartrazine for 2 min.
10. Rinse in Cellosolve, clear and mount as desired.

Results

HBs antigen, elastic fibres and copper-associated protein	dark brown
Background	yellow

REFERENCES

Bertarelli G, Volpino G 1906 Weitere Untersuchungen über die Gegenwart der Spirochaete pallida in den Schnitten primärer sekundärer und tertiärer Syphilis. Zentralblatt für Bakteriologie, Parasitenkunde, Infektionskrankheiten und Hygiene 41: 74

Burns P A 1982 Staining intestinal spirochaetes. Journal of Medical Laboratory Sciences 39: 75

Coombs D M 1967 In: Baker F J (ed) Progress in medical laboratory technique No. 4. Butterworths, London

Dieterle R R 1927 Method for the demonstration of spirochaete pallida in single microscopic sections. Archives of Neurology and Psychiatry 18: 73

Faraco J 1938 Bacillos de Mansen e cortes de paraffina; Methodo complementar para a pesquiza de bacillos de Mansen e Cortes de material incluido el paraffina. Revista Brasileira de Leprologia 6: 177

Fite G L, Cambre P J, Turner M H 1947 Procedure for demonstrating lepra bacilli in paraffin sections. Archives of Pathology 43: 624

Gomori G 1946 A new histochemical test for glycogen and mucin. American Journal of Clinical Pathology 16: 177

Gram C 1884 Ueber die isolierte Farbung der Schizomyceten in Schnitt und Trocnenpräparaten. Fortsch Med 2: 185

Gridley M F 1953 A stain for fungi in tissue sections. American Journal of Clinical Pathology 23: 303

Grocott R G 1955 A stain for fungi in tissue sections and smears. American Journal of Clinical Pathology 25: 975

Harada I T 1976 The nature of mycobacterial acid-fastness. Stain Technology 51: 255

Kinyouin J J 1915 A note on Uhlenhuth's method for sputum examination for tubercle bacilli. American Journal of Public Health 5: 867

Macchiavello A 1937 Rickettsia. Revista Chill Hig. Med. Pre., 1: 5

Massignani A M, Malferrari R 1961 Phosphotungstic acid-eosin confirmed with haematoxylin as a stain for Negri bodies in paraffin sections. Stain Technology 36: 5

Neelsen F 1883 Zentralblatt für die Medizinischen Wissenschaften 21: 497

Ollett W S 1947 A method for staining both Gram positive and Gram negative bacteria in sections. Journal of Pathology and Bacteriology 59: 357

Poltz G, Rampey J H, Furmandeau B 1964 A method for staining acid-fast bacilli in smears and sections of tissue. American Journal of Clinical Pathology 42: 552

Shikata T Uzawa T, Yashiwara N, Akatsura R, Yamazari S 1974 Staining methods of Australia antigen in paraffin sections — detection of cytoplasmic inclusion bodies. Japanese Journal of Experimental Medicine 44: 25

Silver A, Sonnerwirth A C, Alex N 1966 Modifications in the fluorescence microscopy technique as applied to identification of acid-fast bacilli in tissue and bacteriological material. Journal of Clinical Pathology 19. 583

Twort F W 1924 An improved neutral red, light green double stain for staining animal parasites, micro-organisms and tissue. Journal of State Medicine 32: 351.

Warthin A S, Starry A C 19 1920 A more rapid and improved method of demonstrating spirochaetes in tissues. American Journal of Syphilis, Gonorrhoea and Venereal Diseases 4: 97

Weigert C 1887 Fortschr. Med. 5: 228

Wong F T S, Wu P C 1979 The influence of decalcifying fluids on the demonstration of Mycobacterium tuberculosis in paraffin sections. Medical Laboratory Sciences 36: 153–7.

Ziehl F 1882 Zur Farbung des Tuberkelbacillus. Deutsche Medizinische Wochenschrift 8: 451

16

Central and peripheral nervous system

INTRODUCTION

This chapter is concerned with the functional elements which go to make up the nervous system. There are many special techniques capable of demonstrating nervous tissue entities; the majority are silver impregnations of sections or tissue blocks. It is, perhaps, unfortunate that a high percentage of the methods are not only empirical but capricious. This means inevitably, that it is a subjective science where consistent success with a method is largely a matter of expertise and/or experience. Where the rationale of a technique is known it will be given.

Many of the following techniques utilize celloidin sections and some expertise is required in dehydrating and clearing the stained section. The following system is one we have found successful and would commend it to the novice.

1. Take the stained celloidin section from water, through 70% alcohol to 95% alcohol (95 parts 74 O.P. spirit and water 5 parts). Flatten the section using camel hair brushes.

2. Place in absolute alcohol (74 O.P. spirit) and then in a mixture of four parts xylene and one part absolute alcohol to flatten the section by softening the celloidin.

3. Mount on a slide, blot with xylene-soaked blotting paper and then clear in xylene.

4. Brush out any air bubbles under the section (with section wet with xylene). Mount in Canada balsam. Should there be any prominent folds in the section, it sometimes helps to cut away the excess celloidin border using a sharp scalpel blade; this should be done when the section is in xylene just prior to mounting in balsam.

Standard formalin fixation is suitable for most CNS/PNS demonstration techniques, although there are areas, such as myelin and neuroglia for which specialized fixation is required for certain methods. Unless otherwise indicated, frozen or celloidin sections give better results than paraffin, particularly with those techniques employing silver impregnation. The reason for this is not clear. There are silver techniques in which paraffin sections give satisfactory results and some of these will be described.

NEURONES AND THEIR PROCESSES (CNS)

As discussed in chapter 1, when dealing with the normal histology of tissue, neurones may be very large, as in the anterior horn of the spinal cord, or quite small in the granular layer of the cerbellum. The nucleus is often difficult to see due to the scanty chromatin network, but has a prominent nucleolus. The cell body contains varying amounts of discrete granular material known as 'Nissl substance' and also varying amounts of the pigment lipofuscin (see Ch. 11) which increases in amount with advancing age. From the cell body emerges an axon (axis cylinder) and a number of dendrites, and in these may be shown delicate fibrils which pass from the cell body into the processes. These fibrils are the 'neurofibrils'.

Pathology arising from these particular nervous elements is not common. Apart from diseases such as motor neurone disease where there is malformation of the processes, or certain dementias where argyrophilic plaques of neurofibrils are found, there are not many conditions where the various special techniques are of great assistance. However, their employment has, over the years, contributed enormously to our knowledge of nervous tissue structure. The Nissl substance may be lost in neuronal degeneration in trauma, a condition known as 'chromatolysis', although there will be other easily seen changes associated with cell degeneration. The neurone can usually be visualized in a conventional H and E preparation but the processes (and neurofibrils) are only well seen using special techniques (Table 16.1). Formalin fixation gives the best results, although Carnoy fixation is to be recommended for Nissl substance.

Immunocytochemistry can be used in a limited manner to demonstrate neurones by virtue of the presence of Neurone Specific Enolase (NSE). This protein is not confined to neurones and is present in neuroendocrine cells (APUD system).

Table 16.1 Central and peripheral nervous systems. Demonstration of nerve cells and their processes.

Technique	Recommended use
Bielschowsky: block impreg.	Nerve fibres of CNS
Bielschowsky: frozen sections	Nerve fibres of CNS
Formal-thionin	Nerve fibres of CNS
Golgi-Cox	Some nerve fibres of CNS
Von Braunmuhl	Neurofibrils and plaques of CNS
Cresyl fast violet	Nissl substance of CNS
Toluidine blue	Nissl substance of CNS
Glees & Marsland	Nerve fibres of CNS and PNS
Gros-Bielschowsky	Nerve fibres of CNS and PNS
Linder	Nerve fibres of CNS and PNS
Palmgren	Nerve fibres of CNS and PNS
Winklemann & Schmit	Nerve fibres of CNS and PNS
Methylene blue	Nerve endings of PNS
Schofield	Nerve endings of PNS

NISSL SUBSTANCE

Bearing in mind that Nissl substance is composed of coarse aggregates of RNA, it will be appreciated that the component material can be readily demonstrated by the use of most cationic dyes, also techniques designed for RNA demonstration

such as methyl green-pyronin or gallocyanin. Nissl substance will give a strong yellow primary fluorescence. A selection of the more commonly employed techniques is given below.

CRESYL FAST VIOLET FOR NISSL SUBSTANCE

Notes

Two variants will be described one for celloidin sections the other for paraffin. Although, as discussed above, dyes such as thionin, toluidine blue and methyl green-pyronin can be used to demonstrate Nissl substance, undoubtedly cresyl fast violet gives the best results — particularly in the hands of a novice.

Gothard's (1898) differentiator, whilst perhaps giving slightly the better results, is not mandatory as 96% alcohol can be successfully used. It also has a rather pungent odour. Gothard's solution will dissolve celloidin and should only be used in conjunction with the technique for paraffin sections.

Alcohol or Carnoy fixation provide the best results but formalin-fixed material will give results that are quite adequate. The rationale of the technique is a simple acid-base reaction, where the cationic dyes bond with the anionic RNA of the Nissl substance, plus the DNA and RNA of cell nuclei.

CELLOIDIN SECTION TECHNIQUE

Solutions

0.1% aqueous crysyl fast (echt) violet.

Differentiator
95% alcohol	100 ml
Chloroform	2 ml
Acetic acid	8 drops

Technique

1. Place celloidin sections in 70% alcohol overnight at 37°C (this is a degreasing step designed to give even staining).

2. Rinse in distilled water.
3. Place in freshly filtered cresyl fast violet solution and heat to 60–65°C over the pilot flame of a bunsen burner.
4. Cool to room temperature. Wash in water, followed by 70% then 95% alcohol.
5. Differentiate out the excess dye in the alcohol-chloroform-acetic solution. Transfer to 95% alcohol for $\frac{1}{2}$–1 h to complete the differentiation.
6. Dehydrate, clear and mount in Canada balsam.

Results

Nissl substance, nuclei	violet
Background	colourless

PARAFFIN SECTION TECHNIQUE
(Kawamura & Niimi, 1972)

Solution

0.1% aqueous cresyl fast violet acidified by adding 0.7 ml of 10% acetic acid per 100 ml of solution to give a pH of 3.5–3.8.

Technique

1. Take sections to water.
2. Stain for 30 min at room temperature.
3. Wash in water. Differentiate in 95% alcohol until the background is relatively clear.
4. Wash in absolute alcohol, clear and mount in Canada balsam.

Results

Nissl substance, nuclei	violet
Background	colourless

TOLUIDINE BLUE TECHNIQUE FOR NISSL SUBSTANCE

Solutions

0.2% aqueous toluidine blue.

Gothard's solution

Pure creosote	50 ml
Cajuput oil	40 ml
Xylene	50 ml
Absolute alcohol	150 ml

Technique

1. Take sections to water.
2. Stain with toluidine blue for *either*: 6 h at room temperature *or*: 30 min at 56°C.
3. Wash in water.
4. Rinse in 90% alcohol.
5. Differentiate in Gothard's solution or 95% alcohol (see p. 219) controlling microscopically until the Nissl substance is clearly seen in the cell bodies of the larger neurones.
6. Rinse in absolute alcohol, clear in xylene and mount paraffin sections preferably in a DPX-type mountant.

Results

Nucleoli and Nissl substance	dark blue
Nuclei	paler blue

NERVE FIBRES

BIELSCHOWSKY BLOCK IMPREGNATION TECHNIQUE (Bielschowsky, 1904)

Notes

Wherever silver demonstration techniques are concerned the name of Bielschowsky will appear: the father-figure of so many of our argyrophilic fibre demonstration work. In this method the blocks of tissue are impregnated with the sensitizer- ammoniacal silver-reducing solutions and although the method is slow it is, as neurological methods go, a reliable one. When the block is finally sectioned it is always worthwhile cutting a superficial one and then one deeper into the block. In this may both heavily and lightly impregnated areas will be shown.

Solutions

3% aqueous silver nitrate.

Ammoniacal silver

Add 2 drops of 40% aqueous sodium hydroxide to 5 ml of 20% aqueous silver nitrate. Mix and add successive drops of concentrated ammonia with shaking until the formed precipitate is almost dissolved. Make up to a 40 ml volume with distilled water.

Technique

1. Place thin (2–3 mm) blocks of formalin-fixed tissue in pyridine for 2 days (this is said to reduce background silver deposition).
2. Wash in running tap water overnight, followed by washing in several changes of distilled water over 1 day.
3. Treat with the silver nitrate solution for 4–5 days in the dark.
4. Wash well in several changes of distilled water over 2–3 h.
5. Treat with the ammoniacal silver solution for 4–5 h.
6. Wash well in several changes of distilled water for 2–3 h.
7. Reduce in 20% formalin for 12–16 h.
8. Wash well in water for 1–2 h and paraffin process.
9. Cut conventional sections and deparaffinize in xylene. If the background is clear mount in Canada balsam. If not, tone in 0.2% gold chloride. Fix in 5% hypo, dehydrate, clear and mount.

Results

Nerve fibres, neurofibrils	black
Neurones, collagen	brown

FORMOL-THIONIN BLOCK IMPREGNATION TECHNIQUE (Min Chueh Chang, 1935)

Notes

This is quite a simple and ingenious technique which involves simultaneous fixation and staining of the tissue block. When sectioning the block it is as well not to trim in too far as the dye does not penetrate very deeply. Either fresh or formalin-fixed tissue can be used.

Solution

0.4–0.5% thionin in 10% formalin.

Technique

1. If fresh tissue is available, take a thin (2–3 mm) block and treat with formol-thionin for 1 week.
2. If formalin-fixed tissue only is available, take a thin block and wash well in distilled water over 1 day. Treat with formal-thionin for 1 week.
3. Wash in distilled water briefly, then paraffin process (double-embedding may be used, if desired). Dehydration in alcohol should be prolonged, if necessary, until no more thionin diffuses out.
4. Cut sections, deparaffinize and mount as desired.

Results

Neurones	blue
Nerve fibres	red

GOLGI-COX BLOCK IMPREGNATION TECHNIQUE (Golgi, 1878; Cox, 1891)

Notes

Although this technique is one of the slowest of any neurological methods it has the unique facility of impregnating only certain of the neurones and their processes. Examination of single nervous entities is therefore facilitated. Like most of these techniques it is capricious and it is advisable to take through several blocks and vary the fixation-impregnation period. The rationale of the technique is unknown. Only fresh tissue should be used. Celloidin sections are to be preferred as frozen sections tend to fragment during cutting.

Solution

Mix 10 ml of 5% aqueous potassium dichromate and 10 ml of 5% aqueous mercuric chloride. To 8 ml of a stock 5% aqueous potassium chlorate add 20 ml distilled water. Add the solutions together and mix.

Technique

1. Place thin (2–3 mm) blocks of tissue in an ample volume of the fixing-impregnating solution; rest on cotton wool to ensure an even impregnation. Leave for 24 h at 37° C.
2. Change the solution for fresh and leave for a further 24 h at 37° C.
3. Change the solution for fresh, seal the lid of the container with Vaseline petroleum jelly and leave for 1–2 months in a dark place at 37° C.
4 Wash well in several changes of distilled water over several hours. Cut either frozen sections or prepare celloidin sections at a thickness of 50–100μm.
5. Blacken the metallic(?) impregnation with either 5% aqueous sodium carbonate or 10% ammonia for 1 h.
6. Wash well in water. Dehydrate, clear and mount. Conventional mounting in balsam will cause fading; it is recommended that the section be mounted in thick balsam at 40–45° C without a coverslip. Drury & Wallington (1967) state that it is possible to mount successfully in Permount.

Results

Some nerve cells and their processes (blood vessels may also be impregnated)   black

BIELSCHOWSKY TECHNIQUE FOR FROZEN SECTIONS

Notes

The principle of the reaction, (which is the same for most silver reactions for nervous tissue) is that following 'sensitization' in silver nitrate, the section is treated with ammoniacal silver. The ammoniacal silver is formed when ammonia is added to silver nitrate, forming a silver hydroxide precipitate; this is soluble in an excess of ammonia when a solution of ammoniated silver oxides is formed. Subsequent treatment with a reducer, such as formalin, will cause a reduced metallic silver deposit to be selectively laid down. The reason for the silver selectivity (argyrophilia) is unknown. The silver reduction may be followed by toning in gold chloride which is thought to be a simple metallic substitution of gold for silver. This is then followed by treatment with sodium thiosulphate (hypo) which removes any unreduced silver particles preventing subsequent nonspecific blackening by exposure to light under section storage conditions.

This particular technique is reasonably reliable but it does tend to give a somewhat darker background than the Bielschowsky block impregnation technique. Formalin-fixed tissue should be used.

Solutions

4% aqueous silver nitrate.

Ammoniacal silver
  Add six drops of 40% aqueous sodium hydroxide to 5 ml of 20% aqueous silver nitrate. Mix and add conc. ammonia drop by drop with mixing, until the formed precipitate is almost dissolved. Make up to 25 ml with distilled water and filter.

Technique

1. Take 'thin' (15 μm) frozen sections to distilled water and change several times over 1 h.
2. Treat with the silver nitrate solution for 4 h in the dark at room temperature.
3. Rinse briefly in distilled water.
4. Treat with the ammoniacal silver solution for 3–10 min (leave until a brown colour).
5. Wash briefly in distilled water.
6. Treat with 4% formalin in tap water for 10 min.
7. Wash in water. Tone with 0.2% gold chloride, wash and treat with 5% hypo; both treatments for 1–2 min.

8. Wash, mount on a slide and blot. Dehydrate, clear and mount in Canada balsam.

Results

Nerve fibres, neurofibrils   black
Background   light grey

VON BRAUNMUHL'S TECHNIQUE FOR NEUROFIBRILLARY PLAQUES IN ALZHEIMER'S DISEASE (von Braunmuhl, 1957)

Notes

To demonstrate Alzheimer plaques a variety of silver methods can be used, including the standard Bielschowsky, but this variant seems to give particularly good results (Chalk, 1970). It is also a reasonably straightforward type of silver technique (all things being relative). As might be expected, normal neurofibrils and fibres are also demonstrated.

Solutions

20% aqueous silver nitrate.
1% aqueous ammonia.
20% formalin in tap water.
0.25% aqueous gold chloride.
5% aqueous sodium thiosulphate (hypo).

Technique

1. Take 10–30 μm formalin fixed free-floating frozen sections to distilled water and wash well.
2. Place in the silver nitrate solution for $\frac{1}{2}$–1 h (usually the shorter time), at 56° C.
3. Remove dish containing the sections from the incubator and leave at room temperature whilst the following solutions are prepared in separate containers:
   a. 1% ammonia;
   b. distilled water;
   c. 20% formalin.
4. Treat the sections in sequence as follows:
   a. 3 s; b. 1 s; c. 3 s.
   Repeat the sequence a, b, and c once more.

5. Wash in distilled water, tone in the gold chloride for $\frac{1}{2}$–1 min, fix in 'hypo' 1–2 min.
6. Mount sections on slides, blot dry, dehydrate, clear and mount in Canada balsam.

Results

Neurofibrils and plaques   black

MYELIN

The demonstration of myelin can be of definite value when one of the demyelinating diseases, such as multiple sclerosis, or, less commonly, cerebral pontine and medullary myelinolysis, is suspected. For whilst myelinated nerve fibres stain a stronger pink in an H and E solution than the non-myelinated, they are still not easy to discern and any pathological change may easily go unnoticed.

There are two main groups of methods concerned with demonstrating myelin degeneration; the so-called 'negative' techniques where only normal myelin is stained, and the 'positive' techniques where only the degenerate myelin is stained. There are advantages and disadvantages to the use of each. By demonstrating normal myelin only, degenerated myelin sheaths are shown by absence of staining and this may not be easy to distinguish, if only single fibres are involved. On the other hand, the negative method will demonstrate long-standing degeneration (8 weeks or more) when the products of degeneration having been removed would not have reacted with the positive techniques. Techniques which stain degenerate myelin sheaths have an obvious advantage, but they are prone to artefact and show short-term degeneration only (10–60 days). The staining methods are listed in Table 16.2

NORMAL MYELIN

There are many such techniques, e.g. PTAH, osmium tetroxide, Sudan black and iron haematoxylins, but the ones described below give more precise results. Paraffin sections should be cut at 10 μm, as these give better visualization of the

Table 16.2 Demonstration of normal and degenerate myelin

Technique	Normal myelin	Degenerate myelin		
		Early	Later	Long term
Sudan dyes	√		√	
Luxol fast blue	√			√
Loyez	√			√
Weigert-pal	√			√
Iron haematoxylin	√			√
Solochrome cyanine	√			√
Marchi (Swank-Davenport; Busch)		√		

myelin sheaths compared to the normal 5 μm sections. Fresh frozen sections can be stained by Sudan dyes or osmium tetroxide for myelin and, because of the greater retention of myelin lipids compared to paraffin sections, the myelin sheaths will appear thicker with a comparatively narrow nerve fibre lumen.

Note that in addition to the 'specialized' techniques for myelin which follow, it is possible to stain with either Weigert's or Heidenhain's iron haematoxylin (see p. 40 and 74 respectively). These are particularly effective when dealing with celloidin sections of brain.

WEIGERT-PAL TECHNIQUE (Weigert, 1885; Pal, 1886)

Notes

This is very much a hybrid technique as it employs Weigert's mordant, Pal's differentiator, and usually, Kultschitzky's (1889) haematoxylin!

The conventional rationale of the method is preliminary mordanting in chrome salts forms a chromium dioxide complex so that normal myelin will subsequently form a lake with haematoxylin. Only long-standing myelin degeneration will show lack of staining. Due to the fact that· the chrome salts act as fat fixatives the resultant myelin sheaths appear more substantial following processing, than say, those demonstrated by Loyez or Luxol fast blue where conventional formalin fixation precedes processing. With these latter techniques resultant myelin sheaths appear much more slender, presumably due to loss of myelin fats.

Paraffin processing can be carried out with this technique but sectioning is difficult and they become easily detached from the slide. Celloidin processing is to be preferred.

Solutions

Weigert's primary mordant
Dissolve 5 g potassium dichromate in 2.5 g fluorchrome (chromic or chromium fluoride) in 100 ml distilled water.

Kultschitzky's haematoxylin

10% alcoholic haematoxylin (allow to ripen at least 4 weeks)	10 ml
2% acetic acid	90 ml

Pal's differentiator A
0.25% aqueous potassium permanganate.

Pal's differentiator B
Equal parts of 1% aqueous oxalic acid and 1% aqueous potassium sulphite.

Technique

1. Take thin (2–3 mm) pieces of formalin-fixed tissue and treat with the primary mordant 4–7 days.
2. Wash in two changes of alcohol over 30 min. Process through either paraffin or celloidin.
3. Cut 10 μm paraffin or 20 μm celloidin sections and take to water.
4. Stain with the haematoxylin solution overnight at 37° C.
5. Wash in water and blue in any weak alkali such as lithium or sodium carbonate.
6. Prepare three containers; one containing the permanganate solution, one distilled water and the other the oxalic-sulphite mixture. The section is differentiated as follows:

Permanganate	15–20 s (agitate)
Distilled water	1–2 s
Oxalic-sulphite	4–5 min

This sequence is repeated until the background is reasonably clear and the myelin a blue-black colour.

7. Wash well in distilled water. Counterstain, if

desired, in 1% aqueous neutral red solution for 2–3 min. Wash in water.
8. Dehydrate, clear and mount in Canada balsam.

Results

Red blood cells, normal myelin sheaths   blue-black
Nuclei (if counterstained)   red
Background   unstained

LOYEZ TECHNIQUE (Loyez, 1910)

Notes

A simple method and one that can be carried out on routinely fixed, paraffin processed sections. As mentioned previously, the myelin sheaths stained by this method are considerably more 'anaemic' than those demonstrated by techniques using lipid fixatives.

Differentiation may be initiated in either iron alum or 1% acid-alcohol. We prefer the former as it is quicker and gives a clearer background.

Solutions

Haematoxylin
10% alcoholic haematoxylin (ripened by standing for several weeks)
Distilled water
Saturated aqueous lithium carbonate

Preliminary differentiator
4% aqueous iron alum.

Final differentiator
Dissolve 2 g sodium tetraborate (borax) and 2.5 g potassium ferricyanide in 200 ml distilled water.

Technique

1. Take paraffin sections to water.
2. Treat with the iron alum solution overnight at room temperature.

3. Wash in water for several minutes.
4. Stain with the haematoxylin solution for either 2–4 h at 56° C, or overnight at room temperature.
5. Wash in water. Differentiate excess background dye in the iron alum solution. Wash in water. Continue differentiation in the borax-ferricyanide solution until the background is clear. Counterstaining may be carried out in 1% aqueous eosin for 1 min.
6. Wash in water. Dehydrate, clear and mount in Canada balsam.

Results

Red blood cells, normal myelin, nuclei   blue-black
Background   colourless if not counterstained, pink if counterstained

MODIFIED LUXOL FAST BLUE TECHNIQUE (Kluver & Barrera, 1953; Ainge et al, 1969)

Notes

Luxol fast blue is one of the copper phthalocyanin dyes (along with alcian blue and methasol fast blue), and according to Pearse (1955) has a strong affinity for phospholipids and choline bases; hence presumably its affinity for myelin.

It is a popular method owing to the fact that routinely fixed, paraffin processed sections can be successfully stained and moreover, a rather pleasing colour.

The following modification has the twin advantages of simplicity and short staining times. Luxol fast blue staining can be followed by oil red O or similar dye, to show degenerate myelin in a contrasting colour.

Solution

Luxol fast blue   0.1 g
Methanol   100 ml
1.5 M hydrochloric acid   0.5 ml
Mix and filter.

Technique

1. Take paraffin or frozen sections to water.
2. Stain in Luxol fast blue for 1 h at room temperature.
3. Wash in water.
4. Differentiate in 0.05% aqueous lithium carbonate for 20 s or so (a saturated solution diluted to 1 : 20 will serve) until the background is clear.
5. Wash in water. Counterstain in 1% aqueous neutral red for 5 min.
6. Wash in water. Dehydrate and differentiate the neutral red in alcohol, clear and mount as desired.

Results

Red blood cells, myelin	blue to purple depending on the amount of counter-stain remaining
Nuclei and Nissl substance	red
Background	colourless

SOLOCHROME CYANINE TECHNIQUE
(Page, 1965, 1970)

Notes

This method is both simple and quick, and has the advantage, unlike Luxol fast blue which also stains collagen, of being equally suitable for PNS or CNS myelin demonstration in paraffin sections. The finished result tends to be rather more delicate than the Loyez or Luxol fast blue techniques. Fresh frozen sections can be stained with this technique and should be finally mounted in an aqueous mountant for best results.

Solution

Add 0.5 ml conc. sulphuric acid to 0.2 g solochrome cyanine RS in a flask. Stir well with a glass rod until the dye goes into solution. Add 96 ml distilled water and 4 ml 10% aqueous iron alum. Mix and filter; the solution keeps well.

Technique

1. Take paraffin sections to water.
2. Treat with the solochrome cyanine solution for 10–20 min.
3. Wash well in running water.
4. Differentiate in 10% aqueous iron alum solution for 10–30 min until the background and nuclei lose the stain (the myelin will be relatively unaffected).
5. Wash in running water for several minutes.
6. Counterstain with 1% aqueous neutral red solution for 5 min. (van Gieson's stain is an alternative counterstain and will intensify the myelin staining effect.)
7. Differentiate the counterstain and dehydrate in alcohol. Clear and mount as desired.

Results

Red blood cells, myelin, muscle	blue
Nuclei, Nissl substance	red
Background	colourless

DEGENERATE MYELIN

Certain methods may be used to demonstrate relatively early degeneration when the period of survival of the patient between occurrence of the lesion and death does not exceed 60–80 days. In such a period the degeneration products may be found in situ. From 75–250 days survival the products will be intracellular (microglial cells.). After 250 days there are unlikely to be demonstrable degeneration products.

The original and most well-known technique for early myelin degeneration is that of Marchi & Algeri (1885) although this is rather prone to artefacts. The so-called 'pseudo-granulations' and the Swank-Davenport (1935) variant is considered superior (Fraser, 1972). Another technique, the Busch (1898) has given good results in our hands and will also be presented.

After 75 days, intracellular degeneration material can be shown with one of the oil-soluble dyes as previously mentioned, either following Luxol fast blue staining for normal myelin, or one of the silver techniques for microglia. The Sudanophilic intracellular material is rich in cholesterol esters.

Whatever the method chosen, the occurrence of artefact, i.e. false positive black material, will be considerably reduced by minimizing trauma to the gross material. In other words, handling with care the untreated tissue.

MARCHI TYPE TECHNIQUES

SWANK-DAVENPORT TECHNIQUE (Swank & Davenport, 1935)

Notes

The rationale of the method is the tissue is treated with an oxidant, in this case potassium chlorate, in the presence of osmium tetroxide. Normal myelin is readily oxidized and will not subsequently reduce osmium tetroxide. Early degenerate myelin contains oleic acid which is not oxidized and is therefore able to reduce the osmium tetroxide to lower black oxides. Degenerate myelin is shown black against a relatively colourless background. According to Adams (1958) the rationale depends on the hydrophilic normal myelin lipids being permeable and preferentially reducing the potassium chlorate rather than the osmium tetroxide. In degenerate myelin the hydrophobic cholesterol esters are impermeable to potassium chlorate permitting reduction of the osmium tetroxide which is absorbed.

Solutions

1% potassium chlorate.

Impregnating solution

1% aqueous osmium tetroxide	20 ml
1% aqueous potassium chlorate	60 ml
Conc. formalin	12 ml
Acetic acid	1 ml

Technique

1. Take thin (3 mm) slices of formalin-fixed tissue and leave in the aqueous potassium chlorate solution for 10 min–1¼ h.
2. Transfer to the impregnating solution for 7–10 days in the dark (turn blocks frequently).
3. Wash in running water for 24 h.
4. Either cut frozen sections, or use the paraffin or celloidin process. If the paraffin process is used, deparaffinize and mount in Canada balsam (cut at 10 μm thickness).

Results

Degenerate myelin	black
Background	yellow

BUSCH TECHNIQUE (Busch, 1898)

Notes

This method is similar in results to the Swank-Davenport technique but tends to give a rather lighter background. The rationale is the same, excepting that in this case the oxidant used is sodium iodate.

Solution

Sodium iodate	3 g
Osmium tetroxide	1 g
Distilled water	300 ml

Technique

1. Take thin (3 mm) blocks of formalin-fixed tissue and wash in running water for several hours.
2. Treat with the impregnating solution for 5–7 days in the dark.
3. Wash in running water overnight.
4. Paraffin process and cut 10 μm thick sections. Deparaffinize and mount in Canada balsam.

Results

Myelin	black
Background	almost colourless

NEUROGLIA

Strictly speaking there are only four types of neuroglial cells; these are derived from the neuro-ectoderm: fibrous astrocytes, protoplasmic astro-cytes, oligodendrocytes and ependymal cells. There is a fifth cell which is commonly found in CNS tissue and, although of mesenchymal origin, is similar in terms of morphology and in the type of demonstration technique used. This cell has various names; the Gitter cell, rod cell or, as it is more popularly known, the microglial cell.

The astrocytes possess, as their name implies, many processes and have a supportive and nutri-tive function. The oligodendrocytes are small cells, with very few processes and are concerned with myelin formation. The ependymal cells line the ventricles of the brain and choroid plexuses, and vary from flattened to cuboidal, from ciliated to non-ciliated form. Ependymal cells are of little significance from a pathological or demonstration point of view and will not be considered further. The microglial cells are small cells with a typically elongated body having short processes; their func-tion is analagous to that of the reticulo-endothelial-type connective tissue cells in that they are phagocytic.

From a diagnostic point of view, the special techniques concerned with neuroglial demonstra-tion are not in great demand outside the specialist neruopathology laboratory. Malignant tumours of neurological cells (gliomas) are not uncommon in CNS tissue, but are usually readily identified in an H and E preparation. The main use for special techniques is probably that concerned with showing gliosis. Gliosis is a proliferation of the astrocytes and their processes to form the 'scar' tissue of the CNS. This type of lesion is particu-larly well shown in the demyelinating diseases.

In an H and E preparation the neuroglial cells are not shown to great advantage as the processes are not seen. It is usually the nuclei that are to be discerned and only the experienced worker can say with any certainty which nucleus belongs to which type of cell. For example, as previously described in the chapter dealing with normal histology of tissue, it will be found that the astrocytes have a medium-sized spherical vesicular-type nucleus, the oligodendrocytes have a small semipyknotic nucleus (not unlike that of a lymphocyte) whilst microglia have a small vesicular nucleus which is typically kidney-shaped in appearance.

Regarding fixation as a general rule it is safe to use formalin, although for the Cajal and Hortega techniques the formal-ammonium-bromide solution is considered to give superior results. The tissue should be fresh for best results.

In addition to the techniques to be described, one may use the PTAH method which demon-strates the processes rather than the cell bodies, also Anderson's Victoria blue technique and numerous modifications of the Hortega technique. We propose confining ourselves to those tech-niques with which we have experienced good results. For further details regarding the neuroglia and their demonstration, the reader may like to consult Cox (1973).

Astrocytic processes exhibit a weak birefrin-gence which is attributed to the presence of a myosin-like protein. Immunohistochemistry can be invoked for neuroglial identification in that there is a protein specific to astrocytes, the Glial Fibrillary Acidic Protein (GFAP), which can be demonstrated with immunoperoxidase techniques (Elias, 1982).

Table 16.3 Demonstration of glial elements

Technique	Element demonstrated
PTAH	Astrocyte processes
Holzer	Astrocytes and processes
Cajal	Astrocytes and processes
Scharanberg (mod. of Hortega)	Astrocytes and processes
Weil & Davenport	Oligodendroglia and microglia
Marshall (mod. of Weil & Davenport)	Oligodendroglia and microglia
Penfield (mod. of Hortega)	Oligodendroglia and microglia
Naoumenoki & Feigin	Microglia

ASTROCYTES

The following techniques demonstrate both types of astrocyte. The professional neurological worker will doubtless be able to distinguish between the two types. We find it exceedingly difficult. However, a useful guide to the identification of protoplasmic astrocytes is the greater branching of their processes compared to fibrous astrocytes.

CAJAL'S GOLD-SUBLIMATE TECHNIQUE
(Cajal, 1913, 1916)

Notes

This is probably the most well-known of all techniques for neuroglia and although it does not give the clarity of 'staining' of some of the Hortega techniques it is reasonably reliable. We prefer to use yellow gold chloride as opposed to brown gold chloride as on occasion we have experienced better results with the former substance.

Fixation is best carried out in FAB (formal-ammonium-bromide) or, if already fixed in formalin, the cut sections may be treated with ammonia-hydrobromic acid ('bromuration' treatment).

Solutions

FAB fixative
  Formalin   15 ml
  Ammonium bromide 2 g
  Distilled water   85 ml

Bromurator
  1% ammonia
  5% aqueous hydrobromic acid

Gold chloride-sublimate
  Add 0.5 g mercuric chloride to 60 ml distilled water and gently warm to dissolve. Add 10 ml 1% aqueous yellow gold chloride and mix. Prepare fresh before use.

Technique

1. Fix thin slices of fresh tissue in the FAB fixative for 24 h at 37° C. Cut thin (15–25 μm) frozen sections and place in 1% formalin.
   Alternatively, cut frozen sections from formalin-fixed tissue and leave in 1% ammonia overnight at room temperature. Transfer direct to hydrobromic acid for 1 h at 37° C. Wash in three short changes of distilled water.
2. Place several sections flat in the gold chloride-sublimate for 4–8 h at room temperature in the dark, removing sections at varying intervals (4 h will often suffice). Impregnation is usually complete when the sections turn a deep purple macroscopically.
3. Rinse in distilled water for several min.
4. Fix in 5% hypo for 5 min. Wash in water.
5. Dehydrate, clear and mount in Canada balsam.

Results

Astrocytes and their processes	purple to black
Neurones and their processes	varying shades of grey to light purple

HOLZER TECHNIQUE (Holzer, 1921)

Notes

Good results are given with abnormal astrocytic proliferation (gliosis) in paraffin sections, particularly when demonstrating long-term (8 weeks or more) lesions. Normal C.N.S. sections tend to be unspectacular and show neuroglial fibres poorly. The rationale is obscure although presumably the potassium bromide acts as a 'trapping agent' for the previously applied dye.

Helly's fixation gives improved results even when used as a secondary fixative.

Solutions

Alcoholic phosphomolybdic acid solution
  0.5% aqueous phosphomolybdic acid   10 ml
  95% alcohol   20 ml

Alcohol-chloroform solution
  Ethanol   2 ml
  Chloroform   8 ml

Stain

0.5% crystal violet in alcohol-chloroform solution.

10% aqueous potassium bromide.

Differentiator

Aniline oil	6 ml
Chloroform	9 ml
25% ammonia	1 drop

Technique

1. Take 10 μm paraffin sections to water.
2. Treat with the alcoholic phosphomolybdic acid solution for 3 min.
3. Drain slide and flood with the alcohol-chloroform solution.
4. Drain slide and stain with the crystal violet solution for 30 s.
5. Rinse quickly in the alcohol-chloroform solution then take through absolute alcohol and 95% alcohol to distilled water.
6. Treat with the potassium bromide solution for 1 min.
7. Wash in distilled water and blot dry.
8. Differentiate in the aniline solution until the neuroglial fibres only are blue-purple.
9. Dehydrate, clear and mount as desired.

Results

Neuroglial fibres (mainly astrocytic)	deep blue-purple
Background	light-purple

SCHARANBERG'S 'TRIPLE HORTEGA'
(Scharanberg, 1954)

Notes

This method is a variant of the Hortega technique for astrocytes and is sometimes known as the 'triple Hortega' due to the impregnation employed. The results given by this technique can be very good in terms of clarity for neuroglial demonstration and we would rate the results superior to those obtained with the better known Cajal gold-sublimate technique. Either FAB fixation or the bromuration treatment should be carried out.

Solutions

Sensitizer

2% aqueous silver nitrate	50 ml
Pyridine	20 drops

Silver-carbonate

To 10 ml of 10% aqueous silver nitrate add 30 ml of 5% aqueous sodium carbonate. Mix, add conc. ammonia, with mixing, until the formed precipitate is just dissolved. Make up to a total volume of 70 ml with distilled water.

Ammoniacal silver

Add conc. ammonia to a 2% aqueous solution of silver nitrate with frequent mixing, until the formed precipitate is just dissolved.

Technique

1. Take 15–20 μm frozen sections to distilled water.
2. Treat with the silver nitrate-pyridine solution for 15 min at 60° C.
3. Drain and transfer direct to the silver-carbonate solution to which have been added 20 drops of pyridine. Allow to stand for 15 min at 60° C.
4. Drain and transfer direct to the ammoniacal silver solution for 5 min at room temperature (this stage may sometimes be omitted without affecting the final result).
5. Reduce in 1% formalin for 2–3 min.
6. Wash in water and tone if desired in 0.2% gold chloride.
7. Wash in water and fix in 5% hypo.
8. Wash in water and mount the section on a slide. Blot dry.
9. Dehydrate, clear and mount as desired.

Results

Both types of astrocyte and their processes	black
Background	purple-red

OLIGODENDROCYTES AND MICROGLIA

As a rule both types of cell are demonstrated concomitantly by the popular techniques in this group. Oligodendrocyte fibres, in particular, are not easily visualized in normal human material. They are best seen in proliferative lesions in animal tissue such as cat. The two techniques presented are similar; Marshall's is in fact a variant of the Weil and Davenport method. Each technique has something to offer as will be discussed.

WEIL AND DAVENPORT TECHNIQUE
(Weil & Davenport, 1933)

Notes

Good demonstration of both oligodendrocytes and microglia is given by this technique with usually a reasonably clear background. It is sometimes possible to demonstrate sparse oligodendrocytic processes in normal human material.

Better results are obtained if toning is omitted. Conventional formalin fixation is satisfactory.

Solution
Ammoniacal silver

To 2–3 ml of concentrated ammonia add 10% aqueous silver nitrate with mixing until the solution becomes slightly opalescent (usually 18 ml or so).

Technique

1. Take 15 μm frozen or 5 μm paraffin sections to distilled water; give several changes.
2. Treat with the ammoniacal silver solution for 15–20 s.
3. Drain and transfer direct to 15% formalin in distilled water and gently agitate until the sections turn a coffee brown colour (usually several minutes).
4. Rinse well in distilled water. Fix in 5% hypo for 5 min and wash in water.

5. Mount on a slide, blot, dehydrate. Clear and mount as desired.

Results

| Oligodendrocytes, microglia | black (astrocytes are also impregnated but to a less well-marked degree) |
| Background | yellow-brown |

MARSHALL'S TECHNIQUE (Marshall, 1948)

Notes

Whilst oligodendrocytes are also shown by this technique, it is the microglia that are particular well demonstrated. The background is usually rather 'dirtier' than that of the preceding technique.

Formalin fixation is suitable and both paraffin and frozen sections can be utilized. Better results are said to be obtained if the frozen sections are left in 10% ammonia overnight, prior to carrying out the technique.

Solution
Ammoniacal silver

To 2 ml of concentrated ammonia add 5% aqueous silver nitrate until a slight opalescence is obtained.

Technique

1. Take 15–20 μm frozen or 5 μm paraffin section to distilled water; the paraffin sections should be loose (unmounted).
2. Treat with the ammoniacal silver solution for 4–5 s
3. Transfer sections to 3% formalin and agitate for approximately 30 s until they are a reddish brown colour.
4. Wash well in distilled water. Tone in 0.2% gold chloride, this will help clear the background.
5. Wash in water and fix in 5% hypo for 5 min. Wash in water and mount on a slide.
6. Blot, dehydrate, clear and mount as desired.

Results

Oligodendrocytes, microglia   black
and, to a lesser degree, astrocytes

PENFIELD'S MODIFICATION OF THE HORTEGA TECHNIQUE FOR OLIGODENDROGLIA AND MICROGLIA (Penfield, 1928)

Notes

This is one of the classic methods for oligodendroglia and microglia, both cells being demonstrated so that distinction is made on morphological grounds.

Formalin ammonium bromide fixation is preferred, although formalin fixation followed by hydrobromic acid treatment of the sections will give acceptable results.

The impregnating solution is a silver carbonate one, in contrast to the silver hydroxide solution normally employed in histological silver methods.

Solutions

1% aqueous ammonia.

5% aqueous hydrobromic acid ('bromurator').

5% aqueous sodium carbonate.

Impregnating solution

10% aqueous silver nitrate   5 ml
5% aqueous sodium carbonate   20 ml
Mix, and add conc. ammonia drop by drop with frequent mixing until the formed precipitate is *almost* redissolved. Make up to a final 75 ml volume with distilled water. Filter.

1% formalin.

0.2% aqueous gold chloride.

5% aqueous sodium thiosulphate (hypo).

Technique

1. Place free-floating frozen sections in the weak ammonia solution overnight at room temperature.
2. Transfer direct to hydrobromic acid solution for 1 h at 37° C.
3. Wash sections in three changes of distilled water (several minutes in each).
4. Sensitize in the sodium carbonate solution for 1 h at room temperature.
5. Drain slide and place in the impregnating solution for 3–5 min or until sections are a light brown colour.
6. Reduce in the formalin solution with gentle agitation; the sections should turn a uniform grey colour. This will usually take 1–2 min.
7. Wash in water, and tone if desired in gold chloride for 1–2 min.
8. Wash in water and fix in hypo for 1–2 min.
9. Wash in water, mount sections on slides, blot well, dehydrate, clear and mount as desired.

Results

Oligodendroglia and microglia   black
Background   light grey

NAOUMENKO AND FEIGIN TECHNIQUE FOR NEUROGLIA (Naoumenko & Feigin, 1962)

Notes

It is virtually a modification of a Hortega silver technique and demonstrates microglia rather than oligodendroglia. To avoid loss of sections from the slide during the technique they should be mounted using a section adhesive. Either formalin or formalin-ammonium-bromide fixed tissue can be used.

Solutions

3% hydrochloric acid.

5% aqueous sodium carbonate.

0.2% formalin in distilled water.

0.2% aqueous gold chloride.

5% aqueous sodium thiosulphate (hypo).

Impregnating solution

20% aqueous silver nitrate   25 ml
5% aqueous sodium carbonate   200 ml
Mix, and add concentrated ammonia drop by drop with constant mixing, until the formed

precipitate redissolves but the solution remains very faintly turbid. Filter before use.

Technique

1. Take 15–20 μm thick paraffin sections to distilled water washing well in several changes.
2. Treat sections with the hydrochloric acid solution for $1\frac{1}{2}$ h.
3. Rinse briefly (one quick dip) in each of two jars of distilled water.
4. Place sections in the sodium carbonate solution for 2 h.
5. Place sections in the impregnating solution for 1 min.
6. Drain slides and place in two changes of the dilute formalin solution agitating until the section is a light brown-grey colour (this takes approximately 10 s in each change).
7. Wash well in distilled water.
8. Tone in gold chloride for 1 min, wash and fix in hypo for 1 min.
9. Wash in water, dehydrate, clear and mount in Canada balsam.

Results

Microglia   black

PERIPHERAL NERVOUS SYSTEM

The demonstration of peripheral nerve fibres, both myelinated and non-myelinated, and nerve endings is something of a specialized art and there are more than a few techniques to be considered. A major point to be appreciated is techniques which are successful on purely CNS material, may well not be successful when dealing with PNS material. This is largely due to the fact that various other tissues, such as muscle and collagen, may also stain strongly — a complication that does not arise to any extent in CNS tissue.

PNS pathology, unless for example it is gross traumatic pathology of major nerve trunks, is a somewhat esoteric science and practised by few. As a rule the only requirement in the routine laboratory is for nerve fibre demonstration in some of the benign neurogenic tumours or in glomus tumours in order to assist in their identification.

Formalin fixation preferably lengthy, is usually satisfactory for most P.N.S. methods although osmium tetroxide-containing fixatives are of use when dealing with myelinated fibres. Prompt fixation in formalin is to be aimed at with the exception of muscle, which should be allowed to stand for at least 30 min at room temperature before fixing. This will prevent artefacts due to muscular contraction.

In addition to the techniques to be described there are others such as the solochrome cyanine (see p. 226) and the traditional Ranvier (1889). For further discussion and details on P.N.S. technique in general see Page (1970, 1971) and Bone (1972).

SCHOFIELD TECHNIQUE FOR NERVE ENDINGS IN MUSCLE AND SKIN
(Schofield, 1960)

Notes

Although peripheral nerve fibres are also demonstrated, it is the delineation of motor end plates in muscle which is the forte of this technique. Like most silver methods it can be capricious, and it is as well to take through several sections of the same material to enable a subsequent choice to be made. Prolonged formalin fixation gives better results.

Solutions

20% aqueous silver nitrate.

Ammoniacal silver
  Add concentrated ammonia with mixing to 20% aqueous silver nitrate until the formed precipitate is almost dissolved.

Technique

1. Cut thick (50–80 μm) formalin-fixed frozen sections and take to distilled water.
2. Leave overnight at 37° C in 50% alcohol to

which is added 15 drops of pyridine per 50 ml volume (defatting bath?).

3. Rinse in two changes of distilled water.
4. Place in the silver nitrate solution for 15 min at room temperature in the dark.
5. Take up the sections on a glass rod and gently blot dry.
6. Take sections through three baths of 10% formalin in tap water for 10–15 s in each (change solution for each new section).
7. Repeat, but use three baths of 2% formalin.
8. Rinse in two changes of distilled water.
9. Treat with the ammoniacal silver solution for 30–60 s. Should the eventual result be too weak the temperature of the solution may profitably be raised to 27° C.
10. Take up the sections on a glass rod and gently blot dry.
11. Treat with 1% formalin, agitate for approximately 1 min until the sections appear a dark brown colour.
12. Wash in water, fix in 5% hypo.
13. Wash in water, mount sections on a glass slide. Blot dry, dehydrate, clear and mount as desired.

Results

Motor end plates in muscle, nerve endings in skin, and nerve fibres	black
Background	yellow-brown

GROS-BIELSCHOWSKY TECHNIQUE FOR CELLOIDIN AND FROZEN SECTIONS

Notes

This popular technique can show inconsistent results and it is important to leave the sections in the initial silver nitrate solution until they are a light brown in colour. When transferring sections from the formalin bath to the ammoniacal silver, the amount of formalin carried over will influence the degree of silver blackening; consequently if the final impregnation is too weak a repeat section carrying over more of the formalin may prove successful.

Solutions

20% aqueous silver nitrate.
20% formalin in tap water.
10% ammonia.

Ammoniacal silver
  Slowly add concentrated ammonia to 15 ml of 20% aqueous silver nitrate with frequent mixing until the resultant precipitate just dissolves. Add a further 15 drops of concentrated ammonia and mix.

Technique

1. Take celloidin or frozen sections to distilled water, washing well in several changes.
2. Treat with 20% silver nitrate for 20–60 min in the dark at room temperature.
3. Transfer sections to 20% formalin. Give several changes over 5 min.
4. Transfer sections to the ammoniacal silver solution and observe the silver impregnation under a low power objective on a microscope. When the nerve fibres are black against a reasonably clear background (up to 10 mins) transfer the sections to 10% ammonia for 5 min to halt impregnation.
5. Wash in 1% acetic acid for a few minutes, tone in 0.2% gold chloride. Wash in water then fix in 5% hypo.
6. Dehydrate, clear and mount in Canada balsam.

Results

Nerve fibres etc	black
Background	often a grey colour

MODIFIED WINKLEMANN-SCHMIT TECHNIQUE FOR FROZEN SECTIONS
(Winklemann-Schmit, 1957; Frommer, 1964)

Notes

The main advantages of this technique lie in its simplicity and the fact that it may be used for

P.N.S. as well as C.N.S. tissue. Unfortunately, it does tend to produce a rather 'dirty' background. Formalin or Bouin fixation is suitable.

Solutions

20% aqueous silver nitrate.

0.2% hydroquinone in 1% aqueous sodium carbonate (prepare fresh).

Technique

1. Take 15–20 μm frozen sections to distilled water. Wash in three changes for 10 min each time.
2. Treat with the silver nitrate solution for 20 min.
3. Take sections through three dishes of distilled water for 1 s in each.
4. Treat with the hydroquinone reducer for 5 min.
5. Wash in water, tone in 0.2% gold chloride for 2 min.
6. Wash in water, treat with 5% hypo for 5 min. Wash in water, mount on a slide.
7. Dehydrate, clear and mount in Canada balsam.

Results

| Nerve fibres etc. | black |
| Background | grey |

'GLEES AND MARSLAND' TECHNIQUE
(Marsland et al, 1954)

Notes

Although this method for paraffin sections is prone to be capricious it is capable of giving excellent results. It is worthwhile taking through several duplicate sections and positive control sections of CNS material. The sections must be celloidinized using 1% celloidin to give a thick protective coat. This is done not just to keep the sections on the slide but so that when the celloidin coat is removed at the conclusion of the technique, much

of the background silver precipitation will be removed also. Without this precaution, it would be very difficult to pick out tissues such as nerve fibres against the very heavy background which occurs in a successful impregnation. Toning will often help suppress a heavy background, but we prefer not to tone if possible as without it, a clearer distinction can be made between nervous elements and collagen. Both P.N.S. and C.N.S. material can be demonstrated.

Solutions

20% aqueous silver nitrate.

Ammoniacal silver
To 15 ml of 20% aqueous silver nitrate add 10 ml of ethanol, mix. Add concentrated ammonia, with mixing, until the formed precipitate is almost dissolved (usually 40–45 drops). Finally add two drops of ammonia and mix.

Technique

1. Take paraffin sections to alcohol, cover with a thick celloidin film (use a 1% solution in ether-alcohol), and harden in water for up to 5 min.
2. Rinse in several changes of distilled water then place in the 20% silver nitrate solution at 56° C (preheated) until the sections turn a light brown colour; this may take from 20 min to 1 h but is essential to the reaction.
3. Rinse in distilled water.
4. Treat with two changes of 10% formalin in tap water for 10 s each.
5. Drain the slide and treat with the ammoniacal silver solution for 30 s.
6. Drain the slide and treat with two changes of 10% formalin in tap water for 1 min each. The slides should turn a black-brown colour. If sufficient impregnation fails to occur rinse the slide well in distilled water and go back to step 5, repeating the impregnation-reduction step.
7. Wash in water, tone in 0.2% gold chloride if desired.
8. Wash in water, fix in 5% hypo.

9. Wash in water, dehydrate in alcohol, remove the celloidin film in ether-alcohol. Rinse in xylene and mount as desired.

Results

Nerve fibres etc	black
Background (ideally)	yellow-brown if untoned

PALMGREN TECHNIQUE FOR PERIPHERAL NERVE FIBRES (Palmgren, 1948)

Notes

This is a popular technique for the demonstration of nerve fibres in paraffin sections.

As with most silver methods for nervous system constituents, practice and perseverance are necessary in order to achieve really good results. To this end, it is advisable to take through several test sections so that slight variations in times of treatment can be achieved and thus afford a measure of choice of result.

In common with the Glees and Marsland technique for nerve fibres in paraffin sections (p. 235) it is advisable to precelloidinize the section thoroughly. This will minimize background silver deposition when the celloidin film is ultimately removed.

Solutions

Acidic formalin

Formalin	25 ml
Distilled water	75 ml
1% nitric acid	0.2 ml

Silver solution
Silver nitrate	15 g
Potassium nitrate	10 g
Distilled water	100 ml
5% aqueous glycine	1 ml

Reducer
Pyrogallic acid	10 g
Distilled water	450 ml

Absolute ethanol	550 ml
1% nitric acid	2 ml
Allow to stand 24 h prior to use.	

Toning bath
Gold chloride	1 g
Distilled water	200 ml
Glacial acetic acid	0.2 ml

Intensifer
50% ethanol	100 ml
Aniline oil	2 drops

Fixing bath
5% aqueous sodium thiosulphate

Technique

1. Celloidinize paraffin sections and take to distilled water.
2. Wash sections in the acidic formalin for at least 5 min.
3. Wash in three changes of distilled water over 5 min.
4. Place in the silver solution for 15 min at room temperature or 4–5 min at 35° C.
5. Drain the slide and place in the reducer which has been heated to 40–45° C agitate gently and leave for 1 min. The sections should be yellow-brown in colour.
6. Rinse in 50% alcohol for 5–10 s then in three changes of distilled water.
7. Examine microscopically, and if there seems to be insufficient impregnation repeat the procedure from the acidic formalin stage, but reducing the time in the silver solution also the temperature of the reducer to 30° C.
8. Tone in gold chloride until the yellow brown colour has faded (several minutes).
9. Drain and place into the intensifier for 15 s.
10. Wash in water, fix in hypo for a few seconds.
11. Wash again in water, dehydrate, clear and mount as desired.

Results

Nerve fibres	black
Background	grey

LINDER'S TECHNIQUE FOR PERIPHERAL NERVES IN PARAFFIN SECTIONS (Linder. 1978)

Notes

This is a highly recommended technique for nerve fibres in P.N.S. Mineralized tissue which has been decalcified in EDTA or formic acid may also be used.

When preparing the physical developer working solution, it is important to constantly stir, as otherwise a white precipitate will form.

Solutions

Buffer stock solution

2.4.6 collidine	6.6 ml
Distilled water	450 ml

Adjust to pH 7.2–7.4 with 10% nitric acid and make up to a total volume of 500 ml with distilled water.

Buffer working solution
Stock solution	8 ml
Distilled water	92 ml

Impregnating solution
Distilled water heated to 60° C	84 ml
1% aqueous silver nitrate	4 ml
0.38% aqueous sodium cyanate	4 ml
Buffer stock solution	8 ml

Add with mixing the constituents in the order indicated.

Physical developer stock solution
Sodium sulphite ($Na_2 SO_3 7 H_2O$)	20 g
Sodium tetraborate	4.75 g
Distilled water	450 ml

Heat the solution to approximately 50° C and add 10 g leaf gelatin

Physical developer working solution
Stock solution	95 ml
2% aqueous hydroquinone	5 ml
1% aqueous silver nitrate	2 ml

Technique

1. Take paraffin sections to water, celloidinizing en route in the usual way.
2. Place in diluted buffer; soft tissues 10–20 min at 60° C; decalcified tissues overnight at 40–45° C.
3. Drain and transfer slides to the silver impregnating solution; soft tissue 10–30 min at 60° C; decalcified tissue 90 min at 40–45° C.
4. Wash in several changes of distilled water over 3 min.
5. Place sections into the physical developer working solution at approximately 25° C. Leave in the solution until optimal results are achieved by washing with distilled water at intervals and examing microscopically.
6. Wash in distilled water, dehydrate, clear and mount as desired.

Results

Nerve fibres, melanin, carcinoid tumour granules   black

SUDAN BLACK FOR NERVE ENDINGS IN MUSCLE (Cavanagh et. al, 1964)

Notes

Myelinated nerve fibres of muscle are well shown by this simple fat-staining method. Muscle fixed for 2 days in formal-saline is ideal (allow initial 30 min for muscle fibres to relax before fixing).

Solutions

Saturated Sudan black B in 70% alcohol. Filter before use.

Technique

1. Cut thick (80 μm) frozen sections and take to water.
2. Wash in 70% alcohol for 1 min.
3. Stain with the Sudan black (preheated) solution for 30 min at 37° C.
4. Rinse in three changes of 50% alcohol for $\frac{1}{2}$ min each.

5. Wash in water. Mount in an aqueous
mountant.

Results

| Myelinated axons | blue-black |
| Muscle | weak blue-black to colourless |

METHYLENE-BLUE TECHNIQUE FOR MUSCLE (Coers & Woolf, 1959)

Notes

The principle of this technique is one of supravital
staining in the presence of oxygen. The staining
effect is subsequently fixed by treatment with
ammonium molybdate. Both Page (1971) and
Bone (1972) have made recommendations regarding
the procedure of the technique and their papers
should be consulted in the event of any difficulty.

Tissues can be left in the ammonium molybdate
solution at 40° C for several days if it is not possible to continue with the technique the following
day.

Solutions

0.015% methylene blue in normal saline (supplied
in 20 ml ampoules).

8% aqueous ammonium molybdate.

Technique

1. The muscle biopsy is laid out on cork so that
the fibres are longitudinally placed, and
pinned at each end.

2. Using a fine-bore needle inject the dye
solution into and along the muscle fibres so
that they are thoroughly suffused and until
the dye solution runs out of the cut ends of
the muscle fibres. Use ample solution.
3. Moisten the tissue with normal saline and lay
flat on Kleenex tissue. Oxygenate the tissue
by placing in a stream of oxygen for 1 h at a
rate of 4 litres per min.
4. Place in the ammonium molybdate solution
overnight at 4° C.
5. Wash in several changes of distilled water
over 30 min.
6. Dissect out into fine fibres and place as flat as
possible on a glass slide. Cover with another
glass slide.
7. Squash by placing under a heavy weight (7 kg)
for 1 h.
8. Place the slides into 70% alcohol for a few
minutes, then remove the top slide and
complete the dehydration in absolute alcohol.
Clear in xylene and mount in a DPX-type
mountant.

Results

Nerve fibres (sensory and motor) and their endings in muscle and skin	blue
Nuclei	dark blue
Background muscle	weak blue

REFERENCES

Adams C W M 1958 Histochemical mechanisms of the Marchi reaction for degenerating myelin. Journal of Neurochemistry 2: 178
Ainge G, Cook J L, Gisby P R 1969 Rapid staining of myelin in paraffin sections with Luxol Fast Blue MBS. Journal of Medical Laboratory Technology 26: 231–2
Bielschowsky M 1904 Die Silberimprägnation der Neurofibrillen. Journal für Psychologie und Neurologie 3: 169
Bone Q 1972 Some notes on histological methods for peripheral nerves. Medical Laboratory Technology 29: 319–24
Busch J M 1898 Ueber eine Farbungsmethode sekundarer Degenerationen der Nervensystems mit Osmiumsaure. Neurol Zeitbl. 17: 476
Cajal S, Ramon Y 1913 Sobre un nuevo proceder de impregnacion de la neurolgia y sus resultados en los centros nerviosos del Lombre y animales. Travaux

du laboratoire de recherches biologiques de l'université de Madrid 11: 219

Cajal S, Ramon Y 1916 El preceder del oro-sublimado para la coloracion de la neuroglia. Travaux du laboratoire de recherches Biologiues de L'université De Madrid 14: 155

Cavanagh J B, Passingham R J, Vogt J A 1964 Staining of sensory and motor nerves in muscles with Sudan black B. Journal of Pathology and Bacteriology 88: 89

Chalk, B T C 1970 Personal communication.

Coers C, Woolf A L 1959 The innervation of the muscle. Blackwell, Oxford

Cox G 1973 Neuroglia and microglia. In: Cook H C (ed) Selected topics. Bailliere Tindall, London

Cox W 1891 Impregnation des centralen Nervensystem mit Quecksilbersalzen. Archiv für mikroskopische Anatomie 37: 16–21

Elias J M 1982 Principles and techniques in diagnostic histopathology. Noyes Publication, New Jersey.

Fraser F J 1972 Degenerating myelin: comparative histochemical studies using classical myelin stains and an improved Marchi technique minimising artefacts. Stain Technology 47: 147–54

Golgi, C 1878 Rc. 1st Lomb. Sci. Lett. 2nd series 12: 5

Gothard E 1898 Quelques modifications au procede de Nissl, pour la coloration elective des cellules nerveuses. C. r. Seanc. Soc. 69: 530

Holzer W 1921 Uber eine neue Methode der Gliafases Farbung. Zentralblatt für die gesamte Neurologie und psychiatrie 69: 354–460

Kawamura S, Niimi K 1972 Counterstaining of Nanta-Gyaz impregnated sections with Cresyl Violet. Stain Technology, 47: 1–6

Kluver H, Barrera A 1953 A method for the combined staining of cells and fibres of the nervous system. Journal of Neuropathology and Experimental Neurology 12: 400

Kultschitzky N 1889 Uber eine neue Methode der Hamatoxylin-Farbung. Anat. Anz. 4: 223

Linder J E 1978 A simple and reliable method for the silver impregnation of soft or mineralized tissues. Journal of Anatomy 127: 543

Loyez M 1910 Coloration des fibres nerveuse par la methode a l'hematoxyline au fer apres inclusion a las celloidine. Compte rendu des seances de la Societe de Biologie 69: 511

Marchi V, Algeri G 1885 Sulle degenerazioni discendenti consecutive a lesioni della corteccia cerebrale. Riv. sper. Freniat. Med. leg. Alien. ment. 11: 492

Marshall A H E 1948 A method for the demonstration of reticulo-endothelial cells in paraffin sections. Journal of Pathology and Bacteriology LX: 3

Marsland T A, Glees P, Erickson L B 1954 Modification of the Glees silver impregnation for paraffin sections. Journal of Neuropathology and Experimental Neurology 13: 587

Chang M C 1935 Formal-thionin method for fixation and staining of nerve cells and fiber tracts. Anatomical Records 65: 437–41. July, 25, 36

Nauomenko J, Feigin U 1962 A modification for paraffin sections of silver carbonate impregnation for microglia. Acta Neuropathologica 2: 402–6

Page K M 1965 A stain for myelin using solochrome cyanin. Journal of Medical Laboratory Technology 22: 224

Page K M 1970 Histological methods for peripheral nerves. Part 1. Journal of Medical Laboratory Technology 27: 1

Page K M 1971 Histological methods for peripheral nerves. Part II, Medical Laboratory Technology 28: 58

Pal J 1886 Ein Beitrag zur Nerventarbe Technik. Medizinische Jahrbuechat 1: 619

Palmgren A 1948 A rapid method for selective silver staining of nerve fibres and nerve endings in mounted paraffin sections. Acta Zoologica 29: 377–92

Penfield W 1928 A method of staining oligodendroglia and microglia. American Journal of Pathology 4: 153

Ranvier L A 1890 Traite technique d'histologie, 2nd edn. F. Savy, Paris

Scharanberg, K 1954 Blastomatous oligodendroglia as satellites of nerve cells: study with silver carbonate. American Journal of Pathology 30: 957–69

Schofield G C 1960 Experimental studies on the innervation of the mucous membranes of the gut. Brain 83: 490–514

Swank, R L, Davenport H A 1935 Chlorate-Osmic formalin method for degenerating myelin. Stain Technology 10: 87–90

von Braunmuhl A 1957 Hdbch. D. Spez. Pathol. Bd. XIII 1 A 337. Springer, Heidelberg

Weigert C 1885 Eine Verbesserung der Haematoxylin-Blutlaungensalzmethode für das Centralnervensystem. Fortschr. Med. 3: 236

Weil A, Davenport H E 1933 Staining of oligodendroglia and microglia in celloidin sections. Archives of Neurology and Psychiatry Chicago 30: 175

Winklemann R V, Schmit R W 1957 A simple method for nerve axoplasm. Proceedings of the Staff Meetings, Mayo Clinic 32: 217

17

A miscellany

BONE

Bone can be termed a special type of connective tissue in which the extracellular components are calcified giving rigidity and elasticity. It is a store of inorganic ions, notably calcium, and participates in the maintenance of body calcium levels. Bone is in a state of growth and resorption at all times. It is composed of specialized cells and an organic extracellular matrix containing glycoprotein ground substance and collagen fibres. Calcium hydroxyapatite crystals form the mineral component of bone matrix. The cells found in bone are of three types:

Osteoblasts are immature forms of bone cells and are responsible for the secretion of the organic component of the matrix of bone osteoid. This substance then undergoes mineralization. Osteoblasts become trapped within the bone and are then termed *osteocytes*. *Osteoclasts* are multinucleate cells actively involved in the resorptive process. The fibrous component of bone is mainly collagen, which reacts in a similar manner to collagen found in other sites. Bone is of two main types. *Woven bone* is immature and shows the woven organization of the fibrous elements. From this type, lamellar bone is formed which is the basis of all bones. It is seen as a solid mass as compact bone or as a spongy form described as cancellous bone. *Compact bone* forms the shafts of long bones and the exterior surfaces of flat bones. It is solid, hard and immensely strong. Spongy, trabecular or cancellous bone is found in the narrow cavities of the long bones, the centre of flat bones and the vertebrae.

PICRO-THIONIN TECHNIQUE (Schmorl, 1934)

Notes

The rationale of the technique is picric acid treatment, following staining with alkaline thionin, causes a precipitate of the dye to form in the canaliculi and lacunae of bone. The method works well with frozen and celloidin sections but gives indifferent results with paraffin. Fixation with mercuric chloride-containing solutions is said to be contraindicated, formalin being the fixative of choice.

Solutions

0.125% aqueous thionin. Add one drop of concentrated ammonia per 100 ml volume.

Saturated (1.22%) aqueous picric acid.

Technique

1. Take sections to distilled water.
2. Filter on the thionin solution for 5–15 min.
3. Rinse in distilled water.
4. Treat with the picric acid solution for $\frac{1}{2}$–1 min with agitation.
5. Differentiate out the excess blue dye in 70% alcohol for 5–10 min or longer if required.
6. Dehydrate, clear and mount in a DPX-type mountant.

Results

Canaliculi, lacunae	dark brown to black
Background bone	yellow to yellow-brown
Nuclei	red-brown

BONE MARROW

The intertrabecular spaces of bones are filled with bone marrow. The marrow contains the primitive stem cells from which the cellular elements of blood are derived. In the young the bone marrow participates in the process of blood cell formation. Active bone marrow is filled with dividing stem cells and the precursors of mature blood cells. The many maturing erythrocytes produce the red colour of active marrow. Less active marrow consists of a reticulin framework which supports the developing blood cells. There are instances in the routine laboratory when it is necessary to demonstrate this framework or the cells present.

DEMONSTRATION OF BONE MARROW CELLS

A bone marrow smear is often far more use than sections in which the cells have suffered from processing. The routine laboratory should be able to cope with smears, aspirates and biopsies. Thin sections are essential. For this reason the trephine biopsies we receive are embedded in resin.

WOLBACH'S GIEMSA STAIN (Lillie, 1965)

Notes

This Romanowsky method works well for bone marrow smears and sections.

Solution

Giemsa stain	1 ml
Methyl alcohol	1.25 ml
0.5% sodium carbonate	0.1 ml
Distilled water	40 ml

Technique

1. Take sections to distilled water.
2. Stain in Giemsa solution for 1 h changing the stain twice.
3. Transfer to third change of stain and leave overnight.
4. Differentiate in 95% alcohol containing a few drops of 10% colophonium in alcohol.
5. Dehydrate in absolute alcohol, clear in xylene and mount in cedarwood oil.

Results

Nuclei	dark blue
Red blood cells	yellow to pink
Cytoplasm of haemopoietic cells	light blue

ACID GIEMSA (Bayley, 1949 from Drury & Wallington, 1980)

Notes

The counterstain is controlled by the proportion of acetic acid, more acid producing stronger eosin staining. The speed of final dehydration controls the blue stain, which is extracted by absolute alcohol. The method works through a coating of celloidin. Any Romanowsky-type stain may be substituted for Giemsa, but the latter is less liable to precipitation.

Solution

Giemsa stain	30 ml
1% acetic acid	20 ml

Technique

1. Stain in Ehrlich's haematoxylin differentiate more than usual.
2. Blue in tap water.
3. Rinse in distilled water.
4. Stain in Giemsa solution (10 min).
5. Rinse in distilled water and blot dry.
6. Differentiate in absolute alcohol.
7. Clear in xylene and mount.

Results

Bone trabeculae	pink
Cartilage	purple
Red blood cells	pink
Nuclei	blue
Eosinophil and basophil granules of myelocytes	clearly seen

LEISHMAN'S STAIN

Technique

1. Take thin paraffin sections to water and leave in buffered water at pH 6.8 for 30 min.
2. Immerse in Leishman's stain diluted with two parts of buffered water at pH 6.8 to one part of stain. Leave for 10–15 min.
3. Wash and differentiate in 50% methyl alcohol in buffered water at pH 5.0.
4. When the nuclei are purple and the granules of polymorphs are clearly seen, the section is blotted until completely dry, cleared in xylene and mounted in green Euparal.

Results

Nuclei	purple
Leucocyte granules	red (eosinophils) to dark purple (basophils)
Red blood cells	pink

METABOLIC BONE DISEASE

Sections for the demonstration of bone mineral and its relationship with the non-mineralized bone are used in the diagnosis of osteomalacia, osteoporosis and Paget's disease. Except for the Tripp and MacKay method, the sections used are from undecalcified pieces of bone, preferably cancellous bone. The calcium salts are demonstrated to show the bulk of the trabeculae and the non-mineralized seams are shown by a collagen stain.

The production of the sections is carried out either by embedding in resin or by double-embedding in paraffin wax and using the 'sellotape technique'. The former technique is to be preferred as the harder embedding medium allows for far better sections to be cut enabling the mineral density to be studied and showing the excellent staining that can be obtained from the cells.

HAEMATOXYLIN AND EOSIN STAINING OF METHACRYLATE SECTIONS (Drury & Wallington, 1980)

Technique

1. Transfer sections from 70% alcohol to distilled water.
2. Stain in Cole's haematoxylin for 60 min.
3. Wash well in tap water.
4. Stain in 1% aqueous eosin for 30 min.
5. Differentiate in tap water until osteoid is pink and calcified bone a deep purplish brown.
6. Dehydrate sections in 70% followed by 90% and then absolute alcohol.
7. Transfer sections to Euparal essence.
8. Place section on a slide, apply a strip of smooth hard paper over the section, and remove wrinkles by rolling a glass rod over the paper. Peel off the paper.
9. Mount in Euparal. A small weight applied to the cover glass helps flattening of the section.

Results

Osteoid tissue	pink
Calcified bone	purplish brown
Nuclei	blue
Erythrocytes	generally remain unstained

MODIFIED VON KOSSA TECHNIQUE (Tripp & MacKay, 1972)

Notes

This method makes use of the principle in the von Kossa reaction that formed silver phosphate does not require decalcification in order that sectioning be carried out.

By subjecting the tissue block to the von Kossa technique and then decalcifying to remove any unchanged calcium salts, sections of decalcified bone can be cut in the normal way. Van Gieson staining can subsequently be carried out.

In order that nonspecific silver nitrate reduction be avoided, it is important to use either alcoholic or conventional formalin fixation followed by thorough washing in distilled water.

When carrying out the decalcification, avoid

using nitric or hydrochloric acids as these tend to dissolve reduced silver salts. For obvious reasons it is not practicable to reduce the formed silver phosphate in the tissue block using light, and recourse is made to a reducing solution. Even so it will be found that the centres of the thicker trabeculae are not fully blackened, but this is not a serious drawback as any osteoid seams are well shown against the blackened perimeters of the trabeculae.

Philpotts (1980) suggested using 3% silver nitrate in 80% alcohol at 37° C for 24 h. It is necessary to dissolve the silver nitrate in water before adding the alcohol. The reducing solution is also used at 37° C but only for 24 h. This modification has worked well in our hands.

Solutions

2% aqueous silver nitrate.

Reducer
Sodium hypophosphite	5 g
0.1 M sodium hydroxide	0.2 ml
Distilled water	100 ml

Van Gieson's solution, see page 41.

Technique

1. Take thin (2mm) blocks of bone fixed in alcohol or conventional formalin solutions.
2. If formalin-fixed, wash well in several changes of distilled water. This is best carried out by washing in a large volume of distilled water using an automatic tissue processor (with agitation), during the day, changing the distilled water two or three times.
3. Place in the silver nitrate solution in the dark for 2–4 days at room temperature or the modified solution for 24 h at 37°C (according to which is more convenient).
4. Wash in three changes of distilled water for 20 s each.
5. Wash in running tap water for 4 h.
6. Treat with the reducing solution for 2 days.
7. Wash in running water for 1 h.
8. Treat with 5% hypo for 24 h.
9. Wash in water for 1 h and decalcify in 5% or 10% formic acid.
10. Wash in water and then paraffin process in the normal manner.
11. Cut (8–10 μm) sections and mount on slides using a plasma adhesive. Heat-dry for a short period.
12. Take the sections to distilled water and stain with van Gieson's solution for 5 min.
13. Drain the slide, dehydrate, clear and mount as desired.

Results

Mineralized bone	black
Canaliculi and lacunae in the central areas of the non-blackened bone trabeculae	black
Osteoid seams	red
Bone marrow	yellow

GOLDNER'S METHOD

Notes

The technique has proved valuable when applied to resin sections mainly because of the excellent staining of cells. Osteoblast and osteoclast activity are easily assessed, an important factor in the diagnosis of such conditions as Paget's disease, renal osteodystrophy and hyperparathyroidism.

Solutions

Weigert's haematoxylin, see page 40.

Ponceau-Fuchsin solution
Ponceau de Xylidine	0.75 g
Acid fuchsin	0.25 g
Acetic acid	1 ml

Mix, and add to 100 ml distilled water.

Azophloxin solution
    Azophloxin   0.5 g
    Acetic acid   0.6 ml
    Mix and add to 100 ml distilled water.

Final staining solution
    Ponceau-Fuchsin solution   5–10 ml
    Azophloxin solution   2 ml
    Acetic acid (0.2 per cent)   88 ml

Light green solution
    Light green   1 g
    Acetic acid   1 ml
    Mix and add to 500 ml distilled water.

Phosphomolybdic acid/orange G solution
    Phosphomolybolic acid   3 g
    Orange G   2 g
    Dissolve in 500 ml of distilled water, and add a
    crystal of thymol.

Technique

1. Stand sections in a solution of 90 ml 80%
   ethanol and 10 ml of 25% ammonia for 1 h.
2. Rinse in water for 15 min.
3. Stain in Weigert's haematoxylin for 1 h.
4. Rinse in water for 10 min.
5. Rinse in distilled water for 5 min.
6. Stain in final Ponceau fuchsin/Azophloxin
   solution for 5 min.
7. Rinse in 1% acetic acid for 15 s.
8. Stain in phosphomolybdic acid/orange G
   solution for 20 min.
9. Rinse in 1% acetic acid for 15 s.
10. Stain with light green for 5 min.
11. Rinse in three changes of 1% acetic acid.
12. Rinse in distilled water, blot dry and mount.

Results

Mineralized bone	green
Osteoid	orange-red
Nuclei	blue-grey
Cartilage	purple

VON KOSSA METHOD FOR CALCIUM SALTS

Notes

This is the oldest and most widely used method for calcium. Silver is substituted for calcium in calcium salts. This silver salt is then reduced to black metallic silver by the use of light or a photographic developer. As with any method for calcium, acid fixatives should be avoided and buffered neutral formalin is recommended.

Solutions

2% silver nitrate.
2.5% sodium thiosulphate.
van Gieson's stain or 1% neutral red.

Technique

1. Take sections to distilled water, two or three
   changes.
2. Transfer sections to a clear glass container
   and expose to bright sunlight or a high
   intensity light source for 20–60 min. If
   exposed to sunlight the time may be less;
   check microscopically.
3. Wash in several changes of distilled water.
4. Treat with 2.5% sodium thiosulphate to
   remove excess silver (5 min).
5. Wash well in tap water.
6. Counterstain as required either in van Gieson
   or 1% neutral red.
7. Dehydrate, clear and mount in DPX.

Results

Calcium deposits	black

SOLOCHROME CYANINE

Notes

Solocrome cyanine is used as a differential stain to demonstrate osteoid and its relationship with mineralized bone. It can also be used to show the calcification front and repeating bands within the wider osteoid borders. The solution of Hyman & Poulding (1961) gives the best staining in our hands.

Solutions

| Solochrome cyanine | 1 g |
| Conc. sulphuric acid | 2.5 ml |

Mix well to incorporate all the dye in the sludge. Add 500 ml of 0.5% aqueous iron alum (ferric ammonium sulphate). Mix and filter.

Technique

1. Transfer sections to distilled water.
2. Stain in Solochrome cyanine solution for 60 min.
3. Differentiate in warm alkaline tap water until the mineralized areas appear blue and other areas light red. Control microscopically as overdifferentiation causes all parts to become blue.
4. Dehydrate, clear and mount.

Results

Mineralized bone	light blue
Calcification front	dark blue
Osteoid	light red-orange
Wide osteoid	light red-orange with pale blue and orange bands
Nuclei	blue

CORPORA AMYLACEA

These are bodies which may be found in three main human tissue sites: prostate, lungs and brain, the significance of which is poorly understood. The name is derived from 'starch-like bodies' due principally to their reaction with iodine. In veterinary pathology there may be found similar bodies in bovine mammary glands.

PROSTATIC CORPORA AMYLACEA

These are of varying sizes, laminated, round structures found mainly in the gland lumina, and are almost certainly concretions of the gland secretion.

Their staining reactions are:

H and E	bright red
Iodine	brown
PAS	magenta
Congo red	red (sometimes exhibiting dichroic birefringence)

PULMONARY CORPORA AMYLACEA

These are mainly found in the alveoli of the lungs and are of variable size and round in shape. They are laminated bodies, but the laminations may not be as marked as those of prostatic corpora amylacea. Unlike corpora amylacea of prostate and CNS, those of lung are only occasionally seen. Their staining reactions are:

H and E	red
Iodine	brown
PAS	variably positive
Congo red	variably positive (but when positive may exhibit dichroic birefringence).

CENTRAL NERVOUS SYSTEM CORPORA AMYLACEA

These occur in brain and spinal cord (particularly the latter) and tend to be smaller in size than the corpora amylacea of prostate and lungs. They are round in shape and non-laminated. A number of workers have studied these structures. Chemically they are predominantly composed of an amylopectin-like polysaccharide (Sakai et al, 1969) and structurally they seem to be composed of fibrillary and granular material forming intra-astrocytic aggregates (Ramsey, 1965). Their staining reactions are:

H and E	blue
Iodine	brown
PAS	positive
Azure A	metachromatic

CRYSTAL IDENTIFICATION

Although in theory it is possible for a wide range of crystals to occur in tissue and fluids, in practice

Table 17.1 Crystal identification.

Technique	Calcium phosphate/calcium carbonate	Calcium oxalate	Calcium pyrophosphate	Urate
H and E	Blue or colourless	Colourless	Blue	Blue
Von Kossa	Positive	Negative	Variably positive	Variably positive
Modified von Kossa	Positive	Positive	Positive	Variably positive
Hexamine silver	Negative	Negative	Variably positive	Positive
Lithium carbonate extraction	Unchanged	Unchanged	Unchanged	Extracted

it is limited both as regards likely occurrence and diagnostic necessity. We have chosen the following four crystals as being representative of the more important in terms of histological demonstration and diagnosis. Much of the following histochemistry is taken from the work of Worsfold. (1982 unpub. data). (See also Table 17.1.)

CALCIUM PHOSPHATE/CARBONATE

Included in this group are mineral salts of bone (a complex group of mainly calcium salts collectively termed hydroxyapatite) and calcium deposits in tissue which are often assocated with necrosis, e.g. caseation necrosis of tuberculosis, atheroma of blood vessels and infarction. Calcium carbonate is often present in both normal and abnormal mineral deposits, but it is the phosphate salt which is of the greater significance as regards histochemical reactivity.

Nonacid fixatives are preferred, e.g. neutral buffered formalin or alcohol. H and E staining is variable: The crystals may appear blue or colourless. Any haematoxylin staining is attributed to trace elements of iron in the calcium salts. Other staining methods for calcium include alizarin red, purpurin, nuclear fast red, naphthochrome green B, alcian blue and the fluorescent morin technique. Unquestionably the method of choice is the von Kossa reaction (see p. 244). There are two points worth noting with respect to this latter technique. Firstly the von Kossa method involves a substitution reaction whereby silver nitrate treatment forms silver phosphate and carbonate with the calcium salts which are subsequently blackened by light reduction. Therefore it is the nonmetallic radicle which is demonstrated rather than the metal. The second point concerns the use of post silver hypo treatment. In this technique it is better omitted as a semi-bleaching effect of the reduced silver salts can occur.

Calcium phosphate and carbonate salts are monorefringent, and in tissue are extremely variable in appearance.

CALCIUM OXALATE

These are relatively uncommon constituents of tissue and may be found in tissues such as kidney, heart and thyroid in primary oxalosis, which is a rare condition caused by an enzyme deficiency in the normal metabolism of glycine residues. Another equally uncommon cause of calcium oxalate formation in tissue, is in ethylene glycol (antifreeze) intake. The crystals form in renal tubules due to the metabolism of ethylene glycol to oxalic acid. Poisoning cases involving oxalic acid will also produce calcium oxalate deposits in tissue such as kidney. Nonacidic fixatives are preferred, e.g. neutral buffered formalin or alcohol.

The crystals are unstained by H and E and using polarizing microscopy appear as birefringent octahedral clusters. The usual methods for calcium salts are negative including the von Kossa reaction. The following modified method is recommended for positive demonstration of calcium oxalate.

MODIFIED VON KOSSA TECHNIQUE
(Pizzolato, 1964)

Notes

Calcium oxalate crystals are not normally von Kossa positive but using this modified version positive results may be obtained. Oxidation by hydrogen peroxide converts calcium oxalate to carbonate which is blackened in the usual way by light reduction of silver nitrate.

Paraffin sections are easily dislodged from the slide during the method. A section adhesive is advisable.

Solution

Mix equal volumes of 30% (100 vols) hydrogen peroxide and 5% aqueous silver nitrate.

Technique

1. Take sections to distilled water.
2. Drain and add the hydrogen peroxide-silver nitrate solution for 15–30 min. If excess bubbling develops replace with fresh reagent.
3. Wash in distilled water and counterstain as desired, e.g. weak eosin or van Gieson.
4. Dehydrate, clear and mount as desired.

Results

Calcium oxalate (and other   black
calcium salts)

CALCIUM PYROPHOSPHATE

These crystals occur in joints in the condition known as pseudogout, but whereas gout is primarily an affliction of males, both males and females are affected in pyrophosphate crystal synovitis. Synovial tissue fixed in formalin or alcohol can be examined histologically, also aspirated fluid from joints. The latter is examined as wet preparations or by concentrating the crystals and then embedding in fibrin clots for histological processing and examination.

From a diagnostic point of view it is important to distinguish pyrophosphate crystals from urates of gout. In our experience the two most reliable means of so doing are (1) to examine the preparations by polarising microscopy with a quartz first order red compensator (pyrophosphates exhibit a *positive* form birefringence whilst urates have a *negative* form birefringence); (2) use of lithium carbonate extraction of urates (see section dealing with urates).

In an H and E preparation calcium pyrophos-

phate crystals appear as blue-stained rectangular plates or rhombohendrons. They are variably von Kossa (unmodified) and hexamine silver positive.

URATES

Crystals of uric acid may occur either as a by-product of excessive purine (DNA) breakdown in renal tubules such as may rarely occur in leukaemia chemotherapy or, more commonly, in gout. Unlike pyrophosphate synovitis, gout tends to affect the smaller joints in the extremities. It is important to distinguish between the two conditions by identifying the component crystals of the affected tissue, although it must be realized that urates and calcium pyrophosphates can uncommonly occur together in crystal synovitis.

Polarizing microscopy using a quartz first order red compensator is a useful procedure showing the urate crystals to possess a negative form birefringence. Another useful technique is to make use of the fact that only urates are extracted by lithium carbonate treatment prior to hexamine silver demonstration.

In an H and E preparation, uric acid crystals stain blue and are typically needle-shaped. They are variably von Kossa (unmodified) positive.

LITHIUM CARBONATE EXTRACTION-HEXAMINE SILVER TECHNIQUE FOR URATES (Gomori, 1946)

Notes

The rationale of the technique is of an argentaffin-type reduction by urates of the hexamine-silver.

The solution should be preheated to the desired temperature and positive control sections taken through to establish its efficacy. For reasons that are not clear, sections containing urates after long storage may show a loss of hexamine-silver reactivity.

Solutions

Hexamine-silver (see p. 212).

Saturated aqueous lithium carbonate.

5% aqueous sodium thiosulphate.

0.2% light green in 0.2% acetic acid.

Technique

1. Take two positive control and two test sections to water.
2. Treat one section of each pair with the lithium carbonate solution for 30 min.
3. Wash all sections well with distilled water, drain, and treat with hexamine silver for 1 h at 45° C.
4. Wash well in distilled water. Treat with hypo for 2–3 min.
5. Wash in water and counterstain in light green solution for 1 min.
6. Wash in water, dehydrate, clear and mount as desired.

Results

Extracted sections	urates only are extracted
Unextracted sections	urates and possibly pyrophosphates are blackened
Background	green

FIBRIN AND FIBRINOID

Fibrin is an insoluble fibrillar protein formed from plasma fibrinogen; it contains basic amino acids which give it its strong acidophilia. In its early stages of development it can be seen as fine threads, later becoming a homogeneous mass. Fibrin is seen in tissues where damage has occurred due to an acute inflammatory reaction, which produces a transfer of fluid and plasma proteins from damaged blood vessels. The plasma fibrinogen polymerizes forming insoluble fibrin. This will be found in areas of tissue damage, such as thrombi, and is also laid down in acute inflammations particularly those of serous membranes, e.g. in peritonitis, empyema and pericarditis. It is frequently found in synovitis.

Fibrinoid in appearance is a similar amorphous eosinophilic material. Its staining reactions are those as for fibrin with only occasional variations. It appears in tissues in different locations from fibrin, in that it is often seen within blood vessel walls where the vessel has undergone necrosis, in renal glomeruli and connective tissues. Fibrinoid deposits are seen in rheumatoid arthritis, polyarteritis nodosa, lupus erythematosus and other related diseases. There is doubt about the true nature of fibrinoid, but the consensus of opinion appears to be that it is a mixture of fibrin with additional proteins from blood plasma; alternatively fibrinoid may be fibrin that has undergone an ageing process (Lendrum et al, 1962).

DEMONSTRATION OF FIBRIN

It can be seen bright red in an H and E preparation; the results with a PAS usually show a positive reaction. Fibrin is orthochromatic, monorefringent and weakly autofluorescent. Due to its tryptophan content it is DMAB-nitrite positive. In practice many staining methods will demonstrate it and some are shown in the Table 17.2. Fibrin itself does not always react to dye in the same way: long-standing deposits tend to stain in a similar manner to collagen. The method of choice is the MSB of Lendrum et al (1962) which is given below. Formalin fixation is usually adequate although better results are obtained with trichrome-type methods if Helly's solution is used.

Table 17.2 Staining reactions of fibrin

Stain	Fibrin
MSB (and other trichromes)	Red
PAS	Magenta
PTAH	Blue
Gram-Weigert	Blue-black
Phloxine tartrazine.	Red
DMAB-nitrite	Blue
Schmorl	Blue
Milling yellow	Red
Acid picro-mallory	Red
Eosin	Red
van Gieson	Yellow

Methods are now available to demonstrate fibrin by immunofluorescence and these are the only truly specific ones.

MARTIUS YELLOW-BRILLIANT CRYSTAL SCARLET-SOLUBLE BLUE (MSB) (Lendrum et al, 1962)

Notes

This technique employs a small molecule yellow dye, which when used with phosphotungstic acid in alcoholic solution will selectively stain red cells. It is possible that early deposits of fibrin will also take up the dye, the phosphotungstic acid blocking the staining of other tissue structures. A medium sized molecule red dye is then used to stain muscle and mature fibrin. The staining of collagen is still prevented by the phosphotungstic acid used earlier. Additional treatment with aqueous phosphotungstic acid removes any red staining from collagen fibres. A large molecule blue dye is then applied and this will stain collagen and old fibrin.

Lendrum et al (1962) strongly recommend the use of mercuric chloride fixation: in its absence post-fixation in mercury is advisable. Thin sections are necessary to achieve satisfactory results with the method which is selective.

Solutions

0.5% martius yellow (synonym: naphthol yellow) in 2% phosphotungstic acid in 95% alcohol.

1% brilliant crystal scarlet 6 R (synonym: crystal ponceau) in 2.6% acetic acid.

1% aqueous phosphotungstic acid.

0.5% soluble blue (synonym: aniline blue ws) in 1% acetic acid.

Technique

1. Take sections to water and stain with a suitable iron haematoxylin solution. Rinse in 95% alcohol.
2. Stain with the martius yellow solution for 2 min. Wash briefly in water.
3. Stain with the brilliant crystal scarlet solution for 10 min. Wash in water.
4. Treat with the phosphotungstic acid solution for 5–10 min. Wash.
5. Stain with the soluble blue solution for 10 min. Wash and blot dry.
6. Dehydrate, clear and mount and desired.

Results

Fibrin	red
Muscle	paler red
Nuclei	blue-black
Collagen	blue
Red blood cells	yellow

MILLING YELLOW TECHNIQUE (Slidders, 1961)

Notes

This is similar in principle to the previous technique. Acid fuschin staining is followed by phosphotungstic acid, but differs in that there is a progressive replacement and counterstaining with the dye milling yellow.

Fibrin is clearly shown against the yellow background; it is also possible to displace much of the red dye in the muscle.

Solutions

1% acid fuchsin in 2.5% acetic acid.

1% aqueous phosphotungstic acid.

2.5% milling yellow 3G in Cellosolve.

Technique

1. Take sections to water and stain the nuclei with a suitable iron haematoxylin solution.
2. Treat with the acid fuchsin solution for 3–5 min.
3. Rinse in water. Treat with the phosphotungstic acid solution for 5 min.
4. Rinse well in Cellosolve.
5. Differentiate and counterstain in the milling yellow solution until only the fibrin is deeply stained red. This usually takes from $\frac{1}{2}$–1 h.
6. Rinse in Cellosolve. Clear in xylene and mount as desired.

Results

Fibrin	bright red
Muscle	very weak red
Nuclei	blue-black
Background (e.g. collagen, red blood cells)	yellow

ACID PICRO-MALLORY TECHNIQUE (Lendrum, 1949)

Notes

This is very similar in principle to the trichrome techniques; it stains fibrin strongly and muscle weakly.

Solutions

0.2% orange G in saturated alcoholic picric acid.

1% acid fuchsin in 3% trichloracetic acid

1% phosphomolybdic acid.

2% aniline blue ws in 2% acetic acid.

Technique

1. Take sections to water and stain the nuclei with a suitable iron haematoxylin solution. Differentiate so that the background in reasonably clear.
2. Rinse in 95% alcohol and stain with the picro-orange solution for 2 min.
3. Wash in water for 5–10 s until only the red blood cells are yellow.
4. Treat with the acid fuchsin solution for 5 min.
5. Wash briefly, then treat with equal parts of the picro-orange solution and 80% alcohol for a few seconds.
6. Differentiate in the phosphomolybdic acid solution for 5–10 min.
7. Wash in water. Stain with the aniline blue solution for 5–10 min.
8. Wash, dehydrate, clear and mount as desired.

Results

Fibrin	bright red
Muscle	paler red
Nuclei	blue-black
Collagen	blue
Red blood cells	yellow-orange

TRYPSIN DIGESTION (Glynn & Loewi, 1952)

Notes

Using trypsin at an alkaline pH, the authors claim that although fibrin is digested, fibrinoid and collagen are not. In our limited experience with the technique, reasonably good results are easily obtained although it may be necessary to extend times of treatment. Formalin-fixed tissue seems perfectly satisfactory.

The usual commercial source of the enzyme is from beef pancreas. In human tissue the sperma- tazoon acrosome is rich in trypsin, where it is largely responsible (with hyaluronidase) for the breakdown of the zona pellucida of the ovum during fertilization.

Solution

Dissolve 0.1% trypsin in pH 8.0 phosphate buffer.

Technique

1. Take two sections of known positive control material and two sections of the test material to water.
2. Rinse well with distilled water.
3. Treat one test and one positive control section with the preheated trypsin solution for 3 h at 37° C. The remaining duplicate sections are treated with pH 8.0 buffer only, for the same time and temperature.
4. Wash all section well in water for 5–10 min.
5. Carry out a suitable technique for fibrin (the MSB technique gives good results).
6. Dehydrate, clear and mount as desired.

Results

If the MSB technique was used subsequent to digestion then:

Fibrin in undigested sections	red
Fibrin in digested section	not stained

GOLGI APPARATUS

This intracytoplasmic entity which was originally described by Golgi in 1898 using tissue from the owl, is of little significance at light microscopy level in diagnostic pathology. Should it be desired to demonstrate the Golgi apparatus, e.g. for normal demonstration purposes, there is a limited range of techniques which may be used. The structure is rich in various lipids and use can be made of this to demonstrate the apparatus with techniques such as osmium tetroxide or Sudan black. There are also a number of silver techniques which can be used with varying degrees of success; two of these are described below. In the standard H and E stain areas of prominent Golgi apparatus appear unstained; the so-called 'negative' staining effect.

Formalin seems to preserve the Golgi apparatus adequately, but special fixation is necessary for the best demonstration. Equally important, fixation needs to be prompt if reasonable results are to be obtained. Kidney or adrenal are suitable tissues for trying out the various techniques.

McDONALD'S MODIFICATION OF LASCANO'S TECHNIQUE FOR THE GOLGI APPARATUS (Lascano, 1959; McDonald, 1964)

Notes

Excellent demonstration of the Golgi apparatus is afforded by this technique. The one minor disadvantage is that a full day is required and fresh tissue needs to be available early in the day.

Solutions

Fixative

Aminoacetic acid (glycine)	1.7 g
Distilled water	85 ml
Formalin	15 ml
Conc. nitric acid	0.5 ml

Reducer

1.5% hydroquinone in 1.5% formalin.

Technique

1. Take thin (1.5–2 mm) pieces of fresh tissue and place in a 100 ml volume of the fixative.
2. Wash in two changes of distilled water for a few seconds.
3. Treat with 1.5% aqueous silver nitrate for 4 h (agitate periodically).
4. Wash in distilled water for a few seconds.
5. Reduce for $1\frac{1}{2}$–2 h with frequent agitation.
6. Wash in several changes of distilled water for 5–10 min.
7. Paraffin process, cut thin sections and take down to water. Tone in 0.2% aqueous yellow

gold chloride. Wash. Counterstain with neutral red.
8. Dehydrate, clear and mount as desired.

Results

Golgi apparatus	black
Nuclei	red

DAFANO-CAJAL TECHNIQUE FOR THE GOLGI APPARATUS (Cajal, 1912; DaFano, 1919–20)

Notes

The results with this method may be unpredictable and this is due to variation in fixation and/or silver impregnation. It is wise to take through more than one block of the tissue to be examined and to vary the times of treatment. Finally, select the block giving the best results.

A rather complex toning solution is usually specified for this technique. We see no obvious advantage in this as against the conventional gold chloride solution.

Solutions

Fixative

Cobalt nitrate	1 g
Formalin	15 ml
Distilled water	100 ml

Reducer

Hydroquinone	2 g
Formalin	15 ml
Distilled water	100 ml
Sodium sulphite	0.5 g

Technique

1. Place thin (1.5–2 mm) slices of fresh tissue in the fixative for 3–8 h (see notes).
2. Rinse in distilled water for 30 s.
3. Treat with 1.5% aqueous silver nitrate for 36–48 h (change the solution after one day).

4. Rinse in distilled water for 30 s.
5. Reduce for 12–24 h.
6. Wash in water for 5 min.
7. Paraffin process and cut thin sections.
8. Either deparaffinize and mount; or take down to water, tone in 0.1% aqueous yellow gold chloride for 5 min and wash. Counterstain with neutral red and dehydrate, clear and mount as desired.

Results

Golgi apparatus	black
Mitochondria	brown
Background	grey if toned, yellow-brown if untoned

JUXTAGLOMERULAR CELLS

Popularly known as 'JG' cells, these are modified smooth muscle cells which are found in the wall of the afferent arteriole where it enters the renal glomerulus. Granules are contained in the cytoplasm of these cells which are thought to secrete renin, a hormone concerned with blood pressure regulation. They were first described in mouse kidney by Ruyter in 1925. The JG granules are not seen in an H and E stain, and whilst their demonstration is at present of little diagnostic importance, their histochemical delineation is of some interest, particularly in research. There is a marked species difference in the size of JG cells and in their histochemical behaviour. Mouse kidney gives the best results whilst those of human tissue are often unsatisfactory. Formalin-containing fixatives lead to the best staining results, and both paraffin and fixed frozen sections can be used. Fresh, unfixed cryostat sections are not successful (Szokol & Gomba, 1971).

One of the more popular techniques is that of Bowie and this is described in detail. Other techniques, all of which give variable results, are as follows:

PAS (see p. 102).

Aldehyde fuchsin (Harada, 1966) (see p. 55).

Thioflavine T fluorescence (Harada, 1969; Szokol & Gomba, 1971)

0.5% crystal violet in 70% alcohol for 1–3 min (Harada, 1970).

BOWIE'S NEUTRAL STAIN TECHNIQUE
(taken from Cowdry, 1952)

Notes

This technique, like those quoted above, is not specific for JG cells but is sufficiently selective to afford reasonably clear-cut demonstration. The preparation of the neutral dye is rather time-consuming and tedious, but the actual technique is reasonably straightforward. As with any technique for JG cells some degree of practical experience with the stain is necessary before really good results are obtained. Fixation in Helly's fluid (see Appendix 1) is recommended as is the use of rat or mouse kidney tissue.

Solutions

2.5% aqueous potassium dichromate.

Bowie's solution
Dissolve 1 g biebrich scarlet in 250 ml distilled water and filter. Dissolve 2 g ethyl violet in 500 ml distilled water. Filter a small amount at a time of the latter solution into the biebrich scarlet solution with constant stirring until a precipitate is formed. The end point is reached when a small amount of the mixture placed on a No. 1 filter paper shows no coloration other than that of the precipitate. Filter the mixture and dry the precipitate in the filter paper. Finally, dissolve 0.2 g of the dried precipitate in 20 ml of 95% alcohol and use. There is normally enough precipitate formed to make 100 ml volume of stain.

Technique

1. Take paraffin sections to water and remove any mercuric chloride precipitate present with the usual iodine/hypo sequence.
2. Mordant in the potassium dichromate solution overnight at approximately 40° C.
3. Wash well in tap water, then in distilled water.

4. Stain with Bowie's solution, diluted by adding 10–15 drops to 100 ml of 20% alcohol. Leave overnight at room temperature.
5. Drain and blot dry. Remove excess stain by dipping two or three times in two changes of acetone.
6. Differentiate in equal parts of xylene and clove oil until the section is an overall red or reddish-purple colour, with any elastin picked out as blue-purple fibres.
7. Rinse in xylene and mount as desired.

Results

JG granules, elastin	blue-purple
Renal parenchyma	red to magenta

KERATIN

Keratin, a type of protein, forms structures such as finger nails, hair shafts (in animals, hooves and antlers) and also forms the stratum corneum of the thicker skin surfaces. From a pathological point of view, keratin is found particularly in skin lesions such as warts, keratin horns, leukoplakia, squamous cell papillomata, also as keratin 'pearls' in well differentiated squamous cell carcinomas.

The need to demonstrate keratin as such in diagnostic pathology is usually fairly small. However, it is occasionally useful to be able to demonstrate hair shafts in inflammatory lesions such as the pilonidal sinus where degenerate hair shafts may often be found in the sinus track and are the causative irritating factor.

Fixation is not usually important, most fixatives are satisfactory and the need for prompt fixation is not very great.

DEMONSTRATION

In addition to the two techniques described below, keratin is stained red by the phloxine-tartrazine method (see p. 64), is usually Gram-positive, also Congo red positive and stains brightly with orange G or picric acid. Hair shafts are strongly ZN positive whilst the Schmorl reaction (see

p. 148) is often positive to the presence of the contained SH groups. In addition, keratin is birefringent with the polarizing microscope and gives a yellow fluorescence with thioflavine T (see p. 94).

AURAMINE-RHODAMINE FLUORESCENT TECHNIQUE FOR KERATIN

Notes

The technique utilizes the auramine-rhodamine fluorescent technique for tubercle bacilli but uses a post-treatment toluidine blue step to quench any background fluorescence. Good results can be obtained but are unfortunately rather variable. Auramine is considered to be potentially carcinogenic and should be handled with care.

Solutions

Auramine-rhodamine solution (see p. 208)

4% aqueous toluidine blue.

Technique

1. Take sections to water and stain with heated auramine-rhodamine, differentiating in acid-alcohol as for the tubercle bacilli technique (2–3 min).
2. Following acid-alcohol treatment, wash well in water.
3. Stain with the toluidine blue solution for 20 s.
4. Wash in water, blot dry. Dehydrate, clear and mount in a DPX-type mountant.

Results

Keratin	yellow fluorescence

PERFORMIC ACID-METHYLENE BLUE-ALCIAN BLUE TECHNIQUE FOR KERATIN (Lake, 1974)

Notes

Disulphide groups in the keratin form cysteic acid upon oxidation with performic acid. The contained sulphonate radicals of the cysteic acid will form salt linkages at a low pH with cationic dyes such as methylene blue and alcian blue to give highly selective staining of the keratin.

Solutions

Performic acid solution
  98% formic acid   4 ml
  30% (100 volumes) hydrogen peroxide   15.5 ml
  Conc. sulphuric acid   0.11 ml
  Allow the solution to stand for 2 h before use to allow the full formation of performic acid.

0.02% methylene blue (pH 2.5).

0.1% alcian blue
  Dissolve 0.1 g alcian blue in 1 ml conc. sulphuric acid using a glass rod for stirring. Add 9 ml glacial acetic acid and mix. Make up to a 100 ml volume with distilled water, mix and filter.

Technique

1. Take sections to distilled water.
2. Treat with the performic acid solution for 30 min.
3. Wash well in distilled water.
4. Stain with the methylene blue solution for 15 min or alcian blue for 1 h.
5. Wash in water and blot dry. Dehydrate quickly, clear and mount in a DPX-type mountant.

Results

  Keratin (hair shafts)   blue
  Background   colourless

MALLORY BODIES (Alcoholic Hyaline)

Mallory bodies were first described by Mallory in 1911 who considered them to be peculiar to liver tissue in alcoholic cirrhosis. Whilst there are some reservations about this, it is undoubtedly true that Mallory bodies are usually found in the more active episodes of hepatic cirrhosis due to excessive alcohol intake. Other conditions in which they

may be found include primary biliary cirrhosis and Wilson's disease.

The bodies are protein intracytoplasmic hyaline bodies of somewhat irregular shape, and are found in a proportion of cells of the affected liver. They are usually peri- or juxtanuclear in position and the electron microscope has shown them to contain both mitochondria and lysosomes.

For more detailed information see Horvath et al (1972) and Lyon & Christoffersen (1971).

The following is a list of the more popular techniques for demonstrating alcoholic hyaline, but is must be said these may not offer any great advantage over standard H and E preparations. Frozen sections are considered to give better staining results than paraffin.

  H and E   eosinophilic (p. 18)
  PTAH   blue (p. 45)
  Congo red   red (weak) (p. 92)
  Baker's acid haematein   blue (not extracted
                           by pyridine) (p. 136)
  Luxol fast blue   blue (p. 225)
  Phloxine-tartrazine red (p. 64)

VITAMIN C (ASCORBIC ACID)

The following technique is based upon the reduction of acidified silver nitrate in the dark by ascorbic acid which is then demonstrated. It must be borne in mind that other argentaffin substances such as melanin and inorganic phosphates may also react.

Ascorbic acid is found in greatest amount in both liver and adrenal cortex.

VITAMIN C DEMONSTRATION TECHNIQUE (from Giroud & Leblond, 1934)

Notes

Tissues should be as fresh as possible and should not be allowed to dry before fixation in the acidified silver nitrate. The pre-silver nitrate treatment with laevulose is to remove any excess chlorides from the tissue which could otherwise give non-specific silver reduction.

A MISCELLANY 255

The authors recommend that all stages of the technique, from washing with laevulose to the post-hypo washing in water, be carried out in the dark to avoid any non-specific light reduction.

Solutions

5.4% aqueous laevulose (D(–) fructose).

10% aqueous silver nitrate to which are added 2 drops of acetic acid per 1 ml volume.

5% aqueous sodium thiosulphate (hypo).

Technique

1. Thin (2 mm) pieces of tissue are washed for 2–3 min in ample quantities of laevulose. Wash briefly in distilled water.

2. Treat with acetic-silver nitrate for 30 min.
3. Rinse in several changes of distilled water over 5–10 min.
4. Treat with 5% hypo for 15–30 min.
5. Wash in water, paraffin process and cut 5 μm sections.
6. Sections are deparaffinized, taken to water and counterstained with 1% aqueous neutral red for 2–3 min.
7. Wash in water, dehydrate, clear and mount in a DPX-type mountant.

Results

Ascorbic acid	black granules
Nuclei	red

REFERENCES

Cajal Ramon Y 1912 Trab. Lab. Invest. biol. Uni. Madr. 10: 209
Cowdry E V 1962 Laboratory techniques in biology and medicine, 3rd edn. Williams and Wilkins, Baltimore
Da Fano C 1919–1920 Method for the demonstration of Golgi's internal apparatus. Journal of Physiology 53: 92
Drury R A B, Wallington E A 1980 Carleton's histological technique, 5th edn. Oxford University Press, London
Giroud A, Leblond C P 1934a Etude histochimique de la vitamine C dans la glande surrenale. Archs. Anat. microsc. Morph. exp. 30: 105
Glynn L E, Loewi G 1952 Journal of Pathology and Bacteriology 64: 329
Gomori G 1946 A new histochemical test for glycogen and mucin. Americal Journal of Clinical Pathology 16: 177
Harada K 1966 Fixative stain sequences for selective demonstration of juxtaglomerular cells. Stain Technology 41: 83
Harada K 1969 Staining juxtaglomerular granules with basic fluorescent stains. Stain Technology 44: 293
Harada K 1970 Rapid demonstration of juxtaglomerular granules with alcoholic crystal violet. Stain Technology 45: 71
Horvath E, Kovacs K, Ross R C 1973 Subcellular features of alcoholic liver lesions: alcoholic hyalin. Journal of Pathology 110: 245
Hyman J M, Poulding R H 1961 Solochrome cyanin-iron alum for rapid staining of frozen sections. Journal of Medical Laboratory Technology 18: 107
Lake B 1974 Manual of histological demonstration techniques. Butterworth, London
Lascano E F 1959 A new silver method for the Golgi apparatus. Archives of Pathology 68: 499
Lendrum A C 1949 Staining of erythrocytes in tissue sections; a new method and observations on some of the modified connective tissue stains. Journal of Pathology and Bacteriology 61: 442

Lendrum A C, Fraser D S, Slidders W, Henderson R 1962 Studies on the character and staining of fibrin. Journal of Clinical Pathology 15: 401
Lillie R D 1965 Histopathologic technic and practical histochemistry, 3rd end. McGraw-Hill, New York
Lyon H, Christoffersen P 1971 Histochemical studies of Mallory bodies. Acta Pathologica Microbiologica Scandinavica 74A: 649
McDonald D M 1964 Silver impregnation of the Golgi apparatus with subsequent intracellulose embedding. Stain Technology 39: 345
Philpotts C J 1980 Personal communication
Pizzolata P 1964 Histochemical recognition of calcium oxalate. Journal of Histochemistry and Cytochemistry 12: 333
Ramsey H J 1965 Ultrastructure of corpora amylacea. Journal of Neuropathology and Experimental Neurology 24: 25
Sakai M, Austin J, Witmer F 1969 Studies of corpora amylacea (1) Isolation and preliminary characterization by chemical and histochemical techniques. Archives of Neurology 21: 526
Schmorl G 1934 Die Pathologisch-Histologischen Untersuchungsmethoden, ch. 14. Vogel, Berlin, p. 259
Slidders W 1961a The Fuchsin-Miller method. Journal of Medical Laboratory Technology 18: 36
Slidders W 1961b the OFG and Br AB-OFG methods for staining the adenohypophysis. Journal of Pathology and Bacteriology 82: 532
Szokol M, Gombo S Z 1971 Subsequent staining of juxtaglomerular cells in frozen sections. Stain Technology 46: 102
Tripp E J, MacKay E H 1972 Silver staining of bone prior to decalcification for quantitative determination of osteoid in sections. Stain Technology 47: 129
Worsfold D 1982 Unpublished data

Appendix 1

Fixative solutions

Acetic alcohol formaldehyde (AAF)

Formaldehyde 40%	10 ml
Glacial acetic acid	5 ml
Absolute alcohol	85 ml

Acetone
Absolute acetone at 4°C

1% Acrolein

Acrolein	1 ml
0.1M phosphate buffer, pH 7.4	99 ml

The final pH of this fixative should be checked and adjusted to 7.2–7.6 if necessary.

Alcohol
Alcohol 80–100% at 4°C

Bouin's fixative

Picric acid (saturated aqueous)	75 ml
Formaldehyde 40%	25 ml
Glacial acetic acid	5 ml

Carnoy's fixative

Ethyl alcohol	60 ml
Chloroform	30 ml
Glacial acetic acid	10 ml

Clarke's fixative

Absolute alcohol	75 ml
Glacial acetic acid	25 ml

Flemming's fixative

1% chromic acid	60 ml
2% osmium tetroxide	16 ml
Glacial acetic acid	4 ml

10% Formalin

Formaldehyde 40%	10 ml
Distilled water	90 ml

Formol alcohol

Formaldehyde 40%	10 ml
Absolute alcohol	80 ml
Distilled water	10 ml

Formol ammonium bromide

Formalin	15 ml
Ammonium bromide	2 g
Distilled water	85 ml

10% Formol calcium

Formaldehyde 40%	10 ml
Distilled water	90 ml
Calcium chloride	1.1 g
	(or until pH reaches 7.0)

10% Formol saline

Formaldehyde 40%	100 ml
Sodium chloride	9 g
Distilled water	900 ml

Formol sublimate

Mercuric chloride (saturated aqueous)	90 ml
Formaldehyde 40%	10 ml

Formol sucrose

Formaldehyde 40%	10 ml
Sucrose	7.5 g
0.2M Phosphate buffer, pH 7.4	90 ml

Gendre's fixative

Picric acid (saturated in 95% alcohol)	85 ml
Formaldehye 40%	10 ml
Glacial acetic acid	5 ml

6% glutaraldehyde

Glutaraldehyde (25%)	24 ml
0.1 M phosphate buffer, pH 7.4	76 ml

On storage, the glutaraldehyde will become acidic, pH 2.5–3.0. The final pH of the above fixative should be checked and adjusted to 7.0–7.2 if necessary with sodium hydroxide.

Heidenhain's 'Susa'

Distilled water	76 ml
Mercuric chloride	4.5 g
Sodium chloride	0.5 g
Trichloracetic acid	2 g
Acetic acid	4 ml
Formaldehyde 40%	20 ml

Helly's fixative

Distilled water	95 ml
Mercuric chloride	5 g
Potassium dichromate	2.5 g
Sodium sulphate	1 g
Formaldehyde 40% is added before use	5 ml

10% Neutral buffered formalin

Formaldehyde 40%	10 ml
Distilled water	90 ml
Sodium dihydrogen phosphate (anhydrous)	0.35 g
Disodium hydrogen phosphate (anhydrous)	0.65 g

10% Neutral formalin

Formaldehyde 40%	10 ml
Distilled water	90 ml
Calcium carbonate chips to cover bottom of container	

Newcomer's fixative

Isopropanol	50 ml
Propionic acid	25 ml
Petroleum ether	8.3 ml
Acetone	8.3 ml
Dioxane	8.3 ml

Paraformaldehyde fixative

Dissolve paraformaldehyde in distilled water to make a 40% solution by heating in a fume cupboard, stirring constantly until only a faint cloudiness persists. Clarify this solution by adding 10N NaOH drop by drop until the solution is clear. Cool to room temperature and then to 4°C in a refrigerator. Filter after cooling to 4°C. If the solution is being used only for subsequent paraffin sections, the longevity of the 40% paraformaldehyde can be increased by adding sodium pyrophosphate until the solution is a 0.02 M solution of sodium pyrophosphate in the 40% paraformaldehyde solution.

Regaud's fluid

3% potassium dichromate	80 ml
Formalin (40% formaldehyde)	20 ml

(Regaud's fluid does not keep, and the solutions should only be mixed immediately before use).

Rossman's fluid

100% ethanol saturated with picric acid	90 ml
Neutralised commercial formalin	10 ml

Fix for 12–24 h and wash several days in 95% ethanol

Zenker's fixative

Distilled water	95 ml
Mercuric chloride	5 g
Potassium dichromate	2.5 g
Sodium sulphate	1 g
Glacial acetic aicd	5 ml

Appendix 2

Preparation of molar and normal solutions

Preparation of 1 litre of a molar solution

1. Calculate the gram molecular weight (using atomic weights) of the solute
2. Weigh out 1 g molecule of the solute
3. Measure out 1000 ml of distilled water
4. Dissolve the solute in a small quantity of the water
5. Add the remaining distilled water, to make the solution up to 1 litre.
   For solutions of different molarity: e.g. 2M and 0.1 M
   2 M solution = 2 × gram molecular wt in 1000 ml water

Example

Sodium β-glycerophosphate
Molecular weight of sodium β-glycerophosphate = 315.13
Molar solution (M) = 315.13 g in 1000 ml distilled water
    0.1 M = 31.513 g in 1000 ml distilled water.
The chemical is dissolved in a small quantity of the water and the volume is made up to one litre.

PREPARATION OF MOLAR SOLUTIONS OF LIQUIDS

1. Calculate the molecular weight of the liquid   2. Find the liquid's a. valency
            b. specific gravity
            c. concentration
3. Using the formula:
   No. of ml of liquid per 1000 ml of distilled water =

   $$\frac{\text{molecular weight}}{\text{valency} \times \text{specific gravity} \times \text{concn}}$$

   Substitute the values found in (2) to the formula to find the volume of liquid required to make up a molar solution.
4. Measure out the required volume of liquid and make up to 1000 ml by adding distilled water.
   For solutions of different molarity adjustments have to be made to the volume of liquid used.

Example

For a 2 M solution, the volume required for a 1 m solution has to be doubled, then made up to a litre with distilled water.

For an 0.1 M solution the volume required for a 1 M solution has to be divided by 10, then made up to a litre with distilled water.

PREPARATION OF NORMAL SOLUTIONS

A normal solution contains one gram molecular weight of the substance, divided by the hydrogen equivalent of the substance.

Example

(a) Sodium hydroxide, NaOH
    Molecular weight of sodium hydroxide = 40.0. Valency = 1.
    Normal solution = 40.0 g in 1000 ml distilled water divided by 1
        = 4.0 g in 100 ml distilled water.
(b) For liquids, the following formula may be used:
    ml of fluid per 1000 ml of distilled water

    $$\frac{\text{mol. wt}}{\text{valency} \times \text{specific gravity} \times \text{concn}}$$

Example: Hydrochloric acid, HCl

Valency 1, specific gravity 1.18, concn. 36 per cent, mol. wt 36.4

$$\frac{36.4}{1 \times 1.18 \times 0.36} = 85.6 \text{ ml}$$

N HCl = 85.6 ml HCl + 914.4 ml distilled water.

Example: Sulphuric acid, H₂SO₄

Valency 3, specific gravity 1.835, concn. 98 per cent mol. wt 98.08

$$\frac{98.08}{2 \times 1.835 \times 0.98} = 29.1 \text{ ml}$$

N H$_2$S$_2$O$_4$ = 29.1 ml H$_2$SO$_4$ + 970.9 ml distilled water
0.1 NH$_2$S$_2$O$_4$ = 2.91 ml H$_2$SO$_4$ + 997.09 ml distilled water.

Appendix 3
Buffer tables

NOTES RE BUFFER SOLUTIONS

The salts and acids used in the preparation of buffers should be at least laboratory reagent grade. When preparing buffers the molecular weight given on the reagent bottle should be checked, as chemicals are available in different states of hydration.

ACETATE BUFFER (WALPOLE) pH 3.5–5.6

PREPARATION OF STOCK SOLUTIONS

Stock A: 0.2 M acetic acid (mw 60.0)

1.2 ml glacial acetic acid in 100 ml of distilled water.

Stock B: 0.2 M sodium acetate

1.64 g sodium acetate anhydrous (mw 82) or 2.72 g sodium acetate trihydrate (mw 136) in 100 ml of distilled water.

COMPOSITION OF BUFFER

x ml of A + y ml of B made up to 100 ml with distilled water.

pH	x	y
3.6	46.3	3.7
3.8	44.0	6.0
4.0	41.0	9.0
4.2	36.8	13.2
4.4	30.5	19.5
4.6	25.5	24.5
4.8	20.0	30.0
5.0	14.8	35.2
5.2	10.5	39.5
5.4	8.8	41.2
5.6	4.8	45.2

SODIUM ACETATE — HYDROCHLORIC ACID BUFFER (WALPOLE) pH 1.0–5.2

PREPARATION OF SOLUTION

Stock A: M sodium acetate (mw 136.0)

13.6 g sodium acetate in 100 ml distilled water.

Stock B: M hydrochloric acid (mw 36.5).

8.5 ml hydrochloric acid 100 ml distilled water.

COMPOSITION OF BUFFER

50 ml of A + x ml of B made up to 250 ml with distilled water.

pH	x
1.0	75.0
1.2	65.0
1.5	61.0
1.8	54.0
2.0	52.0
2.3	51.0
2.6	50.0
3.0	49.0
3.3	47.5
3.5	46.3
3.8	42.5
4.0	39.0
4.2	35.0
4.4	30.0
4.8	18.0
5.2	10.0

PHOSPHATE BUFFER (SÖRENSEN) pH 5.8–8.0

PREPARATION OF STOCK SOLUTIONS

Stock A: 0.2 M disodium hydrogen orthophosphate (mw 156)

3.12 g sodium dihydrogen orthophosphate in 100 ml of distilled water.

Stock B: 0.2 M disodium hydrogen orthophosphate (mw 142)

2.83 g disodium hydrogen orthophosphate in 100 ml of distilled water.

COMPOSITION OF BUFFER

x ml of A + y ml of B made up to 100 ml with distilled water.

pH	x	y
5.8	46.0	4.0
6.0	43.8	6.2
6.2	40.7	9.3
6.4	36.7	13.3
6.6	31.2	18.8
6.8	25.5	24.5
7.0	19.5	30.5
7.2	14.0	36.0
7.4	9.5	40.5
7.6	6.5	43.5
7.8	4.2	45.8
8.0	2.6	47.4

PHOSPHATE — CITRATE BUFFER (MCILVAINE) pH 3.6–7.8

PREPARATION OF SOLUTIONS

Stock A: 0.2 M sodium dihydrogen orthophosphate (mw 142.0)

2.83 g disodium hydrogen orthophosphate in 100 ml distilled water.

Stock B: 0.1 M citric acid (mw 210.0)

2.1 g citric acid in 100 ml distilled water.

COMPOSITION OF BUFFER

x ml of A+y ml of B

pH	x	y
3.6	32.2	67.8
3.8	35.5	64.5
4.0	38.5	61.5
4.2	41.4	58.6
4.4	44.1	55.9
4.6	46.7	53.3
4.8	49.3	50.7
5.0	51.5	48.5
5.2	53.6	46.4
5.4	55.7	44.3
5.6	58.0	42.0
5.8	60.4	39.6
6.0	63.1	36.9
6.2	66.1	33.9
6.4	69.2	30.8
6.6	72.7	27.3
6.8	77.2	22.8
7.0	82.3	17.7
7.2	86.9	13.1
7.4	90.8	9.2
7.6	93.6	6.4
7.8	95.7	4.3

TRIS — HCl BUFFER pH 7.2–9.0

PREPARATION OF STOCK SOLUTIONS

Stock A: 0.2 M TRIS (mw 121.0)

2.42 g TRIS (hydroxymethyl methylamine) in 100 ml of distilled water.

Stock B: 0.2 M HCI (mw 36.5)

1.7 ml hydrochloric acid in 100 ml of distilled water.

COMPOSITION OF BUFFER

25 ml of A + x ml of B , made up to 100 ml with distilled water.

pH	x
7.2	22.1
7.4	20.7
7.6	19.2
7.8	16.3
8.0	13.4
8.2	11.0
8.4	8.3
8.6	6.1
8.8	4.1
9.0	2.5

TRIS-MALEATE BUFFER pH 5.2–6.8

PREPARATION OF STOCK SOLUTIONS

Stock A: 0.2 M TRIS acid maleate

2.42 g TRIS (hydroxymethyl methylamine) (mw 121), and 2.32 g maleic acid (mw 116) in 100 ml of distilled water.

Stock B: 0.2 M sodium hydroxide (mw 40.0)

0.8 g sodium hydroxide in 100 ml of distilled water.

COMPOSITION OF BUFFER

25 ml of A + x ml of B made up to 100 ml with distilled water.

pH	x
5.2	3.5
5.4	5.4
5.6	7.8
5.8	10.3
6.0	13.0
6.2	15.8
6.4	18.5
6.6	21.3
6.8	22.5

BORIC ACID — BORATE BUFFER (HOLMES) pH 7.4–9.0

PREPARATION OF STOCK SOLUTIONS

Stock A: 0.2 M boric acid (mw 62.0).

1.24 g boric acid in 100 ml distilled water.

Stock B: 0.05 M sodium tetraborate (mw 318.4)

0.159 g Sodium tetraborate in 100 ml distilled water.

COMPOSITION OF BUFFER

x ml of A + y ml of B

pH	x	y
7.4	90.0	10.0
7.6	85.0	15.0
7.8	80:0	20.0
8.0	70.0	30.0
8.2	65.0	35.0
8.4	55.0	45.0
8.7	40.0	60.0
9.0	20.0	80.0

VERONAL ACETATE BUFFER pH 3.6–5.4

PREPARATION OF STOCK SOLUTIONS

Stock A: veronal acetate stock solution

1.94 g sodium acetate trihydrate (mw 136) and 2.94 g sodium barbitone (mw 206) in 100 ml of distilled water.

Stock B: 0.1 M HCI (mw 36.5)

0.85 ml hydrochloric acid in 100 ml of distilled water.

COMPOSITION OF BUFFER

pH	ml of A	ml of B	ml of distilled water
3.6	5.0	14.0	4.0
3.8	5.0	13.0	5.0
4.0	5.0	12.5	5.5
4.2	5.0	12.0	6.0
4.4	5.0	11.0	7.0
4.6	5.0	10.0	8.0
4.8	5.0	9.5	8.5
5.0	5.0	9.0	9.0
5.2	5.0	8.5	9.5
5.4	5.0	8.0	10.0

VERONAL — HCI BUFFER (MICHAELIS) pH 6.8–9.2

PREPARATION OF STOCK SOLUTIONS

Stock A: 0.1 M hydrochloric acid (mw 36.5)

0.85 ml hydrochloric acid in 100 ml distilled water.

Stock B: 0.1 M sodium veronal (mw 206.2)

2.062 g barbitone sodium in 100 ml distilled water.

COMPOSITION OF BUFFER

x ml of A+*y* ml of B

pH	x	y
6.8	19.1	20.9
7.0	18.6	21.4
7.2	17.8	22.2
7.4	16.8	23.2
7.6	15.4	24.6
7.8	13.5	26.5
8.0	11.4	28.6
8.2	9.2	30.8
8.4	7.1	32.9
8.6	5.2	34.8
8.8	3.7	36.3
9.0	2.6	37.4
9.2	1.9	38.1

Appendix 4

Suggested Control Material

Alphafetoprotein — Primary carcinoma of liver
Acetylcholinesterase — motor end plates, axons, neurones
Acid phosphatase — prostate, liver, kidney
Adenosine triphosphatase — muscle, liver
Adrenaline — adrenal medulla
Alkaline phosphatase — kidney, small intestine
Aluminium — lung, skin, (industrial disease)
Arginine — Paneth cells, lymphoid tissue
Ascorbic acid — liver, adrenal cortex

Basement membranes (basal lamina) — kidney, hair follicles, epididymis
Beryllium — lung (industrial disease)
Bilirubin, biliverdin — biliary cirrhosis, cholelithiasis

Calcitonin (C) cells — thyroid (dog)
Calcium oxalate — oxalosis (kidney, thyroid)
Calcium phosphate/carbonate — bone, teeth, atheroma, necrosis
Calcium pyrophosphate — pyrophosphate synovitis
Carcino embryonic antigen (CEA) — colon
Charcot-Leyden crystals — eosinophil granuloma, sputum (asthma)
Chitin — hydatid cysts of liver, lung
Cholesterol — adrenal cortex, atheroma, degenerate myelin
Cholinesterase (nonspecific) — C cells of thyroid, SA and AV nodes of heart
Chromaffin tissue — adrenal medulla
Copper — liver (Wilson's disease, primary biliary cirrhosis)
Cysteine — hair follicles
Cystine — stratum corneum, hair shafts
Cytochrome oxidase — liver, muscle, kidney (mitochondria)

Degenerate myelin — multiple sclerosis, subacute combined degeneration
Dehydrogenases — liver, kidney, heart (mitochondria)
Dopamine — mast cells of rodents

Elastic cartilage — pinna of ear, epiglottis
Elastic fibres — dermis of skin, arteries
Endocrine cells (argentaffin) — appendix, ileum
Endocrine cells (argyrophil) — stomach

Fatty acids (free) — fat necrosis
Fibrin — synovitis, peritonitis, pericarditis
Fibrous astrocytes — CNS white matter, gliosis
Fibrous cartilage — intervertebral discs
Fungi — lungs (*Aspergillus*), skin (*Candida*)

Ganglion cells — intestinal plexus of Auerbach
Glucose-6-phosphatase — colon
Glycogen — liver, voluntary muscle, ectocervix
Golgi apparatus — neurones, kidney
Gram-negative organisms — meningitis, typhoid, colonic abscesses
Gram-positive organisms — gas gangrene, bronchopneumonia, subacute endocarditis

Haematoidin	infarcts, abscesses
Haemosiderin	haemorrhage, haemochromatosis
Haemozoin	malaria (liver)
Herring bodies	pars nervosa of pituitary
Human chorionic gonadotrophin (HCG)	placenta (and tumours of)
Hyaline cartilage	joints
Hyaluronic acid	umbilical cord, skin
Intercellular bridges of epidermis	palmar and plantar skin, squamous cell papilloma
Juxtaglomerular (JG) cells	kidney (mouse)
Keratin	hair shafts, palmar and plantar skin
Lipid (for general staining)	corpus luteum of ovary
Lipofuscin	ganglion cells, heart, Leydig cells
Mallory bodies	liver (active alcoholic cirrhosis)
Mast cells	intermuscular tissue of intestine, breast fibroadenosis
Melanin	negroid skin, naevus tumours
Microglia	CNS grey and white matter, myelin degeneration
Mitochondria	renal tubules, heart, liver
Neurosecretory substance	hypothalamus
Neutral fat	subcutaneous tissue, mesentery
Neutral mucin	stomach
Neutrophils	acute inflammations
Nissl substance	anterior horn cells of spinal cord
Nonspecific esterase	small intestine, liver, kidney
Noradrenaline	adrenal medulla
6-Nucleotidase	thyroid, liver
Oligodendrocytes	CNS grey and white matter
Osteoid seams	trabecular bone in osteomalacia
Oxytalan fibres	periodontal ligaments
Pacinian corpuscles	subcutaneous tissue (e.g. axilla)
Paneth cells	small intestine
Peroxidase	erythrocytes, granulocytes
Phospholipids	myelin, erythrocytes, mitochondria
Plasma cells	rheumatoid synovitis, nasal polypi, lamina propria of intestine
Plasmalogens	adrenal cortex
Protoplasmic astrocytes	CNS grey matter, gliosis
Purkinje cells	cerebellum
Purkinje fibres	subendocardium of heart
Reinke crystals	Leydig cells and ovarian hilar cells
Reticulin fibres	liver, spleen, lymphoid tissue
RNA (cytoplasmic)	plasma cells, neurones, pancreatic exocrine cells
Russell bodies	rheumatoid synovitis
Serotonin	intestinal argentaffin cells, rodent mast cells
Sex chromatin	buccal scrapings
Sialomucin (sialidase-labile)	submandibular salivary gland
Sialomucin (sialidase-resistant)	colon
Starch granules	glove powder contaminants of surgical specimens
Steroids	adrenal cortex, Leydig cells
Sulphated mucin (connective tissue)	cartilage, large blood vessels
Sulphated mucin (epithelial)	colon
Tryptophan	Paneth cells, pancreas
Tyrosinase	melanocytes of skin
Tyrosine	pancreas
Urates	gouty tophi
Vascular fibrinoid	vasculitis (e.g. polyarteritis nodosa)
Virus inclusion bodies	viral warts, herpes simplex, cytomegalovirus

Appendix 5

Index Of Common Dyes

Dye name	Generic name	3rd ed CI No
Acridine Orange	Basic Orange 14	46005
Alcian Blue 8GX	Ingrain Blue 1	74240
Alizarin Red S	Mordant Red 3	58005
Aniline Blue (water sol) (Soluble Blue 3M or 2R, water blue)	Acid Blue 22	42755
Auramine O	Basic Yellow 2	41000
Azophloxine	Acid Red 1	18050
Azur A (McNeal)		52005
Biebrich Scarlet	Acid Red 66	26905
Brilliant crystal scarlet 6R	Acid red 44	16250
Bismarck Brown Y	Basic Brown 1	21000
Carmine	Natural Red 4	75470
Carminic Acid		75470
Celestine blue B	Mordant blue 14	51050
Chromotrope 2R	Acid Red 29	16570
Congo Red	Direct Red 28	22120
Cresyl Fast Violet	—	—
Crystal ponceau 6R (Brilliant Crystal Scarlet 6R, Ponceau 6R)	Acid Red 44	16250
Crystal Violet	Basic Violet 3	42555
Eosin, Yellowish (water & alcohol sol, Eosin Y)	Acid Red 87	45380
Eosin Bluish (Eosin B, Erythrosin B)	Acid Red 51	45430
Fast Garnet GBC salt	Azoic Diazo component 4	37210
Fast Green FCF	Food Green 3	42053
Fast Red B salt	Azoic Diazo component 5	37125
Fast Red TR salt	Azoic Diazo component 11	37085
Fluorescein	Acid Yellow 73	45350
Fuchsin acid	Acid Violet 19	42685
Fuchsin basic	Basic Violet 14	42510
Fuchsin new	Basic Violet 2	42520
Gallocyanin	Mordant Blue 10	51030
Haematein		75290
Haematoxylin	Natural Black 1	75290
Janus Green B	—	11050
Light Green SF	Acid Green 5	42095
Luxol Fast Blue	Solvent Blue 38	—
Malachite Green	Basic Green 4	42000
Martius Yellow	Acid Yellow 24	10315
Metanil Yellow	Acid Yellow 36	13065
Methyl Blue	Acid Blue 93	42780
Methyl Green	Basic Blue 20	42585
Methyl Violet 2B	Basic Violet 1	42535
Methylene Blue	Basic Blue 9	52015
Neutral Red	Basic Red 5	50040
Nile Blue Sulphate	Basic Blue 12	51180
Oil Red O	Solvent Red 27	26125
Orange G	Acid Orange 10	16230
Patent Blue	Acid Blue 1	42045
Phloxine	Acid Red 92	45410
Phosphine	Basic Orange 15	46045
Picric Acid	—	10305
Ponceau 2R (Ponceau de xylidene)	Acid Red 26	16150
Pyronin Y (Pyronin G)		45005
Rhodamine B	Basic Violet 10	45170
Safranin O	Basic Red 2	50240
Solochrome cyanine RS (Eriochrome cyanine R)	Mordant Blue 3	43820
Scarlet R (Sudan IV)	Solvent Red 24	26105
Sudan Black B	Solvent Black 3	26150
Tartrazine	Food Yellow 4	19140
Thioflavine T	Basic Yellow 1	49005
Thionin	—	52000
Toluidine Blue	Basic Blue 17	52040
Victoria Blue B	Basic Blue 26	44045

Index